Ophthalmology

Ophthalmology
Lecture Notes

Thirteenth Edition

Bruce James

MA, DM, FRCS (Ed), FRCOphth
Retired Consultant Ophthalmologist
Department of Ophthalmology
Stoke Mandeville Hospital
Buckinghamshire
and School of Medicine, St. George's University, Grenada, West Indies

Anthony Bron

BSc, FRCOphth, FARVO, FMedSci
Professor Emeritus
Nuffield Laboratory of Ophthalmology
University of Oxford, Oxford
Past Professor of Experimental Ophthalmology,
Vision and Eye Research Unit,
Anglia Ruskin University, Cambridge

Manoj V. Parulekar

MS, FRCS (Ed), FRCOphth
Consultant Ophthalmologist
Birmingham Children's Hospital
and Oxford University Hospitals NHS Trust

WILEY Blackwell

Edition History
1960, 1965, 1968, 1971, 1974, 1980, 1986, 1997, 2003, 2007, 2011, 2017

Registered Offices
John Wiley & Sons, Inc., 111 River Street, Hoboken, NJ 07030, USA
John Wiley & Sons Ltd, The Atrium, Southern Gate, Chichester, West Sussex, PO19 8SQ, UK

For details of our global editorial offices, customer services, and more information about Wiley products visit us at www.wiley.com.

Wiley also publishes its books in a variety of electronic formats and by print-on-demand. Some content that appears in standard print versions of this book may not be available in other formats.

Library of Congress Cataloging-in-Publication Data
Names: James, Bruce, 1957– author. | Bron, Anthony J., author. | Parulekar,
    Manoj V., author.
Title: Lecture notes. Ophthalmology / Bruce James, Anthony Bron, Manoj V.
    Parulekar.
Other titles: Ophthalmology
Description: Thirteenth edition. | Chichester, West Sussex, UK ; Hoboken,
    New Jersey : Wiley-Blackwell, 2024. | Includes bibliographical
    references and index.
Identifiers: LCCN 2023032747 (print) | LCCN 2023032748 (ebook) |
    ISBN 9781119905974 (paperback) | ISBN 9781119905981 (adobe pdf) |
    ISBN 9781119905998 (epub)
Subjects: MESH: Eye Diseases | Eye–anatomy & histology | Handbook |
    Problems and Exercises
Classification: LCC RE50 (print) | LCC RE50 (ebook) | NLM WW 39 | DDC
    617.7–dc23/eng/20231002
LC record available at https://lccn.loc.gov/2023032747
LC ebook record available at https://lccn.loc.gov/2023032748

Cover Design: Wiley
Cover Image: Courtesy of Clifford Bruce James

Set in 8.5/11pt UtopiaStd by Straive, Pondicherry, India

Printed in Singapore
M122350_281223

Contents

Preface to thirteenth edition

Welcome to the thirteenth edition of *Ophthalmology Lecture Notes*! As in the past, our aim has been to make the diagnosis and management of eye disease a palatable process, once again stressing the value of a good history and careful clinical examination. The authors make no apology for starting the book with a chapter on anatomy, which remains key to a proper understanding of eye disease.

The eye is a remarkably accessible organ and optical and digital imaging techniques give increasingly detailed access to its structures at a cellular level. Specular microscopy can image the corneal endothelial cells and optical coherence tomography allows the layers of the retina to be displayed in fine detail and the retinal vasculature to be imaged without the need for fluorescein. The shape of the cornea can be plotted digitally and orbital structures and the visual pathway can be viewed by neuroimaging. The imaging revolution has led to a reduction in the use of more invasive procedures and reduced uncertainty in clinical diagnosis. It has also led to changes in the way that ophthalmology is practiced and introduced the opportunity to hold virtual clinics.

Therapeutically, lasers continue to play an important role in the management of ophthalmic disease. They are used to open up an opaque lens capsule following cataract surgery, to seal retinal holes, to treat angle closure glaucoma and, increasingly, to lower ocular pressure in chronic glaucoma. They now have an established role in reshaping the cornea to treat refractive errors and their role is now extending to their use in cataract surgery itself. Sight-threatening diabetic retinopathy can be treated effectively by retinal lasers to remove the angiogenic stimulus to vasoproliferation.

The development of anti-vascular endothelial growth factor drugs has allowed some forms of macular degeneration to be treated and, together with intraocular steroids, has led to effective treatment of diabetic macular oedema.

These techniques are matched by technological innovations in microsurgery, responsible for dramatic advances in cataract, glaucoma, corneal and vitreoretinal surgery. Optical function in cataract surgery is restored by insertion of a lens which unfolds within the eye. These lenses continue to develop, allowing for the treatment of astigmatism and restoring near and distance vision in some patients without the need for glasses. Vitreoretinal surgery employs inert gases and silicone oil to flatten the detached retina and endoscopic probes allow manipulations within the vitreous and the dissection of microscopic membranes from the retinal surface. Glaucoma surgery continues to advance, using tiny drainage implants to reduce intraocular pressure and reduce dependence on topical drug therapy.

Despite these advances, most ophthalmic diagnoses can still be made from a good history and clinical examination of the eye. Our aim has continued to be, to teach useful skills to anyone engaged in medical practice, not just those with access to advanced diagnostic equipment. Chapter 3 in particular, concentrates on the clinical patterns with which eye disease presents. Many systemic disorders have ocular features which are critical in diagnosis. This book covers the ophthalmic features of systemic hypertension, diabetes, sarcoidosis, endocarditis, demyelinating disease and space-occupying lesions of the brain. It also explains how to recognize iritis, distinguish various forms of retinopathy and understand the difference between papilloedema and papillitis.

As in the twelfth edition, each chapter provides a set of learning objectives and a summary of key points, as well as bullet lists for emphasis. You can test your understanding with the questions and picture quizzes at the end of each chapter. In this edition, we have updated all the chapters and now include a chapter on ocular genetics, to bring this small volume up to date.

Chapter 21 offers classical case histories, which will let you test your diagnostic skills. The final section of the book provides a list of further reading and the details of attractive websites which offer an expanded view of the speciality. Try some of these out.

We hope that you will have as much fun reading these Lecture Notes as we had putting them together.

Bruce James
Anthony Bron
Manoj V. Parulekar

Preface to first edition

This little guide does not presume to tell the medical student all that he needs to know about ophthalmology, for there are many larger books that do. But the medical curriculum becomes yearly more congested, while ophthalmology, still the 'Cinderella' of medicine, is generally left until the last, and only too readily goes by default. So, it is to these harassed final-year students that the book is principally offered, in the sincere hope that they will find it useful; for nearly all eye diseases are recognized quite simply by their appearance, and a guide to ophthalmology need be little more than a gallery of pictures, linked by lecture notes.

My second excuse for publishing these lecture notes is a desire I have always had to escape from the traditional textbook presentation of ophthalmology as a string of small isolated diseases, with long unfamiliar names, and a host of eponyms. To the nineteenth-century empiricist, it seemed proper to classify a long succession of ocular structures, all of which emerged as isolated brackets for yet another sub-catalogue of small and equally isolated diseases. Surely, it is time now to try and harness these miscellaneous ailments, not in terms of their diverse morphology, but in simpler clinical patterns; not as the microscopist lists them, but in the different ways that eye diseases present. For this, after all, is how the student will soon be meeting them.

I am well aware of the many inadequacies and omissions in this form of presentation, but if the belaboured student finds these lecture notes at least more readable, and therefore more memorable, than the prolix and time-honoured pattern, perhaps I will be justified.

Patrick Trevor-Roper

Acknowledgements

Numerous colleagues have provided valuable advice in their specialist areas, for which we are most grateful. We are particularly grateful to Professor Allen Foster at the London School of Hygiene and Tropical Medicine who kindly provided the illustrations for the chapter on Tropical Ophthalmology. We are most grateful for the professional skills of the editorial team at Wiley.

Abbreviations

AIDS	acquired immunodeficiency syndrome	LASIK	laser-assisted *in situ* keratomileusis
AION	anterior ischaemic optic neuropathy	LGB	lateral geniculate body
AMD	age-related macular degeneration	MLF	medial longitudinal fasciculus
ARM	age-related maculopathy	MRA	magnetic resonance angiogram
CCTV	closed circuit television	MRI	magnetic resonance imaging
CMV	cytomegalovirus	NICE	National Institute for Health and Care Excellence
CNS	central nervous system		
CRVO	central retinal vein occlusion	NSAID	non-steroidal anti-inflammatory drug
CSF	cerebrospinal fluid	OCT	optical coherence tomogram
CT	computed tomography	PAS	peripheral anterior synechiae
DCR	dacryocystorhinostomy	PEE	punctate epithelial erosions
ENT	ear, nose and throat	PHMB	polyhexamethylene biguanide
ERG	electroretinogram	PMN	polymorphonuclear leucocyte
ESR	erythrocyte sedimentation rate	PPRF	parapontine reticular formation
GCA	giant cell arteritis	PRK	photorefractive keratectomy
GI	gastrointestinal	PS	posterior synechiae
GPC	giant papillary conjunctivitis	PVR	proliferative vitreoretinopathy
HAART	highly active antiretroviral therapy	RAPD	relative afferent pupil defect
HIV	human immunodeficiency virus	RPE	retinal pigment epithelium
HLA	human leucocyte antigen	TB	Tuberculosis
HSV	herpes simplex	TNF	tumour necrosis factor
ICG	indocyanine green angiography	UV	Ultraviolet
INR	international normalized ratio	VA	visual acuity
IOL	intraocular lens	VEGF	vascular endothelial growth factor
KP	keratic precipitate	VKH	Vogt–Koyanagi–Harada disease
LASEK	laser-assisted subepithelial keratomileusis		

About the companion website

Do not forget to visit the companion website for this book:

www.wiley.com/go/ophthalmology13e

There you will find valuable material designed to enhance your learning, including:

- Interactive MCQs
- Interactive EMQs
- Figures from the book

Scan this QR code to visit the companion website.

Anatomy

Learning objective

✔ The anatomy of the eye, orbit and the third, fourth and sixth cranial nerves, as a background to the medical conditions affecting them.

Introduction

Knowledge of ocular anatomy and function is important to the understanding of eye diseases. An outline is given below.

Surface anatomy

The eyes are disposed symmetrically about the face and their forward-looking arrangement permits a large overlap in visual fields, the basis of stereopsis. Lying within the bony orbits, they are protected from trauma by the orbital walls and rims and by the eyelids, by blinking and eye closure. With the eyes open and looking straight ahead, all but the upper and lower margins of the cornea are exposed in the *palpebral aperture,* together with two small white triangles of bulbar conjunctiva, and the underlying sclera. The medial and lateral ends of the aperture are termed the medial and lateral *canthi* (Figure 1.1).

The lids and the upper and lower orbital rims are overlain by the orbicularis muscle which sweeps over these structures in an ellipse, from a region just medial to the medial orbital rim. It acts as the palpebral sphincter (Figure 1.2). Like all other facial muscles, it is supplied by the *seventh cranial nerve*. Contraction of its orbital part results in protective, forced eye closure, while contraction of its palpebral part is employed in the downstroke of the upper lid during a blink and in light eye closure. The levator palpebrae muscle, the elevator of the upper lid, is concerned with the upstroke of the blink (*third cranial nerve*). The synchronized contractions of the blink are completed within just 300 ms.

The contents of the orbit are separated from the overlying skin by a connective tissue sheet, or orbital septum, which extends from the orbital rim to the tarsal plate, deep to orbicularis.

Sensory innervation of the face: the fifth cranial nerve

The sensory innervation of each half of the face is provided by the *trigeminal nerve* (Figure 1.3). The eye, upper lid, eyebrow, forehead and nose are supplied by its ophthalmic division (V1), via its lacrimal, frontal, and nasociliary branches, which enter the orbit through the superior orbital fissure. The maxillary division (V2), lying inferolaterally to V1 in the cavernous sinus, exits the cranial cavity via the foramen rotundum and, at the inferior orbital fissure, gives rise to the infraorbital and zygomatic nerves. These supply chiefly the lower lid and the upper lip and cheek. The mandibular division (V3), exiting the skull via the foramen ovale, supplies the lower lip, chin and jaw, and the preauricular skin and temporal region. It is also motor to the muscles of mastication.

Centrally, the three divisions of the trigeminal nerve converge upon the trigeminal ganglion, whose sensory roots enter the pons to be distributed to the trigeminal nuclei in the brainstem. The mesencephalic

Ophthalmology: Lecture Notes, Thirteenth Edition. Bruce James, Anthony Bron, and Manoj V. Parulekar.
© 2024 John Wiley & Sons Ltd. Published 2024 by John Wiley & Sons Ltd.
Companion website: www.wiley.com/go/ophthalmology13e

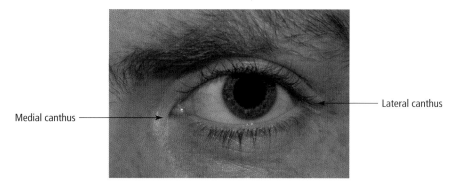

Figure 1.1 The eye, looking straight ahead.

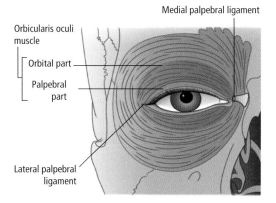

Figure 1.2 Disposition of the orbicularis muscle.

nucleus is concerned with proprioception, the main sensory nucleus with touch and the medullary nucleus of the spinal tract with pain and temperature sensibility. Fibres from the ophthalmic division go to the lowest part of this nucleus, those from the mandibular division to its highest part.

Gross anatomy of the eye

The eye comprises (Figure 1.4):

- A tough, collagenous outer coat which is transparent anteriorly (the *cornea*) and opaque posteriorly (the *sclera*). The junction between them is called the *limbus*. The extraocular muscles attach to the

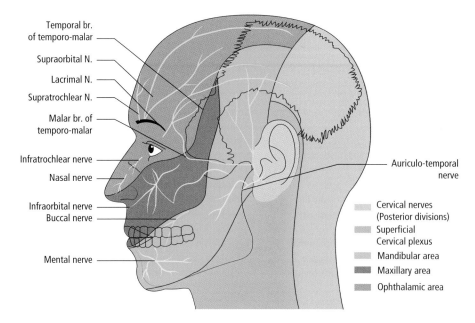

Figure 1.3 Sensory innervation of the face by the trigeminal nerve.

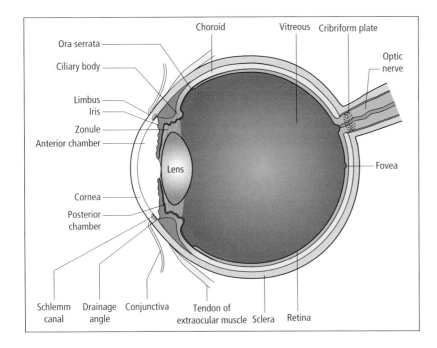

Ora serrata

Ciliary body

Limbus

Iris

Zonule

Anterior chamber

Lens

Cornea

Posterior chamber

Choroid

Vitreous

Cribriform plate

Optic nerve

Fovea

Schlemm canal

Drainage angle

Conjunctiva

Tendon of extraocular muscle

Sclera

Retina

Figure 1.4 The basic anatomy of the eye.

outer sclera, while the optic nerve leaves the globe posteriorly.

- A rich vascular coat (the uvea) forms the choroid posteriorly (lining the inner surface of the sclera) and the ciliary body and iris anteriorly. Internal to the choroid lies the retina, to which it is firmly attached and whose outer third it nourishes.
- The *lens* lies behind the iris, supported by the *zonules,* whose fine fibres run from the lens equator to the ciliary body. The ciliary body contains the smooth *ciliary muscle* whose contraction controls focusing by altering lens shape. When the eye is focused for distance, tension in the zonule is high and maintains the lens in a flattened profile. When the ciliary body contracts, tension is relaxed, the lens takes up a more curved shape and focusing for near objects is achieved.
- The ciliary body also provides attachment for the *iris*, which forms the pupillary diaphragm. It is covered by the *ciliary epithelium*, which secretes *aqueous humour* and maintains the ocular pressure.
- The space between the cornea anteriorly and the iris and central lens posteriorly, filled with aqueous humour, is the *anterior chamber*. Its periphery is the iridocorneal angle or *drainage angle*. The angle gives access to an interlacement of cell-lined collagen beams called the *trabecular meshwork* (Figure 1.24), through which aqueous drains into Schlemm canal and thence into the venous system via the aqueous veins. This is the basis of aqueous drainage.

- Between the iris, lens and ciliary body lies the *posterior chamber*, a narrow space distinct from the *vitreous body* behind. Both the anterior and posterior chambers are filled with aqueous humour. Between the lens and the retina lies the vitreous body, occupying most of the posterior segment of the eye. The posterior segment refers to the posterior two-thirds of the eye, lying behind the anterior vitreous face. The anterior segment comprises all those structures lying *anterior* to the vitreous.

Anteriorly, the *bulbar conjunctiva* of the globe passes from the limbus into the fornices of the conjunctival sac and thence onto the posterior surface of the lids, where it becomes the *tarsal conjunctiva*. A connective tissue layer (*Tenon capsule*) separates the conjunctiva from the sclera and is prolonged backwards as a sheath around the rectus muscles.

The orbit

The eye, or globe, lies within the bony orbit, which has the shape of a four-sided pyramid (Figure 1.5). At its posterior apex is the *optic canal,* which transmits the optic nerve to the chiasm, tract and lateral geniculate body. The *superior and inferior orbital fissures* transmit the blood vessels and cranial nerves that supply the orbital structures. The *lacrimal gland* lies

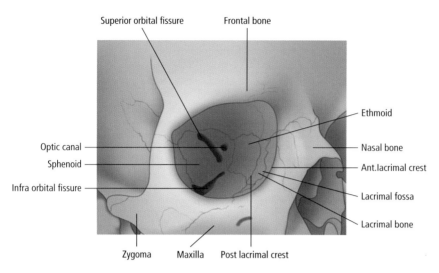

Figure 1.5 The anatomy of the orbit.

anteriorly in the superolateral aspect of the orbit. On the anterior part of the medial wall lies the fossa for the *lacrimal sac*.

The eyelids (the tarsus)

The eyelids (Figure 1.6):

- offer mechanical protection to the globe;
- spread the tears over the conjunctiva and cornea with each blink.

The levator muscle is the main elevator of the upper lid. It passes forwards from an attachment on the sphenoid bone, above the optic foramen, to an aponeurosis which inserts into the tarsal plate. It is innervated by the third cranial nerve. Damage to the nerve or weakening of the aponeurosis in old age results in drooping of the upper eyelid (ptosis). A flat, smooth muscle (the superior tarsal, or Müller muscle) innervated by the sympathetic nervous system, arises from the deep surface of the levator and inserts into the tarsal plate. Müller muscle contributes to a lesser extent to elevation of the lid and if the sympathetic supply is

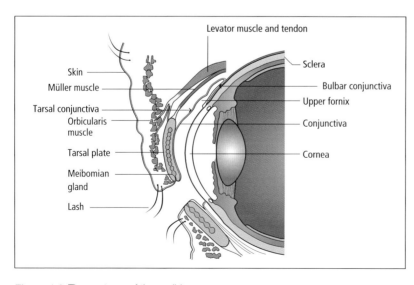

Figure 1.6 The anatomy of the eyelids.

(a) (b)

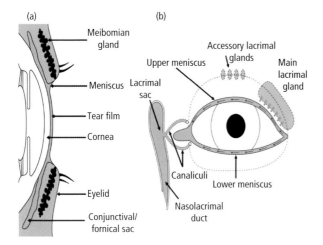

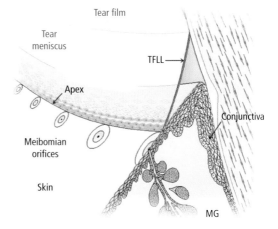

Figure 1.7 Drawing of the eye: (a) in cross section, (b) in frontal view to illustrate the distribution of the tears. (*Source:* Reproduced from Gaffney et al. (2010) / with permission of Elsevier.)

damaged, a slight ptosis results as part of Horner syndrome.

Each eyelid comprises:

- an anterior layer of skin;
- the palpebral part of the *orbicularis muscle*;
- a tough collagenous layer (the *tarsal plate*) which houses the *meibomian oil glands*;
- an epithelial lining, the *tarsal conjunctiva*;
- the lash-bearing, lid margins.

The *tarsal conjunctiva* is reflected at the fornices onto the anterior surface of the globe, where it becomes the *bulbar conjunctiva*. When the eyes are closed, this lining forms the conjunctival sac, which contains the tears. When the eyes open, the tears are spread as a film which covers and protects the exposed cornea and conjunctiva. At the lid margins, the *tear film* is bordered by the tear menisci (Figure 1.7).

The lid margins exhibit a narrow, posterior conjunctival zone, continuous with the tarsal conjunctiva and a cutaneous zone anteriorly, which bears the lashes. These zones are separated by the *mucocutaneous junction* which forms the anterior boundary of each tear meniscus (Figure 1.8). At the medial ends of each lid margin, dipping into a lake of tears at the nasal canthus, are the lacrimal puncta, through which tears drain from the tear menisci into the lacrimal drainage system.

The meibomian oil glands, embedded in the tarsal plates (Figure 1.8), deliver their oil to the skin of the lid margin, just anterior to the mucocutaneous junction. This oil spreads onto the anterior surface of the tear film with each blink, to form a lipid layer, which stabilizes the tear film and possibly retards evaporation.

Figure 1.8 Diagram of lid margin to show meibomian gland (MG) orifices, meniscus and tear film lipid layer (TFLL). (*Source:* Reproduced from Bron et al. (2011) / with permission of Elsevier.)

The lacrimal drainage system

Tears drain into the upper and lower *puncta* and then into the *lacrimal sac* via the upper and lower *canaliculi* (Figure 1.9). They form a *common canaliculus* before entering the lacrimal sac. The *nasolacrimal duct* passes from the sac into the nasal cavity, entering at the *inferior meatus*. Failure of the distal part of the nasolacrimal duct to fully canalize at birth is the usual cause of a watering, sticky eye in an infant. Tear drainage is an active process. Each blink helps to pump tears through the system.

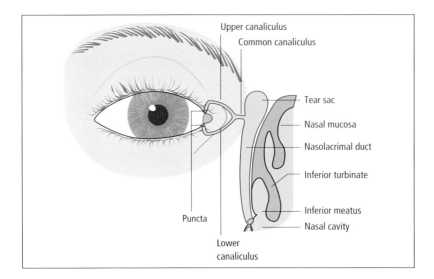

Figure 1.9 The major components of the lacrimal drainage system.

Detailed functional anatomy

The tear film

The eye is bathed constantly by the tears, secreted by the lacrimal gland into the upper, outer fornix of the conjunctival sac. There is a small contribution from the conjunctiva. Tears are lost from the surface in part by evaporation and in part by drainage via the nasolacrimal system. Lacrimal secretion is under parasympathetic control through a feedback loop from the cornea, via the trigeminal nerve, to the superior salivatory nucleus in the brainstem and thence to the lacrimal gland. This ensures that tear production is regulated reflexly in response to signals from the ocular surface, arising from the cooling effect of airflow or from atmospheric particles. This reflex system is referred to as the *Lacrimal Functional Unit*.

The most superficial epithelial cells of the ocular surface express a mucin-rich *apical glycocalyx* in their surface membranes which renders the surface wettable by the tears (Figure 1.10). When the eyes are open, the exposed ocular surface is covered by a tear film, 3 μm thick, which has two layers:

- A thin, superficial *lipid layer* (100 nm) produced by the meibomian glands and delivered to the tear film from the lid margins.
- An underlying *mucoaqueous layer* containing gel mucin from the conjunctival goblet cells and *aqueous tear fluid* from the lacrimal gland, directly in contact with the ocular surface.

Functions of the tear film

- It provides an optically smooth air/tear interface, providing distortion-free refraction of light at the cornea.
- It is replenished with each blink, moistening the eye and preventing dehydration of the exposed ocular surface.
- It removes debris and foreign particles from the ocular surface through the action of the blink and by the flow and drainage of the tears.
- It transmits oxygen to the avascular cornea.
- The tears have antimicrobial properties by means of lysozyme, lactoferrin, defensins and immunoglobulins, particularly *secretory IgA*.

The cornea

The cornea is 0.5 mm thick and comprises (Figure 1.10):

- The *epithelium,* an anterior, non-keratinised squamous layer five cells thick, thickened peripherally at the limbus where it is continuous with the conjunctiva. The limbus houses the germinative *stem cells* which maintain the corneal epithelium.
- An underlying *stroma* which accounts for over 90% of the corneal thickness. On its most anterior aspect is a tough, *anterior limiting layer* (Bowman layer), 20 μm thick, which is free of cells and composed of fine, short, tightly interwoven collagen fibrils. The basal cells of the epithelium are firmly attached to an underlying basal lamina by *hemidesmosomes* and to Bowman layer by *anchoring fibrils*.

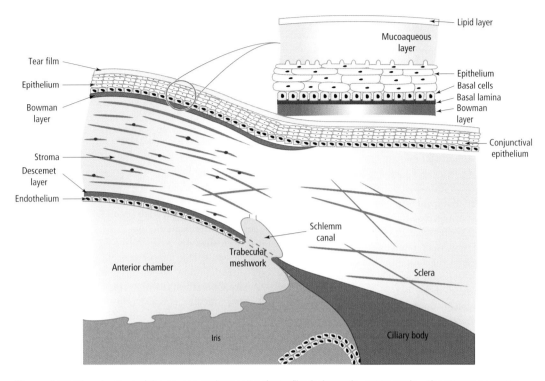

Figure 1.10 The structure of the cornea and precorneal tear film (schematic, not to scale – the stroma accounts for 95% of the corneal thickness).

The main body of the stroma consists of type I collagen fibrils arranged in parallel within multiple lamellae, embedded in a ground substance rich in proteoglycans. Between the lamellae are scattered keratocytes which, like fibroblasts, engage in stromal maintenance and repair. The anterior lamellae lie in the plane of the cornea, while posteriorly they have a more woven arrangement between the lamellae. The extraordinarily regular packing of the stromal collagen fibrils, with a small diameter and narrow separation (in the region of 200 nm), accounts for the almost perfect transparency of the cornea. Backscattered light (towards the source), is obliterated by destructive interference so that over 90% of the incident light is transmitted into the eye.

The stroma is bounded behind by the *posterior limiting layer* (Descemet layer), the basal lamina of the corneal endothelium. It is chiefly composed of type IV collagen.

- The orderly architecture of the cornea, on which transparency depends, is maintained by regulating stromal hydration. The *endothelium,* a monolayer of hexagonal, nonregenerating cells covering the posterior aspect of Descemet' layer (Figure 1.11) actively

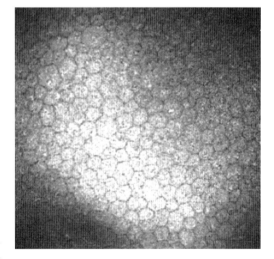

Figure 1.11 Normal corneal endothelium shown by confocal microscopy. (*Source:* Courtesy of Paula Hedges.)

pumps ions from the stroma into the anterior chamber carrying water with them. This controls corneal hydration, thickness and order, and hence transparency. Failure of endothelial pumping leads to corneal oedema and swelling and a loss of transparency as the orderly structure breaks down.

The difference between the regenerative capacity of the epithelium and endothelium is important. Damage to the epithelial layer, by an abrasion for example, is rapidly repaired by cell spreading and proliferation. Endothelial damage by disease or surgery is repaired by cell spreading alone, with a loss of cell density. When cell density falls below a critical level, a loss of barrier and pumping functions leads to corneal overhydration (oedema), stromal swelling, disruption of the regular packing of the collagen fibrils and to corneal clouding. The effect on vision is compounded by an associated *epithelial oedema*.

The cornea is avascular and its nutrition is supplied almost entirely by the aqueous humour, which circulates through the anterior chamber and bathes the posterior surface of the cornea. The aqueous also supplies oxygen to the posterior stroma, while the anterior stroma receives its oxygen from the ambient air. The oxygen supply to the anterior cornea is reduced but still sufficient during lid closure; however, a too tightly fitting contact lens may deprive the anterior cornea of oxygen, causing epithelial oedema and visual loss.

Functions of the cornea

- It protects the internal ocular structures.
- Together with the lens, it refracts and focuses light onto the retina. *The junction between the ambient air and the curved surface of the cornea, covered by the optically smooth tear film, forms a powerful refractive interface.*

The sclera

- The sclera is formed from interwoven collagen fibrils lying within a ground substance and maintained by fibroblasts. Because of the coarse weave and the variation in fibril width, the sclera, in contrast to the cornea, scatters light strongly and appears white and opaque.
- It is of variable thickness, about 1 mm around the optic nerve head and about 0.3 mm, just behind the rectus muscle insertions.

The choroid

- The choroid is a vascular layer formed of arterioles and venules and a dense, fenestrated capillary network, which is fused with the basal lamina of the retina (Figure 1.12).
- It is loosely attached to the sclera.
- It has a remarkably high blood flow similar to that of the cerebral circulation.
- It nourishes the outer third of the retina and may have a role in its temperature homeostasis.
- Its basal lamina, fused with that of the retinal pigment epithelium (RPE), forms the acellular *Bruch membrane* that acts as a diffusion barrier between the choroid and retina and facilitates the passage of selected nutrients and metabolites between the retina and choroid.

The retina

The retina is the thin, light-sensitive, innermost layer of the globe, fused externally with the vascular choroid and closely apposed internally, to the *vitreous gel* (Figure 1.13). On ophthalmoscopy, the retina is the major feature of the *fundus oculi* (Figure 1.14), extending peripherally to its junction with the ciliary body, at the *ora serrata*.

The key landmarks of the fundus oculi are the *optic nerve head* (referred to ophthalmoscopically as the *optic disc*), the retinal *veins and arteries* (actually arterioles) and the *fovea,* the cone-rich centre of the retina, two disc diameters lateral to the temporal margin of the optic disc. At the centre of the fovea is the *foveola*, a declivity marking the thinnest part of the retina, containing only cone photoreceptors. In

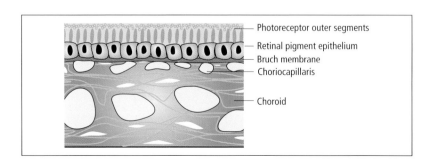

Figure 1.12 The relationship between the choroid, RPE and retina.

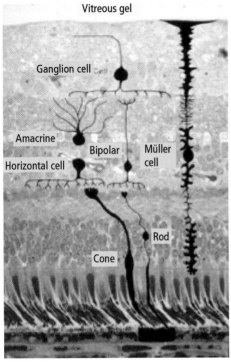

Vitreous gel

Ganglion cell

Amacrine

Bipolar

Horizontal cell

Müller cell

Rod

Cone

Inner limiting membrane
Nerve fibre layer

Ganglion cell layer
Inner plexiform layer

Inner nuclear layer

Outer plexiform layer

Outer nuclear layer

External limiting membrane
Photoreceptor inner segments
Photoreceptor outer segments
Retinal pigment epithelium
Choroid

Figure 1.13 The structure of the retina. (*Source:* Courtesy of John Marshall.)

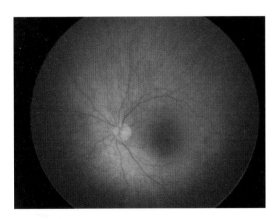

Figure 1.14 Photograph of the fundus oculi.

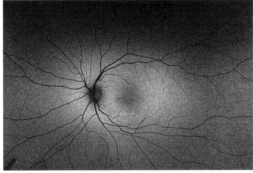

Figure 1.15 Autofluorescence photograph of the macula lutea.

youth, it is visible during ophthalmoscopy as a pin-point reflection of light from the foveal *pit*.

A barely discernible, broad, disc-shaped zone, 5.5 mm in diameter, centred on the fovea and appearing slightly yellow in colour in appropriate lighting conditions, is termed the *macula* or *macula lutea* ('yellow spot'), whose yellow colour is due to the abundant presence of three xanthophyll, carotenoid pigments, *lutein, zeaxanthin* and *meso-zeathanthin*, in the axons of the cone photoreceptors and therefore in the outer plexiform layer. These macular pigments (MPs) are also present to a lesser extent in the inner plexiform layer of the central retina and also in the retinal glial (Müller) cells (Arunkumar et al. 2020). This zone can be imaged by autofluorescence techniques (Figure 1.15). The macula can be the seat of a wide range of inherited, degenerative or toxic disorders which may threaten vision or be responsible for blindness. The most common of these is *age-related macular degeneration*, or AMD (Chapter 12).

The MPs protect the receptors and the underlying RPE from the phototoxicity of high-energy blue light, partly acting as an optical filter, absorbing strongly in the wavelengths 445–450nm, and partly as anti-oxidant, free-radical scavengers, able to quench the damaging action of reactive oxygen species (ROS), such as hydroxyl or peroxyl radicals, or reactive non-radical compounds such as singlet oxygen, peroxynitrite, or hydrogen peroxide.

The retinal MPs are entirely of dietary origin since they cannot be synthesized in the human body; lutein and zeaxanthin are derived from leafy green vegetables and orange and yellow fruits and vegetables. Kale, spinach and broccoli are rich sources of lutein, while corn products are rich in zeaxanthin. Meso-zeaxanthin is a metabolic product of these ingested carotenoids. There is evidence that foodstuffs and nutritional supplements containing lutein and zeaxanthin can reduce the risk of AMD, while ß-carotenoids, such as those contained in carrots, though a source of vitamin A, afford no such protection.

The vascular architecture of the retina is routinely demonstrated during *fluorescein angiography* which permits the capillary systems of the inner retina to be seen at high resolution (Chapter 3, Figure 1.16). The vascular nutrition of the inner two thirds of the retina is supplied by the retinal capillaries while the outer third of the retina is nourished, across the RPE, by the capillary bed of the choroid (the *choriocapillaris*). At the fovea, however, the retina is sufficiently thin that its nutritional needs are supplied entirely by the choroid.

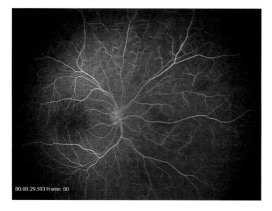

00:00:29.593 Frame: 00

Figure 1.16 A fluorescein angiogram showing the vascular architecture of the retina.

In keeping with this, in terms of its retinal vascular blood supply, the fovea is *capillary-free* (Figure 1.17).

The retina is derived embryologically from the optic vesicle, an outpouching of the forebrain connected to it by the optic stalk, the forerunner of the optic nerve. With development, the optic vesicle invaginates to form the optic cup, whose outermost layer forms the RPE while its innermost layer forms the neuroretina (Figure 1.18). A ventral infolding of the optic stalk forms the choroidal fissure which closes at 5–7 weeks of gestation. Failure to do so may give rise to the congenital defect of *coloboma*.

The layers of the retina

The layers of the retina are, from outside in, the RPE and the neuroretina, the latter consisting of the photoreceptors (rods and cones), the bipolar nerve layer (and the amacrine and horizontal nerve cells) and the retinal ganglion cell (RGC) layer, whose axons give rise to the innermost, nerve fibre layer (Figure 1.13). The RGC axons converge to the optic nerve head, where they form the *optic nerve*. The optic nerve head is visible by ophthalmic examination, when its appearance is referred to as the *optic disc*. The disc displays a small, roughly central depression, the *optic cup*, outside which is the *neuroretinal rim*, which transmits the RGC axons into the nerve. Loss of RGC axons in glaucoma is accompanied by a narrowing of the rim and a widening of the cup in the vertical plane – a diagnostic feature.

Müller cells, the principal glial cells of the retina, extend across its full thickness, from the photoreceptor layer to the RGC layer and are vital for the health of the retinal neurons. The basal lamina of the Müller cells forms the *external limiting membrane* of the retina at the interface of the photoreceptors and outer nuclear layer, and the *internal limiting membrane* (ILM) at the surface of the nerve fibre layer, sometime referred to as the hyaloid membrane. Collagen fibrils of the vitreous inserted into the ILM give attachment between vitreous and retina at selected sites such as the optic disc, fovea and retinal vessels. Insertions at the retinal periphery may transmit forces from the mobile vitreous to the retina that can induce a retinal hole and lead to retinal detachment. This is a particular risk in highly myopic individuals (Chapter 12).

The retinal pigment epithelium (RPE)

- Consists of a single layer of cells.
- Is loosely attached to the neuroretina, except at the periphery (*ora serrata*) and around the optic disc.

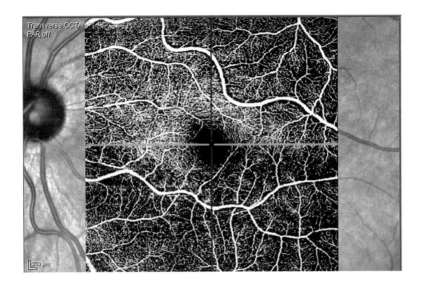

Figure 1.17 An OCT angiogram showing the absence of the capillary network at the fovea. (*Source:* Ambreen Tunio.)

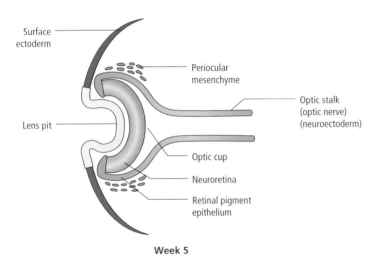

Surface ectoderm

Periocular mesenchyme

Optic stalk (optic nerve) (neuroectoderm)

Lens pit

Optic cup

Neuroretina

Retinal pigment epithelium

Week 5

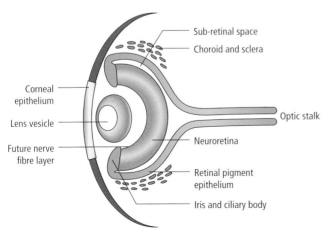

Sub-retinal space

Choroid and sclera

Corneal epithelium

Lens vesicle

Optic stalk

Future nerve fibre layer

Neuroretina

Retinal pigment epithelium

Iris and ciliary body

Week 6

Figure 1.18 The presumptive regions of the human eye at five and six weeks of development (schematic).

- Forms microvilli which project between and embrace the *outer segment discs* of the rods and cones (Figure 1.19).
- Phagocytoses the redundant, pigment-containing discs, which are replaced by new ones.
- Takes part in the regeneration of the photoreceptor visual pigments, rhodopsin and cone opsin and in recycling vitamin A.
- Contains melanin granules which absorb light scattered by the sclera, thereby enhancing image formation on the retina and reducing glare.
- The RPE plays a key role in maintaining the photoreceptors, transferring nutrients and vitamin-A precursors to them and removing waste products. In particular, as new outer segment discs are formed proximally, the older, spent, distal discs are removed by the interdigitating microvilli.

The photoreceptor layer

The photoreceptor layer is responsible for converting light from the image formed on the retina into electrical impulses that are delivered to the visual cortex. These are transmitted via synaptic connections, from the rods and cones to the bipolar cells and thence to the RGCs, lateral geniculate bodies and finally to the visual cortex. Within the retina, the *amacrine* and *horizontal* cells are involved in preliminary processing of the visual signal.

- *Cones* (Figure 1.20) are responsible for daylight and colour vision and have a relatively high threshold to light. Different subgroups of cones are selectively responsive to short, medium and long wavelengths (blue, green and red light). They are packed in greatest density at the foveola, where they provide the high resolution required for detailed vision, as in reading. Their density falls off towards the periphery and with it, the level of visual resolution which may be achieved. During viewing of a visual scene, the eyes are directed so that the image of an object of interest falls upon the fovea so that it is perceived in colour and in the greatest possible detail. By directing the eyes in a series of saccades over the whole of the visual scene, a detailed picture of the visual world is rapidly built up in the visual cortex and visual

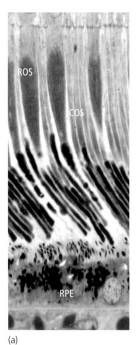
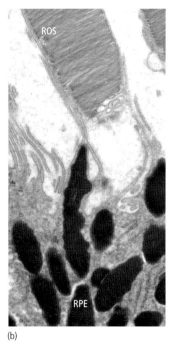
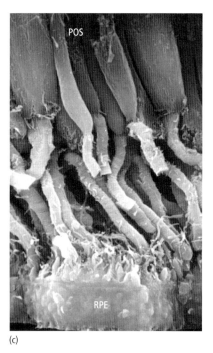

(a) (b) (c)

Figure 1.19 Micrograph showing the interface between the retinal pigment epithelium (RPE) and the rod (ROS) and cone (COS) photoreceptor outer segments (POS). (a) light microscopy (LM), (b) electron microscopy (EM) and (c) scanning electron microscopy (SEM). The EM micrograph shows how RPE microvilli engage with the stack of ROS discs to remove the older, redundant ones. (*Source:* Courtesy of John Marshall.)

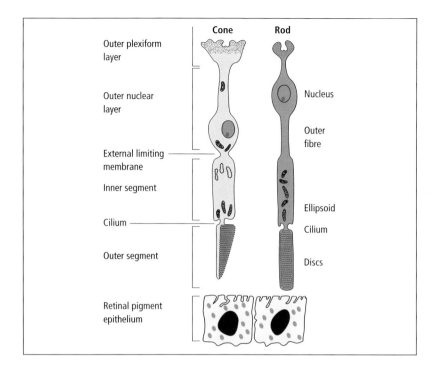

Cone Rod

Outer plexiform layer

Outer nuclear layer

Nucleus

External limiting membrane

Outer fibre

Inner segment

Cilium

Ellipsoid

Cilium

Outer segment

Discs

Retinal pigment epithelium

Figure 1.20 The structure of the retinal rods and cones (schematic).

association areas and brought to consciousness in the mind's eye.

- *Rods* are responsible for night vision. They have a low light threshold and do not signal wavelength information (colour). They form the large majority of photoreceptors in the remaining retina, their density being highest in the periphery and falling off towards the fovea, where they are entirely absent.

The layer of bipolar, amacrine and horizontal cells

These nerve cells are in synaptic connection, permitting a preliminary integration of nerve impulses at this level.

The retinal ganglion cell layer

There are about 1 million RGCs in the retina, each consisting of a *soma*, containing the nucleus and abundant mitochondria and an *axon* which sweeps (in the *nerve fibre layer*) in an arcuate fashion to the optic nerve head, above and below the horizontal, to form the optic nerve (Figure 1.21). In youth, this pattern may be discerned ophthalmoscopically. The topographic arrangement of the RGCs in the retina and nerve head is very precise, and is responsible for a reti-

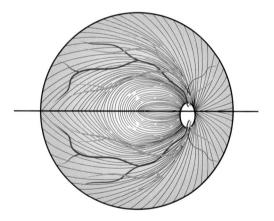

Figure 1.21 Diagram of the retina showing the sweep of the RGC axons towards the optic nerve.

notopic projection onto the visual field, such that loss of a bundle of such nerves gives rise to a characteristic arcuate visual field loss, or *nerve fibre bundle defect*. Such a defect is typically found in chronic glaucoma (Chapter 11) when, as a result of raised intraocular pressure, bundles of nerve fibres are damaged locally at the nerve head. In youth this loss may actually be visible in the retina ophthalmoscopically.

About 1–2% of the RGCs contain the visual pigment *melanopsin*, which, activated maximally by blue light in the range λ 460–480 nm, allows them to signal daily and seasonal, non-image-forming changes in ambient light. These photoreceptor RGCs (pRGCs) thus represent *an additional photoreceptor layer* (Foster 2020). They project, via the retino-hypothalamic tract to the suprachiasmatic nucleus (SCN) of the hypothalamus (Figure 1.22), the *master clock* of the body, which, in turn, projects to about 35 regions of the brain (Nikolaev et al. 2021). Additionally, a sympathetic nervous connection traversing the superior cervical ganglion, extends to the *pineal gland*, where it stimulates the synthesis of the hormone *melatonin*. Melatonin synthesis is triggered by the waning of light at the end of the day, when it is released into the third ventricle and subsequently into the vascular circulation. Its level in the bloodstream rises and falls over a defined period between dusk and dawn, peaking in the early hours of the morning at around 2.00–3.00 hours. Once daylight is established melatonin synthesis ceases. During the night, while its level is raised, it may act immediately on sensitive targets or, after a priming period and a delay, it may act later, when melatonin levels are low. In this way melatonin influences *clock-controlled genes* and cellular time-keepers in the brain, including the SCN and in a range of target tissues, such as the liver, muscle, pancreas, and adipose tissues. Melatonin synchronizes the message of the master clock to control circadian rhythms, sleep and pupillary activity in response to the day/night cycle.

Sleep propensity has a homeostatic component and a time-of-day, or circadian clock, component. Melatonin, acting on MT receptors in the SCN, is

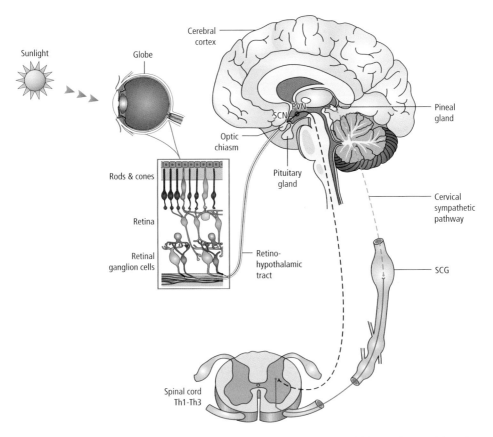

Figure 1.22 Neural pathways concerned with light-dependent biorhythms. Melanopsin-containing photoreceptor RGCs, activated by sunlight, project via the retino-hypothalamic tract to the suprachiasmatic nucleus (SCN) of the hypothalamus which serves as the master clock of the body. Melatonin is produced by the pineal gland under the control of the sympathetic nervous system. Synthesis and release of melatonin is triggered by the waning of light at the end of the day. PVN, para-ventricular nucleus; SCG, superior cervical ganglion. (*Source:* Figure modified from Vasey et al. (2021); and Ptito et al. (2021).)

thought to promote sleep by attenuating the wake-promoting signal of the circadian clock. Because melatonin does not increase the non-Rapid Eye Movement (REM) component of sleep – it is thought to be a marker for homeostatic sleep pressure. It is considered that the sleep-promoting effects of melatonin are due mostly to its action on the circadian component of sleep regulation (Zisapel 2018, Foster 2021).

The vitreous

- The vitreous is a clear gel lying behind the lens and occupying two-thirds of the globe.
- It is 98% water. The remainder is gel-forming hyaluronic acid traversed by a fine collagen network. There are a few cells, or *hyalocytes*.
- It is firmly attached anteriorly to the peripheral retina, *pars plana* and around the optic disc, and less firmly to the macula and retinal vessels.
- It has a physically supportive role and permits the passage of nutrients and metabolites.

In later life, the homogeneous gel structure of the vitreous is replaced by pools of liquefaction. Inward collapse of the remaining gel, away from the surface of the retina (vitreous detachment), is a common occurrence. Occasionally, this puts traction on the retina at points of peripheral attachment, so that the vitreous pulls off a flap of underlying retina, leading to a retinal break or hole. This is a risk factor for subsequent retinal detachment (Chapter 12).

The ciliary body

The ciliary body (Figure 1.23) is subdivided into three parts:

1 the ciliary muscle;
2 the ciliary processes (pars plicata);
3 the pars plana, located posteriorly.

The ciliary muscle

- This comprises smooth muscle arranged in a ring overlying the ciliary processes.
- It is innervated by the parasympathetic system via the third cranial nerve.
- The lens of the eye is suspended from the ciliary muscle by the fibrils of the *ciliary zonule.* Contraction of the ciliary muscle is responsible for changes in lens thickness and curvature during accommodation (see below).

The ciliary processes (pars plicata)

- There are about 70 radial *ciliary processes* arranged in a ring around the posterior chamber. They are responsible for the secretion of aqueous humour.
- Each ciliary process is formed by an epithelium, two layers thick (the outer *pigmented* and the inner *non-pigmented*) and a vascular stroma.
- The stromal capillaries are fenestrated, allowing plasma constituents ready access to the stroma.
- The *tight junctions* between the non-pigmented epithelial cells provide a barrier to free diffusion into the posterior chamber. They are essential for the active secretion of aqueous by these cells.
- The epithelial layers show marked infoldings, which increase their surface area for fluid and solute transport.

The pars plana

- Situated posteriorly to the ciliary muscle, this comprises a stroma covered by an epithelial layer, two cells thick.
- Because it is relatively avascular, it is safe to make surgical incisions through the scleral wall in this region to gain access to the vitreous cavity.

The iris

- The iris diaphragm is attached peripherally to the anterior part of the ciliary body.
- It is perforated centrally by the *pupil,* which is constricted or dilated by contraction of the circular *sphincter* or radial *dilator* muscles, respectively, to control the amount of light entering the eye.
- It has an anterior border layer of fibroblasts and collagen and a cellular stroma in which the sphincter muscle is embedded at the pupil margin.
- The sphincter muscle is innervated by *parasympathetic* nerves.
- The smooth dilator muscle extends from the iris periphery towards the sphincter. It is innervated by *sympathetic* nerves.
- Posteriorly, the iris is lined by a pigmented epithelium two layers thick.

The iridocorneal (drainage) angle

This lies between the iris, the anterior tip of the ciliary body and the cornea. It is the site of aqueous drainage from the eye via the trabecular meshwork (Figure 1.24).

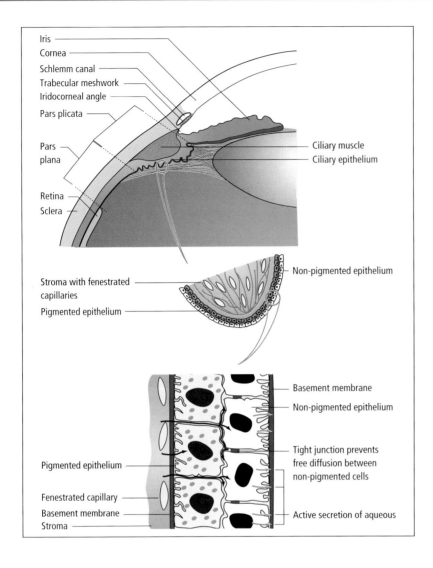

Figure 1.23 The anatomy of the ciliary body.

The trabecular meshwork

This overlies Schlemm canal and is composed of a lattice of collagen beams covered by trabecular cells. The spaces between these beams become increasingly small as Schlemm canal is approached. The outermost zone of the meshwork accounts for most of the resistance to aqueous outflow. Fluid passes into Schlemm canal, both through giant vacuoles in its endothelial lining and through intercellular spaces.

Damage here raises the resistance and increases intraocular pressure in primary open-angle glaucoma. Some of the spaces may be blocked and there is a reduction in the number of cells covering the trabecular beams (see Chapter 11).

The lens

Function

The lens is the second major refractive element of the eye, the cornea being the first. It is a perfectly transparent structure that lies directly behind the iris and pupil, suspended from the ciliary body by the fibres of the ciliary zonule (Figure 1.25). The zonular fibres insert into the lens equator, transmitting forces generated by the ciliary muscle to the lens, to change its shape and refractive power. This allows focusing to be adjusted from distance to near. At rest, during distance viewing, the zonular fibres are under tension, giving the lens a flattened profile. Contraction of the muscle during accommodation for near, relaxes the

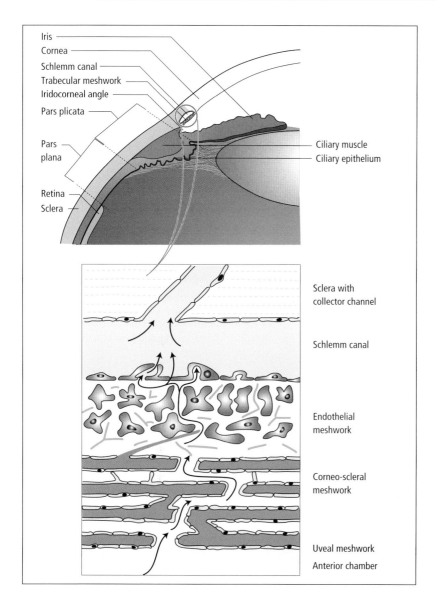

Iris
Cornea
Schlemm canal
Trabecular meshwork
Iridocorneal angle
Pars plicata
Pars plana
Retina
Sclera

Ciliary muscle
Ciliary epithelium

Sclera with collector channel

Schlemm canal

Endothelial meshwork

Corneo-scleral meshwork

Uveal meshwork
Anterior chamber

Figure 1.24 The anatomy of the trabecular meshwork.

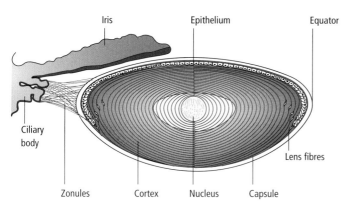

Iris
Epithelium
Equator

Ciliary body

Zonules
Cortex
Nucleus
Capsule
Lens fibres

Figure 1.25 The anatomy of the lens.

zonule and permits the elasticity of the lens to increase its curvature and hence its refractive power. This may seem counterintuitive, but it comes about because the muscle bulges inwards and moves forwards during contraction.

Anatomy

The lens comprises:

- a tough, outer collagenous capsule.
- an anterior epithelium.
- A compact inner mass of lens fibre cells.

The capsule is the basal lamina of the lens epithelium, a monolayer of cells lying between the capsule and the lens fibres anteriorly. The anterior part of the capsule increases in thickness throughout life but synthesis of the posterior part ceases after birth, so that it is thinner and more fragile than the anterior part. This is important during cataract surgery when it may be inadvertently torn.

The epithelial cell sheet extends to a germinative zone at the lens equator, where cell division gives rise to the shells of lens fibres that make up the bulk of the lens. Fibres are elongated, spindle-shaped cells disposed with remarkable regularity in layers which arch over the lens equator (Figure 1.26). Anteriorly and posteriorly, their tips meet to form the lens *sutures,* which increase in complexity as the lens ages.

The high refractive index of the lens is due to the high concentration of lens-specific proteins within the fibres (the *lens crystallins*). Their molecular order, together with the regular packing of the lens fibres, accounts for its near perfect transparency in youth.

The lens grows throughout life, starting *in utero,* as shells of new fibres are laid down at the surface of the fibre mass. Thus, the oldest, central fibres that form the *lens nucleus* represent the foetal lens and the fibres external to this that make up the *lens cortex* are all laid down postnatally. For this reason, the depth of a lens opacity may provide a clue to its time of formation.

With age, the deeper lens fibres lose their nuclei and intracellular organelles and become inert. As a result, the metabolic work required to maintain lens transparency depends entirely on the activity of the lens epithelium and of the youngest, still nucleated, most superficial fibres. It is remarkable that these deeper lens fibres, which are essentially dead, retain their transparency into late life. However, over the life span, there is progressive cross-linking of the lens crystallins, leading to increasing stiffness of the lens and a loss of deformability. The resulting loss of accommodative power, leading to a difficulty in focusing on near objects, reaches a peak at around 50 years and is termed *presbyopia.*

Crystallin cross-linking, formation of high molecular weight aggregates and additional post-translational modifications of proteins, including a yellow or brownish pigmentation, also leads to a steady loss of lens transparency with age, particularly affecting the lens nucleus, which at some point may amount to cataract.

The optic nerve

The optic nerve is formed by *retinal ganglion cell axons* which make up the *nerve fibre layer* of the retina (Figure 1.27), and come together at the *optic nerve head* (Figure 1.21). There are approximately 1 million nerve fibres in each optic nerve (Figure 1.27).

- It passes out of the eye through the cribriform plate of the sclera, a sieve-like structure which permits the passage of the axons.
- In the orbit, the optic nerve is surrounded by a sheath formed by the dura, arachnoid and pia mater, continuous with that surrounding the brain. It is bathed in cerebrospinal fluid (CSF).

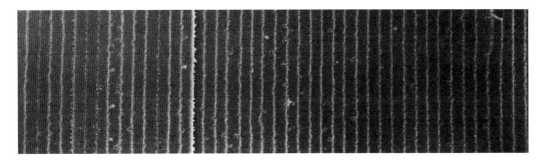

Figure 1.26 Remarkable regularity of rabbit lens fibre packing, shown by surface electron microscopy. (*Source:* Kuzak et al. (2004) / Reproduced with permission from ELSEVIER.)

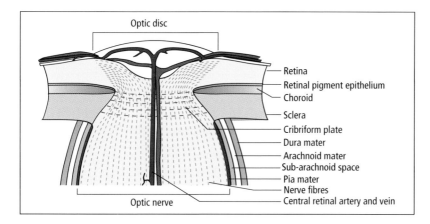

Retina
Retinal pigment epithelium
Choroid
Sclera
Cribriform plate
Dura mater
Arachnoid mater
Sub-arachnoid space
Pia mater
Nerve fibres
Central retinal artery and vein
Optic nerve

Figure 1.27 The structure of the optic nerve head.

The central retinal artery and vein enter and leave the eye in the centre of the optic nerve.

The extraocular nerve fibres are myelinated; *those within the eye are not.*

The ocular blood supply

The eye receives its blood supply from the *ophthalmic artery* (a branch of the internal carotid artery) via the central retinal artery, ciliary arteries and muscular arteries (Figure 1.28). The conjunctival circulation anastomoses anteriorly with branches from the external carotid artery.

The anterior optic nerve is supplied by branches from the ciliary arteries. The inner retina is supplied by arterioles branching from the central retinal artery.

These arterioles each supply a defined area of retina, with little overlap. Obstruction results in ischaemia of most of the area supplied by that arteriole. The fovea is so thin that it requires no supply from the retinal circulation. It is supplied indirectly, as are the outer layers of the retina, by diffusion of oxygen and metabolites across the RPE from the choroidal capillaries.

The endothelial cells of the retinal capillaries are connected by tight junctions, so that the vessels are impermeable to proteins. This forms an *inner blood–retinal barrier,* with properties similar to those of the blood–brain barrier. The capillaries of the choroid, however, are fenestrated and leaky. The retinal pigment epithelium cells are also connected by tight junctions, giving rise to an *external blood–retinal barrier* lying between the leaky choroid and the retina.

Breakdown of these barriers is responsible for the clinical features of many retinal vascular diseases.

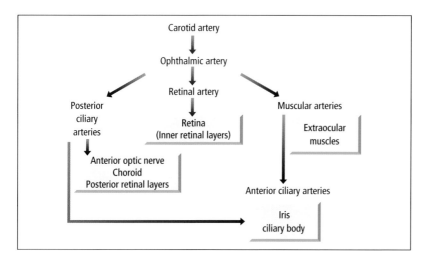

Figure 1.28 Diagrammatic representation of the ocular blood supply.

The third, fourth and sixth cranial nerves

The structures supplied by each of these nerves are shown in Table 1.1.

Central origin

The nuclei of the third (oculomotor) and fourth (trochlear) cranial nerves lie in the midbrain; the sixth nerve (abducens) nuclei lie in the pons. Figure 1.29a–c shows some of the important relations of these nuclei and their fascicles.

Nuclear and fascicular palsies of these nerves are unusual. If they do occur, they are associated with other neurological problems reflecting the accompanying brainstem injury. For example, if the third nerve fascicles are damaged as they pass through the red nucleus, the ipsilateral third nerve palsy will be accompanied by a contralateral tremor. Also, a nuclear third nerve lesion results in an ipsilateral palsy of the muscles supplied by the third nerve, bilateral ptosis and a palsy of the contralateral superior rectus, since both sets of crossing fibres from the nucleus are affected.

Peripheral course

Figure 1.30 shows the intracranial course of the third, fourth and sixth cranial nerves.

Third nerve

The third nerve leaves the midbrain ventrally between the cerebral peduncles. It then passes between the *posterior cerebral* and *superior cerebellar arteries* and then lateral to the *posterior communicating artery*. Aneurysms of this artery may cause a third nerve palsy. The nerve enters the cavernous sinus in its lateral wall and *enters the orbit through the superior orbital fissure.*

Fourth nerve

The nerve decussates and leaves the *dorsal* aspect of the midbrain below the inferior colliculus. It first curves around the midbrain before passing like the third nerve between the *posterior cerebral* and *superior cerebellar arteries* to enter the lateral aspect of the cavernous sinus inferior to the third nerve. It *enters the orbit via the superior orbital fissure.*

Sixth nerve

Fibres leave from the inferior border of the pons. It has a long intracranial course passing upwards along the pons to angle anteriorly over the petrous bone and into the cavernous sinus, where it lies inferomedial to the fourth nerve in proximity to the internal carotid artery. It *enters the orbit through the superior orbital fissure.* This long course is important because the nerve can be involved in numerous intracranial pathologies, including base of skull fractures, invasion by nasopharyngeal tumours and raised intracranial pressure.

The seventh cranial nerve

The seventh cranial nerve arises from a nucleus in the pons, loops over that of the sixth cranial nerve (Figure 1.29c) and leaves the brainstem at the *cerebellopontine angle* where it is joined by the *nervus intermedius*. The two nerves travel together in the

Table 1.1 The muscles and tissues supplied by the third, fourth and sixth cranial nerves.

Third (oculomotor)	Fourth (trochlear)	Sixth (abducens)
Medial rectus	Superior oblique	Lateral rectus
Inferior rectus		
Superior rectus (innervated by the contralateral nucleus)		
Inferior oblique		
Levator palpebrae (both levators are innervated by a single midline nucleus)		
Preganglionic parasympathetic fibres from the Edinger Westphäl nucleus run in the third nerve and end in the ciliary ganglion. Here, postganglionic fibres arise and pass in the short ciliary nerves to the sphincter pupillae and the ciliary muscle		

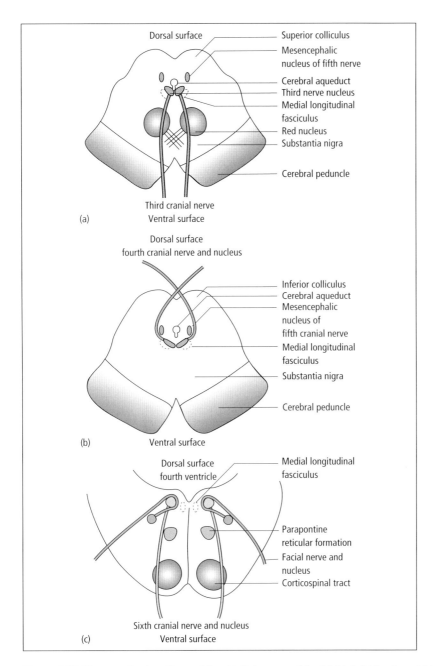

Dorsal surface
Superior colliculus
Mesencephalic
nucleus of fifth nerve
Cerebral aqueduct
Third nerve nucleus
Medial longitudinal
fasciculus
Red nucleus
Substantia nigra

Cerebral peduncle

Third cranial nerve
(a) Ventral surface

Dorsal surface
fourth cranial nerve and nucleus

Inferior colliculus
Cerebral aqueduct
Mesencephalic
nucleus of
fifth cranial nerve
Medial longitudinal
fasciculus
Substantia nigra

Cerebral peduncle

(b) Ventral surface

Dorsal surface
fourth ventricle
Medial longitudinal
fasciculus

Parapontine
reticular formation
Facial nerve and
nucleus
Corticospinal tract

Sixth cranial nerve and nucleus
(c) Ventral surface

Figure 1.29 Diagrams to show the nuclei and initial course of the (a) third, (b) fourth and (c) sixth cranial nerves.

internal auditory canal where they fuse to form the geniculate ganglion. From there, the somatic motor fibres issue from the skull through the stylomastoid foramen, to supply the muscles of the face and scalp. The *nervus intermedius* carries secretomotor fibres to the lacrimal gland via the *nerve of the pterygoid canal,* a mixed autonomic nerve which includes sympathetic fibres from the carotid plexus. The preganglionic, parasympathetic fibres synapse with postganglionic fibres in the *pterygopalatine ganglion* and reach the lacrimal gland via the lacrimal nerve. The nervus intermedius also carries taste

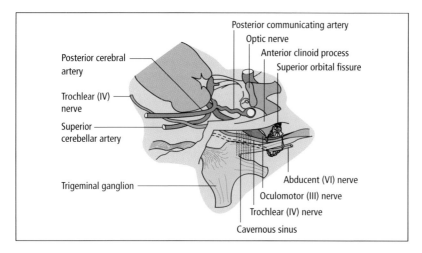

Figure 1.30 The intracranial course of the third, fourth and sixth cranial nerves.

fibres and secretomotor fibres to the submandibular and sublingual glands, which run in the chorda tympani.

Assessment questions
True or False

1. The cornea

a Has an endothelial layer that regenerates readily.
b Has an epithelial layer that fails to regenerate.
c The endothelium actively pumps water from the stroma.
d Is an important refractive component of the eye.
e Has a stroma composed of randomly arranged collagen fibrils.

2. The retina

a Is ten layers thick.
b Has ganglion cells whose axons form the optic nerve.
c Has three types of rods responsible for colour vision.
d The neuroretina is firmly attached to the retinal pigment epithelium.
e The RPE delivers vitamin A for rhodopsin production.

3. The lens

a Grows throughout life.
b Is surrounded by a collagenous capsule.
c Cortex and nucleus are rich in organelles.

d Has a high refractive index owing to its protein content.
e Shape becomes more curved during accommodation for near.

4. The suspensory ligament of the lens (the zonule)

a Attaches the lens to the ciliary body.
b Is part of the iridocorneal angle.
c Is composed of smooth muscle.
d Transmits changes in tension to the lens capsule.

5. The posterior chamber

a Is another name for the vitreous body.
b Lies between the iris, lens and ciliary body.
c Contains aqueous humour, secreted by the ciliary processes.
d Is in communication with the anterior chamber.

6. The tear film

a Is 100 μm thick.
b Tears are drained by the nasolacrimal system.
c The mucoaqueous layer is in contact with the cornea.
d Is important in the refraction of light entering the eye.
e The tears contain lysozyme and secretory IgA.

7. The iridocorneal angle

a Is the site of aqueous production.
b Lies between the cornea and the iris.
c In primary open-angle glaucoma, there is a reduction in the number of cells covering the trabecular meshwork.

d Fluid passes through the trabecular meshwork to Schlemm canal.

8. The optic nerve

a Axons leave the eyeball through the cribriform plate.

b Is not bathed in CSF until it enters the cranial cavity.

c Anteriorly is supplied by blood from the ciliary arteries.

d Axons are not myelinated in the retrobulbar part of the nerve.

e Is formed by axons of the nerve fibre layer of the retina.

9. The third, fourth and sixth cranial nerves

a All originate in the midbrain.

b A nuclear third nerve palsy will cause a contralateral palsy of the superior rectus.

c The fourth nerve supplies the lateral rectus.

d The sixth nerve has a long intracranial course.

e The third nerve may be affected by aneurysms of the posterior communicating artery.

Answers

1. The cornea

a False. The human endothelium does not normally regenerate; dead cells are replaced by the spreading of surviving cells.

b False. The epithelial layer readily regenerates.

c False. The endothelial cells actively pump out ions and the water follows osmotically. Removal of water maintains corneal transparency.

d True. The cornea is a more powerful refractive element than the natural lens of the eye.

e False. The fine, equally spaced, stromal collagen fibrils are arranged in parallel and packed in an orderly manner. This is a requirement for transparency.

2. The retina

a True. See Figure 1.13.

b True. The retinal ganglion cell axons form the retinal nerve fibre layer and exit the eye at the optic nerve head.

c False. The rods are responsible for night vision and three cone types are responsible for daylight and colour vision.

d False. The attachment is loose; the neuroretina separates from the RPE in retinal detachment.

e True. Vitamin A is delivered by the RPE to the photoreceptors and combined with opsin.

3. The lens

a True. It does grow throughout life.

b True. This is of great importance in cataract surgery.

c False. Only the most superficial cortical fibres possess organelles. The older, deeper cortical fibres and nuclear fibres lose their nuclei and other organelles with the passage of time.

d True. The high protein content accounts for its high refractive index.

e True. This increases the power of the lens.

4. The suspensory ligament of the lens (the zonule)

a True. Zonular fibres extend from the pars plicata of the ciliary body to the lens equator.

b False. The zonule lies behind the iris and iridocorneal angle.

c False. The ciliary muscle contains smooth muscle, not the zonule, which is acellular.

d True. Contraction of the ciliary muscle relaxes the zonular fibres allowing the lens to increase its curvature and thus its refractive power (this is 'accommodation').

5. The posterior chamber

a False. The vitreous body is quite separate.

b True. See Figure 1.4.

c True.

d True. Communication is via the pupil, in the gap between iris and lens at the pupil margin. If this gap is narrowed or closed, pressure in the posterior chamber pushes the iris forward and may close the angle (acute closed-angle glaucoma).

6. The tear film

a False. The tear film is about 3 μm thick.

b True. There is a punctum on the medial aspect of both upper and lower eyelids. These allow tears to drain into the nasolacrimal drainage system.

c True. The mucin layer is produced by goblet cells.

d True. It provides a smooth interface for the refraction of light.

e True. These contribute to the antibacterial properties of the tear film.

7. The iridocorneal angle

a False. It is the site of aqueous drainage.

b True. See Figure 1.23.

c　True. This may reduce aqueous drainage.

d　True. Flow depends on the pressure gradient between the anterior chamber and Schlemm canal and there is also an active component.

8.　The optic nerve

a　True. This sieve-like structure provides support for the optic nerve as it leaves the eye.

b　False. In the orbit, outside its pial sheath, the optic nerve is surrounded by cerebrospinal fluid within the subarachnoid space. This is in continuity with that in the intracranial cavity.

c　True. The supply to the anterior part of the optic nerve differs from the supply to the anterior layers of the retina.

d　False. They are myelinated in the retrobulbar optic nerve but not in the eye. Occasionally, patches of myelination occur at the nervehead and within the retina.

e　True. It is made up from retinal ganglion cell axons.

9.　The third, fourth and sixth cranial nerves

a　False. The nuclei of the sixth and seventh nerves lie in the pons.

b　True. The superior rectus is innervated by the contralateral nucleus.

c　False. It supplies the superior oblique.

d　True. This makes the sixth nerve susceptible to trauma, which may cause lateral rectus palsy.

e　True. It passes lateral to the artery.

References

Arunkumar R. *et al*. The macular carotenoids: a biochemical overview. *Biochim Biophys Acta Mol Cell Biol Lipids* 2020; 1865(11): 158617.

Bron *et al*. A solute gradient in the tear meniscus. I. A hypothesis to explain Marx's line. *Ocul Surf* 2011; 9(2): pp. 70–91.

Foster R.G. Sleep, circadian rhythms and health. *Interface Focus* 2020; 10(3): p. 20190098.

Foster R.G. Melatonin. *Curr Biol* 2021; 31(22): pp. R1456–R1458.

Gaffney E.A. *et al*. A mass and solute balance model for tear volume and osmolarity in the normal and dry eye. *Prog Retin Eye Res* 2010; 29(1): pp. 59–78.

Kuzak J.R., Zoltolski R.K. & Sivertson C. Fibre cell organisation in crystalline lenses. *Exp Eye Res* 2004; 78: pp. 673–687.

Nikolaev G. *et al*. Membrane melatonin receptors activated cell signaling in physiology and disease. *Int J Mol Sci* 2021; 23(1): p. 471.

Ptito M. *et al*. The retina: a window into the brain. *Cells* 2021; 10(12): p. 3269.

Vasey C. *et al*. Circadian rhythm dysregulation and restoration: the role of melatonin. *Nutrients* 2021; 13(10): p. 3480.

Zisapel N. New perspectives on the role of melatonin in human sleep, circadian rhythms and their regulation. *Br J Pharmacol* 2018; 175: pp. 3190–3199.

2

Genetic disorders and the eye

Learning objectives

✔ To understand the difference between, and inheritance of, autosomal dominant, recessive and X-linked disorders.
✔ To understand the difference between phenotype and genotype.
✔ To understand the advantages and disadvantages of genetic counselling.

Introduction

Development of the eye depends on the normal functioning of multiple genes. The eye can therefore be affected by a great range of genetic disorders, some confined to the eye and others affecting many organ systems. Some of these, such as keratoconus and age-related macular degeneration, are multifactorial, dependent on the interaction of an array of genes and environmental factors. Others are determined by single gene alterations (monogenic disorders) and are inherited on strict Mendelian principles. These include albinism, retinoblastoma and retinitis pigmentosa where the gene defect can determine disease development and severity and may even be accessible to treatment by genetic manipulation.

The human genome is composed of 46 chromosomes (23 pairs). Twenty-two pairs of which are autosomes and the 23rd pair are sex chromosomes (XX in the female and XY in the male). Various genes are located on these chromosomes (loci). There are two copies of every gene (alleles). An alteration in the allele which adversely affects the function of the gene is referred to as a mutation.

Autosomal recessive disorders

Here, affected individuals carry two abnormal copies of the gene, one on each chromosome (biallelic defects). An affected individual can be homozygous for the mutation, where both alleles carry the same mutation, or they may be a compound heterozygote, when each copy carries a different mutation. Affected individuals are born to two *asymptomatic carrier* parents who are heterozygotes, carrying one normal and one mutant gene copy. Parents are unaffected since one normal copy of the gene is sufficient for normal function. With each pregnancy, there is a 25% chance of producing an affected child, 25% of producing a normal child and 50% of producing a child who is a carrier. A major risk factor is parental consanguinity (e.g. union between second cousins or closer) or where parents are from a small gene pool, (e.g. from an isolated community), where the risk of each parent carrying the mutated gene is increased (Figure 2.1a, b).

Ophthalmology: Lecture Notes, Thirteenth Edition. Bruce James, Anthony Bron, and Manoj V. Parulekar.
© 2024 John Wiley & Sons Ltd. Published 2024 by John Wiley & Sons Ltd.
Companion website: www.wiley.com/go/ophthalmology13e

Autosomal dominant disorders

Here, affected individuals carry one normal and one abnormal (mutated) copy of a gene. In this heterozygous state, a single copy of the mutation is sufficient to cause disease. Although the mutation responsible for the condition may arise spontaneously during development (sporadic event), it may also be inherited from a parent. In this case, the affected person has at least one affected parent; the condition is passed on to successive generations, and affected individuals are found in multiple generations. There is a 50% chance of passing the mutated gene to an offspring (i.e. of having an affected child) in each pregnancy (Figure 2.1c).

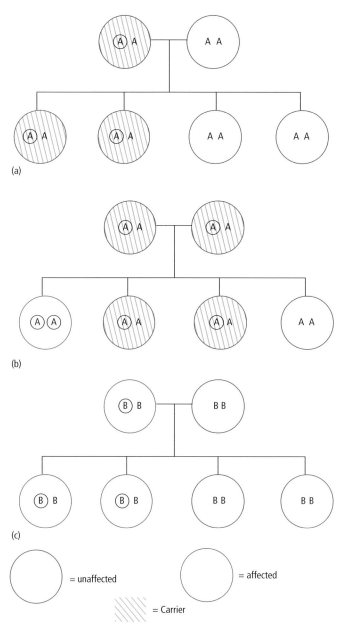

Figure 2.1 (a) Recessive trait, the circled A, is not expressed in the next generation if there is one carrier parent. (b) Recessive trait is expressed in 25% of the next generation if each parent is a carrier. Fifty percent of that generation will be carriers. (c) Dominant trait, the circled B, is expressed in 50% of the next generation if one parent has the trait on one chromosome.

X-linked disorders

X-linked disorders are caused by a mutation of a gene carried on the X chromosome. Males have only one X chromosome so that the mutated allele is not balanced by a normal allele in the Y chromosome and the mutation will manifest in disease. Females have two copies of a given allele, but in individual cells of the female body, only one copy of a given gene is active; the other (usually the abnormal copy) is suppressed in a process called Lyonisation. Thus, X-linked recessive conditions generally do not result in disease in females as the normal copy is sufficient for normal function (Figure 2.2).

The presence of affected males only in a pedigree, with females either unaffected or mildly affected, is suggestive of X-linked disease and *lack of father-to-son (male-to-male) transmission* is the defining feature. Mothers of affected males are obligate carriers and have a one in two chance of passing the mutation to their offspring. Each son therefore has a 50% chance of being affected and each daughter a 50% chance of being a carrier.

Classically, X-linked recessive conditions only affect males e.g. X-linked retinoschisis and Norrie disease. Rarely there may be mild disease (phenotypic) manifestations in heterozygous females e.g. X-linked retinitis pigmentosa.

Phenotyping and genotyping

The phenotype of an individual is the set of anatomical, biochemical and physiological characteristics that characterize that individual. The phenotype results from the expression of an organism's genetic code (genotype), and the influence of environmental factors.

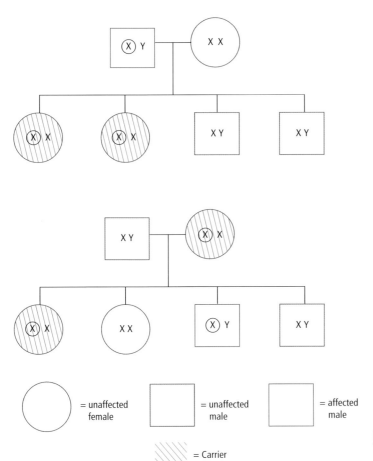

Figure 2.2 X-linked inheritance. The circled X chromosome contains the mutation.

Penetrance and expressivity

In dominant disorders, not all carriers of the mutation will manifest disease. Some individuals may carry a mutation but have no signs of the disorder. This is referred to as incomplete penetrance. Examples in ophthalmology include juvenile glaucoma, retinoblastoma and retinitis pigmentosa.

Two individuals with identical mutations will not necessarily have the same disease manifestations. Despite having the same genotype, the phenotype differs. This is termed variable expressivity of the genotype and is seen, for example, in neurofibromatosis.

Both variable expressivity and incomplete penetrance result from the impact of other modifying genes or environmental factors that affect the function of the primary gene.

Mitochondrial inheritance

Mitochondria contain a small genome (16,500 bases) that is distinct from the nuclear genome (3,200,000,000 bases). As with mutations carried on the nuclear chromosomes, mutations in the mitochondrial DNA can be associated with disease; a notable example is Leber hereditary optic neuropathy. Mitochondria are inherited exclusively from the ovum and a mitochondrial DNA mutation can only be passed on from a mother to her child.

In some mitochondrial disorders, only a proportion of mitochondria carry mutations, and the clinical severity can vary (heteroplasmy).

Heterogeneity in genetic disorders

Locus heterogeneity occurs when mutations in different genes result in the same clinical disease phenotype, as in some forms of congenital cataract.

Phenotypic heterogeneity occurs when mutations in the same gene, in the same environment, produce two or more distinct disorders in different individuals. SOX2 mutations can cause microphthalmia, (a small eye), anophthalmia (an absent eye), or coloboma (failure of part of the eye to develop).

Multifactorial disorders

Many ophthalmic conditions e.g. glaucoma, age-related macular degeneration are likely to be caused by a complex interplay of multiple genes (polygenic) and the environment.

Genetic counselling

The decision to have a genetic investigation requires careful consideration by the affected adult or the parents of the affected child.

Genetic testing can bring benefits to those living with genetic ophthalmic disorders. A molecular diagnosis is helpful to affected individuals as it confirms the clinical diagnosis and gives a name to the disease, clarifies the mode of inheritance, and provides prognosis for vision. There may however be a psychological impact of genetic diagnosis such as guilt, stigma, denial and anxiety. It may also cause problems in obtaining some types of insurance. The possibility of incidental findings on testing that may have major implications on the individual and family must also be considered.

Syndromes and the eye

Developmental defects in children can be part of a syndrome. There may be clues from the family. A full medical and general examination, including family members, is always important in these cases.

Gene therapy

Molecular diagnosis is a prerequisite for accessing potentially new gene treatments, participation in clinical trials, and inclusion in disease registries. Retinal gene therapy uses adeno-associated viral (AAV) vectors that escape the human immune system to deliver DNA encoding a therapeutic protein rather than giving the protein by direct injection. Current retinal gene therapy clinical trials using AAV2 have started for Retinitis pigmentosa replacing RPE65 and X-linked retinitis pigmentosa replacing RPGR as well as other rarer retinal diseases (Figure 2.3).

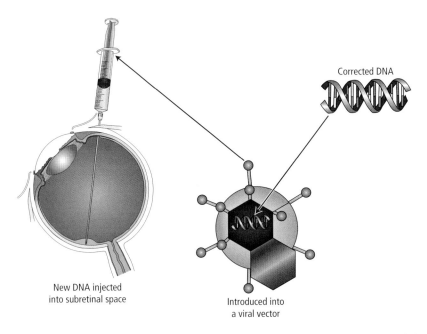

Figure 2.3 Gene therapy for retinal disease. The corrected DNA is introduced into a viral vector and then injected into the sub-retinal space to reach the target cells.

🔑 KEY POINTS

- Many eye diseases have a genetic component. Understanding the different modes of inheritance is important in diagnosis and counselling.
- Mitochondrial DNA mutations may also cause eye disease.

Assessment question
True or False

1. In an autosomal dominant condition

a   There are two copies of the mutation.
b   Affected individuals many not express the disease identically.
c   Mitochondrial DNA is affected.

Answer

1. In an autosomal dominant condition

a   False. There is only one copy of the mutation in a dominant condition. Recessive conditions require two copies of the mutation.
b   True. There may be incomplete penetrance and variable expressivity of the condition.
c   False. Mitochondrial DNA is inherited only from the mother but is not part of the autosomal DNA.

3

History and examination

Introduction

Ophthalmic diagnosis is heavily dependent on a good history and a thorough examination. The majority of ophthalmic diagnoses do not require additional tests. The sequence of history and examination is described below.

It is imperative that hands are washed before and after each examination. If ocular infection is suspected, then it is necessary to disinfect the slit lamp and other handheld equipment. Equipment making contact with the eye, for example a diagnostic contact lens, is either disposable or routinely disinfected.

General ophthalmic history

A good history must include details of:

- Ocular discomfort and symptoms of visual loss, with time of onset, eye affected and associated non-ocular symptoms (Table 3.1).
- Past ocular history (e.g. poor vision in one eye since birth, recurrence of previous disease, particularly inflammatory).
- Past medical history (e.g. of *hypertension,* which may be associated with some vascular eye diseases such as central retinal vein occlusion, *diabetes,* which may cause retinopathy, and systemic *inflammatory* disease such as sarcoidosis, which may cause ocular inflammation).
- Drug history (including drug allergies), since some drugs such as isoniazid and chloroquine may be toxic to the eye.
- Family history (e.g. of ocular diseases known to be inherited, such as retinitis pigmentosa, or of disease where family history may be a risk factor, such as glaucoma).
- Presence of allergies.

Ophthalmology: Lecture Notes, Thirteenth Edition. Bruce James, Anthony Bron, and Manoj V. Parulekar.
© 2024 John Wiley & Sons Ltd. Published 2024 by John Wiley & Sons Ltd.
Companion website: www.wiley.com/go/ophthalmology13e

Table 3.1 Key points in the ophthalmic history.

Consider the symptoms carefully:
How long have they been present?
Are they continuous or intermittent?
What precipitated them?
What makes them better or worse?
How are they changing? Are there associated symptoms?
Is there a history of previous eye, or relevant systemic disease?
Is there a relevant drug history, family history or social history (alcohol, smoking, exposure to chemicals)?

Table 3.2 Red eye: causes and symptoms.

Major causes	Trauma
	Infection
	Acute glaucoma
	Uveitis and other forms of inflammation
Associated symptoms	Discharge
	Pain
	Photophobia
	Blurred vision

Specific ophthalmic history

The symptoms associated with specific eye diseases are brought together here to provide an overview of the important questions to ask. A more detailed description of each disorder is given in later chapters, and you should review this section when you have read more about the specific conditions.

Red eye

A red eye is one of the most common presenting complaints in ophthalmology. It means redness of the white of the eye, that is the exposed bulbar conjunctiva and underlying sclera. It may also involve the lid margins, and eversion of the lids may reveal redness of the tarsal conjunctiva. Redness implies vessel dilatation, often inflammatory but sometimes due to congestion alone. It can accompany infection, inflammation, trauma, and acute elevation of intraocular pressure and also obstruction to the venous drainage of the eye (Table 3.2). Determining associated symptoms will help establish the diagnosis (Table 3.3). The term 'conjunctival *injection*' is also used to describe redness due to dilatation of the conjunctival vessels (Figure 3.1a).

Trauma

A traumatic cause is usually obvious, and you should note the precise details of the event. Was it due to a blunt injury to the eye, a sharp object, or a high-speed projectile? High-speed metal fragments, thrown off during hammering, may penetrate the

Table 3.3 Red eye: differential diagnosis.

Deep red, sclera obscured	Subconjunctival haemorrhage
Diffuse bulbar and tarsal injection	Infective conjunctivitis
	Allergic conjunctivitis
	Angle closure glaucoma
	Reaction to topical medication
	Dry eyes
	In association with orbital cellulitis
Diffuse/focal bulbar injection	Episcleritis
	Scleritis
	Chemical injury
	Endophthalmitis
	Pingueculae
	Pterygia
	Eyelid malposition
	Blepharitis
	Cavernous sinus thrombosis
limbal injection/ciliary flush	Anterior uveitis (iritis)
	Keratitis
	Corneal abrasion
	Corneal ulcer
	Corneal foreign body

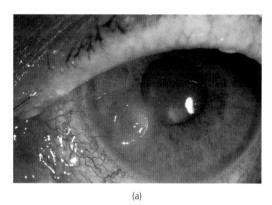 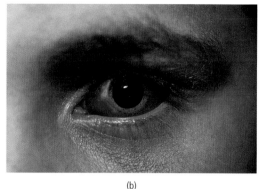

(a)   (b)

Figure 3.1 (a) Injected bulbar conjunctiva associated with a corneal ulcer. (b) A subconjunctival haemorrhage.

globe and threaten sight. When the fragment is tiny, the *patient may be entirely unaware that their red eye is due to an ocular injury*. Was there any contact with chemicals such as domestic cleaners or hair spray?

Here are some causes of a red eye due to trauma:

- A *subconjunctival haemorrhage* (Figure 3.1b) is bright red due to exposure of the blood to ambient oxygen which has diffused through the conjunctiva – the blood is fully oxygenated. It obscures the white of the sclera and therefore, if traumatic, may hide the site of an entry wound. The cause of spontaneous subconjunctival haemorrhages may not be found, but it can be caused by systemic hypertension or blood clotting disorders including anticoagulant therapy. The international normalized ratio (INR), a measure of the prothrombin time, may need checking if the patient is on anticoagulants.
- *Corneal injury:* The sensory innervation of the cornea is chiefly nociceptive, and its innervation density, 400 times greater than in the fingertip, is higher than in any other part of the body. Any injury or inflammation of the cornea therefore causes extreme pain and watering of the eye (epiphora). *Corneal foreign bodies* and *abrasions* are typical examples of such injuries. They stimulate reflex antidromic vasodilatation of limbal episcleral vessels, resulting in a patch of redness at the limbus, termed a *limbal* or *ciliary* flush, close to the site of injury and thereby aiding its detection. Where trauma is associated with iritis, the ciliary flush may surround the limbus. Trauma can also cause conjunctival *injection*.
- *Chemical injury* may be associated with generalized or local conjunctival inflammation, but alkali burns may cause ischaemic whitening, signifying severe tissue damage.

Infection

The commonest site of infection is the conjunctiva itself.

- *Conjunctivitis* is a generalized inflammation of the conjunctiva and therefore associated with redness of both the bulbar and the tarsal conjunctiva. There are symptoms of discharge and mild discomfort rather than pain. Any visual blur due to discharge *is cleared on blinking*. Bacterial infections are associated with a purulent discharge that may stick the lids together. Viral infections cause a more watery discharge. In severe cases, where the cornea is affected in addition to the conjunctiva (e.g. in adenovirus *keratoconjunctivitis*), the patient experiences pain, photophobia and blurred vision. Chlamydial infections can produce a chronically red eye.
- *Corneal infection* may be peripheral or central. A peripheral lesion does not affect vision but may be heralded by a tell-tale localized ciliary flush. A central lesion affecting the visual axis is more often accompanied by a circumcorneal flush which becomes more generalized with increased severity of the infection. The eye is painful, and the vision reduced. There may be a mucopurulent discharge. A history of contact lens use is common as an initiating factor.
- *Intraocular infection* (endophthalmitis) may occasionally occur within hours or days, following intraocular surgery. It causes a ciliary flush and a marked, generalized conjunctival inflammation. The eye is painful (unusual after routine intraocular surgery) and the vision reduced. A history of recent surgery is the clue. The condition may advance rapidly and such a patient requires *immediate referral* to an eye unit. Endophthalmitis is a frequent outcome of a penetrating injury to the eye

and, more rarely, may be the consequence of septicaemia.

- An *infection of the orbit,* orbital cellulitis, presents with swollen and often erythematous lids. The globe is pushed forward (*proptosed*) by the swollen orbital contents, the conjunctiva is oedematous *(chemotic)* and the eye is diffusely red, due to both conjunctival and episcleral vessel dilatation. *Eye movements are reduced.* This is a *medical emergency,* since vision may be lost rapidly and permanently, due to optic nerve damage.

Acute glaucoma

The sudden rise in ocular pressure associated with acute angle closure glaucoma and other causes of acute glaucoma, result in a generalized red eye, corneal clouding, reduced vision and severe pain. It needs urgent treatment (Chapter 11). This does not happen with chronic glaucoma where the pressure rises over an extended period.

Other forms of inflammation

A number of other inflammatory diseases may present with a red eye, of which the commonest, mainly seen in primary care, is allergic eye disease.

- *Seasonal allergic conjunctivitis*, or hay fever conjunctivitis, is a common disorder, particularly in the spring and summer when exposure to allergens is at its height. The conjunctiva is injected and may be chemosed; the eye itches and waters and there is accompanying sneezing (due to allergic rhinitis) as part of the overall picture of hay fever. Vision is unaffected, other than by the presence of mucus, but the eye may be photophobic. *Vernal keratoconjunctivitis* is a more severe and chronic form of allergic eye disease, which also presents with a red, itching, irritable eye, frequently with a mucus discharge. Vision may be affected. The upper tarsal plate exhibits typical broad elevations called *'cobblestone' papillae,* which are rich in eosinophils and other inflammatory cells (Figure 3.2). There may be a history of atopy, including eczema and asthma.
- In *episcleritis,* the episcleral tissues are inflamed. This may result in focal or diffuse inflammation and may or may not be painful. There is no discharge, and the vision is not reduced.
- In *scleritis,* inflammation of the sclera is associated with the collagen vascular diseases. Focal or generalized inflammation and swelling of the sclera is seen through the conjunctiva, which is also swollen. Pain is deep and boring.

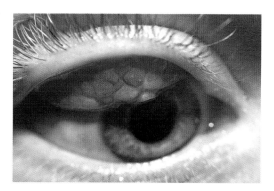

Figure 3.2 The appearance of giant (cobblestone) papillae in vernal keratoconjunctivitis.

- In anterior uveitis (iritis), an inflammation of the iris, there is circumlimbal injection.

Miscellaneous causes of a red eye

- *Dry eyes* may also be associated with a mild redness and irritation of the eye. In severe cases, the vision may be blurred.
- *Malposition of the lid margins* (e.g. inturning or entropion) and misdirection of the lashes (trichiasis) may cause a localized redness of the globe where the lashes make contact with the bulbar conjunctiva. A ciliary flush may be added in response to a localized keratitis where the lashes impinge on the cornea (Figure 3.3).
- *Lid margin inflammation* (blepharitis), whether anterior or posterior, leads to thickening and redness of the lid margins, sometimes with telangiectasia. The distinctive features are described in Chapter 6.
- Other conjunctival or corneal lesions, for example pterygia and pingueculae, may present with focal redness. They are easily visible.
- A red eye may be associated with topical medication. This may be due to the preservatives in the drops or the drug itself.
- Elevation of venous pressure and dilation of conjunctival and scleral venules associated with a cavernous sinus thrombosis or a carotid-cavernous sinus fistula.

Sudden visual loss

Sudden *uniocular loss of vision* is caused either by a sudden clouding of the ocular media or by a problem with the retina or optic nerve. It is important to determine the onset and duration of the visual loss and

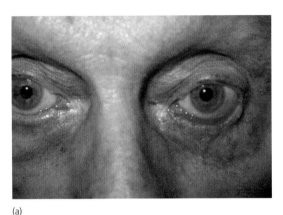
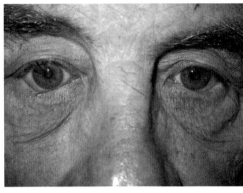

(a)   (b)

Figure 3.3 (a) The appearance of an ectropion. (b) The appearance of an entropion.

whether there has been any progression or recovery. It is essential to establish whether this is truly a *sudden* loss of vision or whether it is a longstanding loss which had gone unnoticed and has been revealed when the fellow eye was covered. It is always important to identify any associated symptoms, whether visual or of pain (Table 3.4), which preceded visual loss.

A general medical history is vital. For example, is the patient diabetic or hypertensive?

Opacities of the transparent media of the eye

- The sudden onset of corneal oedema and clouding in *acute angle closure glaucoma,* resulting from intraocular pressure building up over minutes or hours, causes blurred vision, accompanied by severe pain and redness of the eye. There may be a history of past attacks of blurred vision and eye pain or headache which then subsided. Such prodromal attacks may be precipitated in the dark, or by pupil dilation, which cause a subacute attack of angle closure glaucoma.
- Visual loss may also occur quite rapidly with *keratitis* or a *corneal ulcer,* again with redness, and severe pain.
- *Anterior uveitis (iritis)* may cause some blurring of vision when inflammatory cells adhering to the back of the cornea (*keratic precipitates*), or pupillary *synechiae* (where the iris becomes adherent to the lens), lie on the visual axis.
- In *posterior uveitis,* visual loss may be caused by a *vitritis,* when the vitreous is invaded by inflammatory cells. This may be secondary to a local retinitis or choroiditis, with further visual loss due to retinal damage. The eye is slightly painful and

photophobic. *Endophthalmitis* is an extreme form of posterior uveitis, usually due to an intraocular bacterial infection following intraocular surgery or penetrating injury to the globe. It presents with rapidly escalating pain and a profound visual loss. The vitreous is opacified by a massive infiltration by polymorphonuclear leucocytes (PMNs) and by exudative inflammatory products. This is an ocular emergency requiring immediate treatment.

- *Haemorrhage into the vitreous* is a common cause of sudden, painless visual loss and may result from a rupture of abnormal fine capillary vessels growing from the surface of the retina (proliferative diabetic retinopathy) or be associated with central retinal vein occlusion or 'wet' age-related macular degeneration. It may also follow a posterior vitreous detachment, when it is caused by a retinal tear which may precede a retinal detachment.

Retinal abnormalities

- *Total occlusion* of the central retinal vein or retinal artery results in a *sudden painless loss of vision* involving the whole visual field. A branch occlusion causes a partial loss of vision.
- *Wet, age-related macular degeneration* can cause a sudden loss or distortion of vision. Central vision is lost but peripheral vision is retained. Other acute disorders affecting the macula include *macular oedema* and *central serous retinopathy.* A *macular hole* may cause sudden central visual loss.
- A *retinal detachment* results in a curtain-like loss of the visual field, which starts at the top of the visual field in the case of an inferior detachment, or at the bottom of the field if the detachment is superior. It may be preceded by vitreous floaters, either due to a

Table 3.4 Sudden visual loss or disturbance: causes.

Painful		Angle closure glaucoma
		Corneal ulcer/keratitis
		Anterior uveitis(iritis)
		Endophthalmitis
		Retrobulbar optic neuritis
		Orbital cellulitis
		Giant cell arteritis
Painless	Fleeting visual loss	Embolic retinal artery occlusion
		Migraine – migraine headache usually follows the visual symptoms
		Raised intracranial pressure
		Prodromal, in giant cell arteritis
	Persistent visual loss	Vitreous haemorrhage
		Retinal artery occlusion
		Retinal vein occlusion
		Retinal detachment
		Age-related macular degeneration
		Other macular disease
		Optic neuritis
		Ischaemic optic neuropathy
		Orbital disease affecting the optic nerve
		Intracranial disease affecting the visual pathway

small vitreous bleed (see above) or to a vitreous detachment and condensations in the vitreous gel. Vitreous detachment also puts traction on the retina, giving rise to the key symptom of flashing lights.

- Inflammation of the retina associated with a *posterior uveitis* may cause visual loss, particularly if the macula or optic nerve is involved.
- A transient loss of vision, lasting minutes and described as 'a shutter' coming quickly across the vision, is typical of *amaurosis fugax*. It is caused by platelet emboli passing through the retinal circulation.
- A proportion of patients who suffer from migraine headaches experience a prodromal visual aura (fortification spectra or scintillating scotomata) due to transient ischaemia of the visual cortex. It precedes the headache and lasts between 20 and 30 minutes.

Optic nerve abnormalities

- *Optic neuritis*, due to focal demyelination of the optic nerve, causes a loss of vision developing over a few days. When the lesion affects the optic nerve behind the globe (*retrobulbar neuritis*), the optic nerve head appears normal. When the optic sheath is involved, the patient complains of pain on eye movement. Anterior optic neuritis is accompanied by nerve head swelling or *papillitis*.
- *Anterior ischaemic optic neuropathy* (AION) results from an acute decrease in blood supply causing infarction of the optic nerve head. It presents with sudden loss of vision. It may be caused by *giant cell arteritis* (GCA), with associated symptoms of pain in the temple, jaw claudication, shoulder pain and tiredness. There is usually a profound loss of vision in the affected eye. GCA is a *medical emergency* requiring urgent treatment with steroids. AION may also be seen in patients with vascular disease accompanying ageing, diabetes or hypertension. The risk is increased in those with small optic discs, which accommodate axonal swelling less readily. The loss of visual field is painless. Symptoms are often first noticed in the morning, perhaps

reflecting the fall in blood pressure and optic nerve head perfusion that occurs during sleep. Visual loss commonly affects the upper or lower visual field.

- Episodes of visual loss lasting only a few seconds are typical of *raised intracranial pressure* in the presence of papilloedema. These visual 'obscurations' are often induced by a change in posture.
- The optic nerve may be compressed in orbital cellulitis, resulting in rapid visual loss.

Visual loss involving both eyes

This usually suggests disease of the visual pathway from the optic nerves to the visual cortex. Occasionally, an ocular cause may be found, for example if both eyes are affected by uveitis.

Gradual visual loss

Patients may adjust to a gradual loss of vision, so there may be a lengthy delay before they seek medical help. This is particularly so in older patients with cataract. Also, in chronic glaucoma, because of its slow evolution, the patient may be unaware of a considerable degree of visual field loss until it is detected by chance or investigated when glaucoma is diagnosed at a routine assessment.

- Cloudy ocular media, due to the gradual development of corneal oedema, cataract or, rarely, vitreous opacity, are possible causes of a gradual, painless reduction in vision (Table 3.5).
- In patients with clear media, retinal abnormalities, particularly those affecting the macula, may be

present. Retinal dystrophies often cause a gradual reduction in vision. Dry macular degeneration may also result in a slow decline in central vision, sometimes accompanied by visual distortion.

- Compressive optic nerve disease is usually associated with gradual visual loss, which may also be caused by intracranial disease such as a pituitary tumour. Associated symptoms such as headache, nausea and double vision and an unsteady gait may suggest the presence of a space-occupying lesion.

Ocular pain

The presence of pain can be very useful in deciding the cause of other ocular symptoms. It is seldom the only presenting feature of eye disease, and most causes have already been discussed. They are summarized in Table 3.6.

Diplopia

The onset of diplopia or double vision can be a worrying symptom, both for the patient and for the clinician! It is important, as ever, to obtain a full history (Table 3.7). It is important to establish if the diplopia

Table 3.5 Gradual visual loss: causes.

Media cloudy	Corneal opacity
(Opacities in the cornea, lens or vitreous appear black against the red reflex)	Cataract
	Vitreous haemorrhage
Media clear	
Retinal disorder	Age-related macular degeneration
	Macular oedema/retinal dystrophy
Optic nerve/pathway disorder	Optic neuropathy
	Central nervous system disease affecting visual pathways (e.g. visual cortex)

Table 3.6 Causes of ocular pain.

Discomfort	Blepharitis
	Dry eye
	Conjunctivitis
	Allergy
	Dysthyroid eye disease
Pain on eye movements	Optic neuritis
Pain around the eye	Giant cell arteritis Migraine
	Orbital cellulitis
	Causes of 'headache'
Severe pain	Keratitis
	Corneal abrasion/ulcer/foreign body
	Uveitis
	Angle closure glaucoma
	Endophthalmitis
	Scleritis
	Myositis of extraocular muscles

Table 3.7 **Establishing the history in a patient with diplopia.**

Does the diplopia disappear when either eye is covered (to confirm a binocular cause)?

Was the onset sudden or gradual?

Is there a history of trauma?

Is the double vision present all the time?

Is it worse when the patient is tired?

Are the two images horizontally, vertically or diagonally displaced?

What are the associated symptoms (abnormalities of the pupils, other neurological symptoms)?

Are there any clues in the general medical history (diabetes, hypertension, thyroid disorders)?

Table 3.8 **Binocular Diplopia: causes.**

Neurogenic	III, IV, VI nerve palsies
	Inter- and supranuclear gaze palsies
	Failure to control a longstanding squint
	Associated with field defects (bitemporal hemianopia)
Myogenic	Thyroid eye disease Myasthenia Myositis Myopathy
Orbital	Trauma
	Space-occupying lesions
	Carotid-cavernous sinus fistula
Monocular	Corneal disease Cataract

is monocular (seen with one eye when the other eye is covered) or binocular (seen only with both eyes open). Where the diplopia persists despite covering one or other eye, the diplopia (sometimes polyopia) has a refractive cause such as cataract.

Binocular diplopia results from a loss of binocular alignment of the two eyes in a particular direction of gaze. The most common cause is an extraocular muscle paresis due to disease of the third, fourth or sixth cranial nerve (Table 3.8), but it may also result from a physical restriction of eye movements. Onset is usually acute and painless and the symptom constant. Testing eye movements reveals the type of palsy present. Inter- and supranuclear palsies may also present acutely (Chapter 16). The nature of the disorder in eye movements usually helps locate the site of the lesion.

- Myasthenia may cause intermittent diplopia where the symptoms are worse as the patient tires.

- If thyroid eye disease is suspected (Graves disease), look for the systemic features of that condition as well as the characteristic proptosis, restricted eye movements and acute inflammation over the insertion of the extraocular muscles.
- Trauma may cause a *neurogenic diplopia* if the cranial nerves are damaged, and a *restrictive diplopia* when orbital tissue becomes trapped in an orbital fracture of the floor or medial wall of the orbit. Once again a good history will suggest the most likely diagnosis.
- Diplopia may result from decompensation of a longstanding well-controlled squint. Here again the symptoms may be intermittent.

Examination

Both structure and function of the eye are examined.

Physiological testing of the eye

Visual acuity

Adults

Visual acuity (VA) tests the visual resolving power of the eye. The standard test is the Snellen chart, consisting of rows of letters (known as optotypes) of decreasing size (Figure 3.4a). Each row is numbered with the distance in metres at which each letter width subtends 1 minute of arc at the eye. Acuity is recorded as the reading distance (e.g. 6 m) over the row number of the smallest letter seen. If this is the 6 m line, then VA is 6/6; if it is the 60 m line, then VA is 6/60. Snellen acuities are thus recorded as 6/5, 6/6, 6/9, 6/12, 6/18/, 6/36/ and 6/60. Visual resolution is ten times greater at 6/6 than 6/60. Some countries (e.g. the United States) use a different scale, with the foot as the unit of distance. On this scale 20/20 equates to 6/6.

Increasingly, the logMAR VA chart is being used, both in research and clinically (Figure 3.4b). It is particularly useful in more accurately assessing vision and change in vision in patients with poorer acuity. Unlike the Snellen chart, which shows uneven jumps in size from row to row, the logMAR letter sizes change in smooth, log-linear steps. The number of letters on each line is equal, so that the lines of letters form a distinctive V-shaped pattern on the chart. The chart also allows accurate scoring of incompletely seen lines, where each letter reported accurately contributes to the score. Scores are recorded as a decimal, 0.00 equating to 6/6 (see Appendix A).

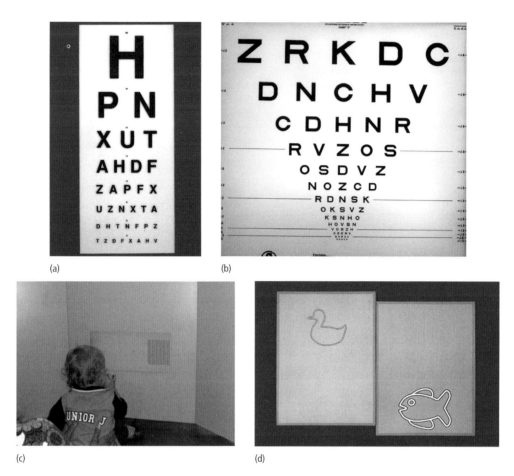

(a) (b)

(c) (d)

Figure 3.4 Methods of assessing visual acuity. (a) The Snellen chart. (b) A logMAR acuity chart. (c) Teller cards. (d) Cardiff cards.

Whatever chart is used, best vision is tested with spectacles if worn. Viewing through a pinhole will correct for moderate refractive error.

Children

In children, various age-appropriate methods are used to assess VA:

- Very young children are observed to see if they can follow objects or pick up scattered 'hundreds and thousands' cake decorations.
- A consistent tendency to object to occlusion of one eye may indicate poor vision in the fellow eye.
- Teller acuity cards can also be used. This is a *preferential looking test* based on the finding that children prefer to look at complex rather than plain targets (Figure 3.4c). The cards have alternate black and white stripes of reducing size, and are presented simultaneously with a grey card.

The children are observed to see whether they prefer to look at the patterned card. The bandwidths define the acuity at the test distance. As the width of the bands decreases, the pattern becomes harder to resolve against the grey background.

- The Cardiff Acuity Test (Figure 3.4d) can be used to assess vision in 1–3 year olds. The gaze of the child is observed and the examiner estimates whether the object seen is at the top or bottom of the card. When the examiner is unable to identify the position of the object from the child's gaze, it is assumed that the child cannot see the picture and the resolution of the eye is inferred.
- Older (verbal) children are able to identify or match single pictures and letters on charts which they hold in their hands, with those, of varying size, presented to them at a distance (*Sheridan–Gardiner test*).

Visual fields

The visual fields map the peripheral extent of the visual world. Each field can be represented as a series of contours or *isopters,* representing the ability to resolve a target of given size and brightness at a particular location. The field is not flat; towards the centre of fixation, the eye is able to detect much smaller objects than at the periphery. This produces a *hill of vision* in which objects which are resolved in finest detail are at the peak of the hill (representing the *fovea*) and acuity falls towards the periphery (Figure 3.5). On the temporal side of the field is the blind spot, which corresponds to the position of the optic nerve head, where there are no photoreceptors.

The visual field may be tested in various ways.

Confrontation tests

In this simple test, the examiner compares his own field with that of the patient. It is presumed that the examiner's visual field is normal. One eye of the patient is covered and the examiner sits opposite, closing his eye on the same side, that is if the patient's left eye is covered, the examiner closes his own right eye. The test object, traditionally the head of a large red hat pin, is then brought into view from the periphery and moved centrally. The patient is asked to report when he first sees the object. Each quadrant is tested and the location of the blind spot is determined, as well as the outline of the field of vision. With practice, hemianopias, quadrantinopias and central *scotomas* can also be identified (Figure 3.6).

A scotoma is a focal area of decreased sensitivity within the field, surrounded by a more sensitive area.

Other tests for hemianopic or quadrantic defects

- This can be useful in picking up a bitemporal hemianopia in patients with a chiasmal lesion. Sit facing the patient and hold your hands up, palms forwards, one on either side of the midline. Ask the patient to cover one eye and look directly at your face. Enquire if the two palms appear qualitatively the same. Repeat the test with the fellow eye. The patient may notice that the outer (temporal) palm appears duller on each side. Such patients may also miss the temporal letters on the Snellen chart when their VA is measured.

- Ask the patient to count the number of fingers which you show in each quadrant of the visual field.

A useful way to identify a neurological field defect is to use a red target. Sensitivity to red may be greatly depressed in optic nerve lesions. A red-topped pin is used to perform a confrontation test, the patient being asked to report when he first sees the pin top as red (not when he first sees the pin top). More simply, a red object can be held in the centre of each quadrant or hemifield and the patient asked to compare the quality of red in each location. In a hemianopic field defect, the red would appear washed-out or 'less red' in the affected field.

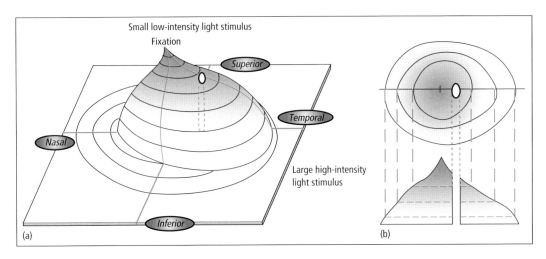

Figure 3.5 The hill of vision: (a) shown diagrammatically; (b) a normal plot of the visual field of the left eye. The different lines (isoptres) correspond to different sizes or intensities of the target. (*Source:* Anderson et al. (1982)/with permission of Elsevier.)

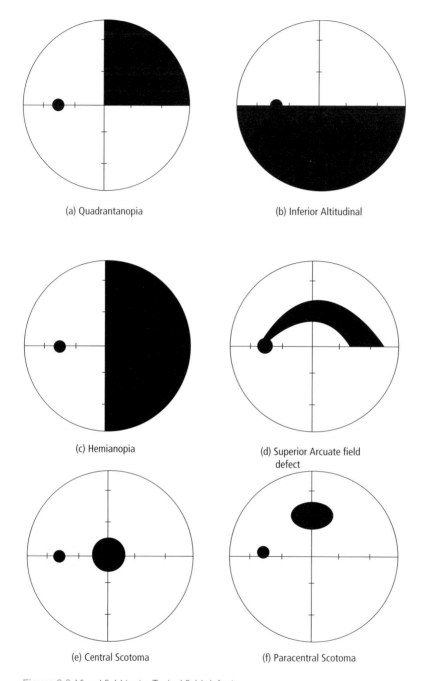

(a) Quadrantanopia

(b) Inferior Altitudinal

(c) Hemianopia

(d) Superior Arcuate field defect

(e) Central Scotoma

(f) Paracentral Scotoma

Figure 3.6 Visual field tests: Typical field defects.

Perimeters

These machines permit more accurate plotting of the visual field. There are two types:

- *Kinetic perimeters:* For example, the Goldmann perimeter, in which the patient indicates when he/ she first sees a light of a specific size and brightness, brought in from the periphery. This is rather like the moving pinhead of the confrontation test (Figure 3.7).

- *Static perimeters*: Spots of light, of varying brightness, are presented in sequence at fixed points any-

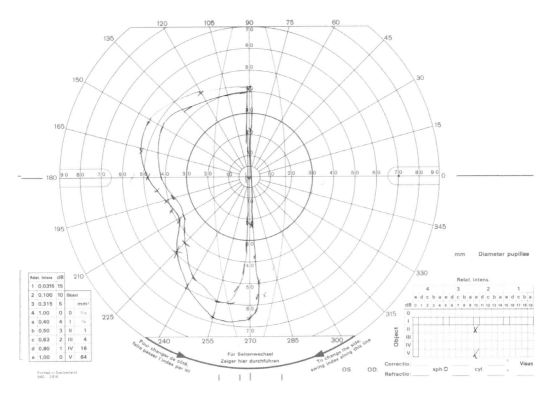

Figure 3.7 Example of a Goldmann kinetic visual field plot showing a right hemianopic field defect. The red and blue lines or isoptres represent different size and brightness of light stimuli.

where in the visual field. The patient indicates when a light is first seen at each location, and this information is used to plot a threshold map of visual sensitivity across the field (Figure 3.8). The threshold is the dimmest light of a prescribed size that the subject can see 50% of the time.

These techniques are particularly useful in chronic ocular and neurological conditions, to monitor changes in the visual field (e.g. in glaucoma or compressive lesions of the visual pathway).

Increasingly sophisticated perimeters are being developed using computer programs that enable the time it takes to perform an accurate threshold visual field to be reduced. The intensity of light is recorded in decibels: the higher the number, the dimmer the light (Figure 3.8).

Perimeters that test different pathways in the visual system have also been developed. For example, a flickering target tests the M-cell pathway, responsible for motion detection. These may be important in diseases that may selectively affect one pathway, such as glaucoma.

Colour vision

This is the ability of humans and other animals to distinguish objects based on the wavelengths (or frequencies) of the light they reflect, emit or transmit. Colour perception is a subjective process and is subserved by several types of cone cells in the eye.

The Ishihara colour blindness test, devised early in the last century, remains one of the best-known colour vision deficiency tests (Figure 3.9). It was devised to check for congenital red–green colour blindness, but can be used for testing acquired colour vision loss as well. Other tests include HRR (Hardy-Rand-Rittler) plates. The Farnsworth Munsell 100 Hue test and the D-15 panel are arrangement tests where the subject has to arrange coloured blocks in the correct sequence. Those with colour vision deficiencies will make predicable mistakes.

A useful bedside test for checking optic nerve dysfunction (which affects the ability to see the colour red at an early stage) is to look for red desaturation by comparing the two eyes, the eye with optic nerve disease sees a bright red object as a washed-out colour (see also confrontation testing of the visual field).

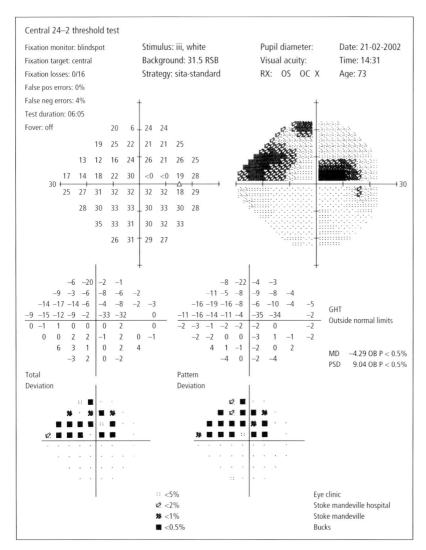

Figure 3.8 Example of a threshold field plot from an automated perimeter. The upper left diagram shows the threshold values for each test location. This is pictorially represented in the upper right picture. The middle diagrams compare the subject's field with that of a normal age-matched population. The lower diagrams indicate how likely it is that the value of each location differs from this control population. In this plot of the right eye, there is a field defect (scotoma) affecting part of the superior field, the patient has glaucoma.

Contrast sensitivity

This is a very important measure of visual function, especially in situations of low light or glare. In simple terms, *contrast sensitivity* refers to the ability to distinguish between an object and its background. For example, imagine a black cat against a white snowy background (high contrast) versus a grey cat against a grey background (low contrast). It is measured using charts such as the Pelli Robson chart (Figure 3.10). VA tests e.g. Snellen and logMAR use uniform high contrast, black letters on a white background (Figure 3.4a,b) while the Pelli Robson chart presents successive groups of letters in progressively fainter shades of grey. Contrast sensitivity is reduced in certain conditions, for example cataract and optic nerve disease (e.g. optic neuritis, chronic glaucoma).

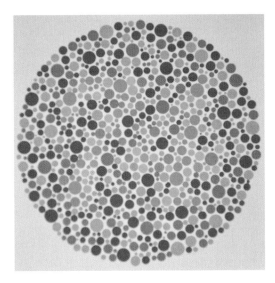

Figure 3.9 Example of an Ishihara colour vision plate.

Intraocular pressure

Intraocular pressure is measured by a contact technique, with a Goldmann applanation tonometer (Figure 3.11a, b). A clear plastic cylinder is pressed against the anaesthetized cornea. The ring of flattening, viewed through the cylinder, is made visible by the presence of fluorescein in the tear film (see below). A horizontally disposed prism, within the cylinder, splits the ring of contact into two hemicircles. The force applied to the cylinder can be varied to alter the amount of corneal flattening and thus the size of the ring. It is adjusted so that the two hemicircles just interlock. This is the end point of the test and the force applied, converted into units of ocular pressure (mmHg), can now be read from the tonometer.

Optometrists use an instrument which supplies a puff of air of varying intensity to produce corneal flattening rather than the prism of the Goldmann tonometer. Various other tonometers are also available, including small, handheld electronic devices. An example is rebound tonometry, where a rapidly vibrating probe is brought close to the cornea. The force required to indent the cornea is converted into a pressure reading. The I-care tonometer is an example which is particularly useful in children.

With all contact techniques, the thickness of the cornea has a significant effect on the measurement of intraocular pressure, affecting the accuracy of measurement. These tonometers underestimate the pressure where the cornea is thin and easier to deform. A *thicker cornea* requires more force for the same deformation, leading to an *overestimation* of

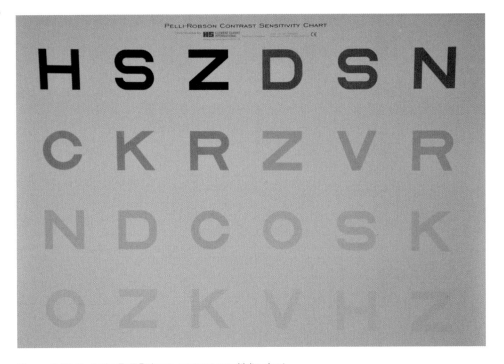

Figure 3.10 Part of a Pelli Robson contrast sensitivity chart.

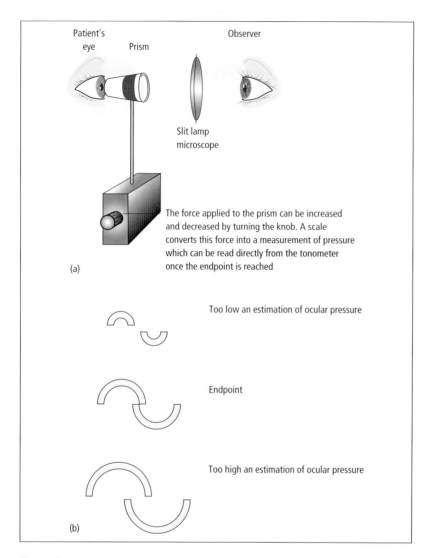

Patient's eye Prism

Observer

Slit lamp microscope

The force applied to the prism can be increased and decreased by turning the knob. A scale converts this force into a measurement of pressure which can be read directly from the tonometer once the endpoint is reached

(a)

Too low an estimation of ocular pressure

Endpoint

Too high an estimation of ocular pressure

(b)

Figure 3.11 (a) Measurement of intraocular pressure with a Goldmann tonometer. (b) Two hemicircles are seen by the examiner. The force of contact is increased until the inner borders of the hemicircles just touch. This is the endpoint, at which a fixed amount of flattening of the cornea is achieved.

intraocular pressure. Measurement of corneal thickness can now readily be performed with small handheld ultrasonic pachymeters, which are used increasingly to make the appropriate correction.

The Ocular Response Analyser (ORA) is able to measure IOP, compensated for corneal thickness. A 25 msec pulse of air is used to indent the cornea which then regains its original shape. The change in shape is recorded, much like the traditional air puff tonometers mentioned above but the technique here analyses the inward and outward movement of the cornea as well as the degree of indentation of the cornea (hysteresis). This allows the machine to compensate for the individual's corneal biomechanics.

Pupillary reactions

The size of the pupils (*miosis*, constricted; *mydriasis*, dilated) and their response to light and accommodation give important information about:

- the function of the afferent pathways controlling pupil size (the optic nerve and tract) (see Chapter 14);

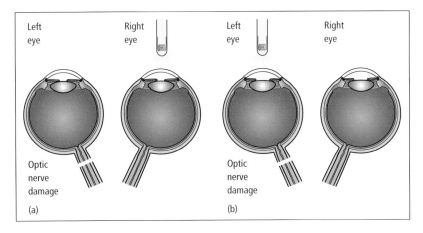

Figure 3.12 The *swinging flashlight test* for a relative afferent pupil defect (RAPD) in a diagnosis of left optic neuritis. (a) A light directed at the right eye causes the pupils to constrict equally. (b) When the light is moved rapidly to the left eye, both pupils dilate because of the lack of afferent drive to the light reflex from the damaged left optic nerve. This is a left relative afferent pupillary defect.

- the function of the efferent pathway;
- the action of drugs on the pupil.

Examination of the pupils begins with an assessment of the size and symmetry of the pupils in a uniform light (resting pupil size). If there is asymmetry (*anisocoria*), it must be decided whether the smaller or larger pupil is abnormal. A pathologically small pupil (after damage to the sympathetic nervous system) will be more apparent in dim illumination since dilation of the normal pupil will be greater. A pathologically large pupil (seen in disease of the parasympathetic nervous system) will be more apparent in bright light since the fellow pupil will be small.

Some healthy individuals show pupil size asymmetry unassociated with disease (physiological anisocoria) – this tends to be more prominent in dim illumination. Remember that inflammation of the anterior segment (*iritis*), trauma or previous ocular surgery may cause structural iris changes or posterior synechiae, which mechanically alter pupil shape or response (see Chapter 10).

In order to test the efferent limb of the pupil reflex, the patient is asked to look at a near object. Normal pupils constrict in conjunction with accommodation and convergence. This is termed *the near reflex*.

To look for a defect in optic nerve function, the *swinging flashlight test* is used. This is a sensitive index for an afferent conduction defect. The patient is seated in a dimly illuminated room and views a distant object. A penlight is directed at each eye in turn while the pupils are observed. The light is directed from the side to avoid stimulating the near

reflex. A unilateral defect in optic nerve conduction is demonstrated as a relative afferent pupil defect (RAPD) (see Figure 3.12 for full description, Figure 3.13 for the pathway involved in the reflex and Chapter 15 for clinical importance).

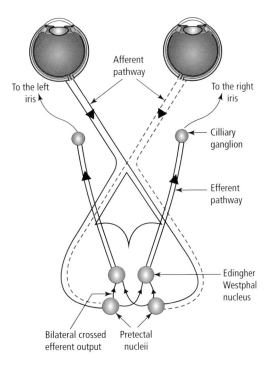

Figure 3.13 The pathway involved in the relative afferent pupillary defect.

Eye movements

These are assessed while sitting facing the patient who is asked to look at a penlight held directly ahead. In the absence of squint and with the eyes in forward gaze (the 'primary position'), the reflection of light from the corneas will be symmetrically placed. If a squint is present and only one eye is fixated on the light, then the reflection from the non-fixating eye is displaced to one side. The direction of displacement indicates the nature of the squint (see Chapter 16).

Record the following:

- the position of the eyes;
- the result of the cover test (see chapter 16);
- the range of eye movements;
- any abnormal eye movements.

An abnormal direction of gaze of one of the eyes, with the eyes in the primary position, may suggest a squint. This can be confirmed by performing a cover test (see Chapter 16).

The range of eye movements is assessed by asking the subject to follow a moving object. Horizontal, vertical and oblique movements are checked from the primary position of gaze, asking the patient to report any double vision (*diplopia*). The presence of any abnormal eye movements e.g. oscillating eye movements (*nystagmus*) (see Chapter 16) is also noted.

Movement of the eyes when following an object is recorded. Such movements (*pursuit* movements) have the angular velocity of the target. They are usually smooth but may be altered in disease. The ability to direct gaze from one object to another is called a *saccadic* eye movement. These are extremely rapid eye movements whose speed is predetermined and not under voluntary control. Saccades can be tested by asking the patient to look, back and forth, at targets (such as the fingers) held at either side of the head. These movements should be fast, smooth and accurate (i.e. they should not overshoot or undershoot the target). In children, use a toy or other interesting object to assess eye movements while gently steadying the child's head.

Eyelids

These are usually symmetrically arranged, with the upper and lower lid margins just crossing the upper and the lower limbus of each eye. The margin of the lid is applied closely to the globe in the healthy eye. If the lid margin is turned away from the globe, an *ectropion* is present; if the lid margin is turned in an *entropion* is present and the lashes may rub against the globe.

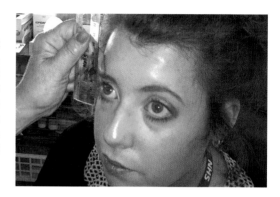

Figure 3.14 Assessment of ptosis. The examiner holds a ruler to measure the extent of lid movement while compressing the frontal muscle with a finger to prevent it contributing to lid elevation. Note the difference in brow position that this causes.

A drooping lid (*ptosis*) may reflect:

- an anatomical disorder (e.g. a congenital weakness of the levator muscle or age-related dehiscence of the levator tendon from the tarsal plate);
- an organic problem (e.g. weakness of the levator muscle in myasthenia gravis or impairment of its nerve supply in third nerve palsy).

In assessing ptosis, the distance between the upper and lower lids is measured with the patient looking straight ahead. The excursion of the upper lid from extreme downgaze to extreme upgaze is then recorded. The examiner's finger compresses the frontal muscle to prevent it contributing to elevation of the lid (Figure 3.14). In myasthenia, repeated up and down movements of the lids will increase the ptosis by fatiguing the levator muscle (see Chapter 6).

Anatomical examination of the eye

Lids and anterior segment

Simple examination of the eye and adnexae can reveal a great deal about pathological processes within the eye.

Ophthalmologists use a biomicroscope (*slit lamp*) to examine the eye and lids. This provides a magnified, stereoscopic view. The slit of light permits a cross section of the transparent media of the eye to be viewed. By adjusting the angle between this beam and the viewing microscope, the light can be used to highlight different structures and pathological processes within the eye. Each structure is carefully examined, starting with the lids and working inwards.

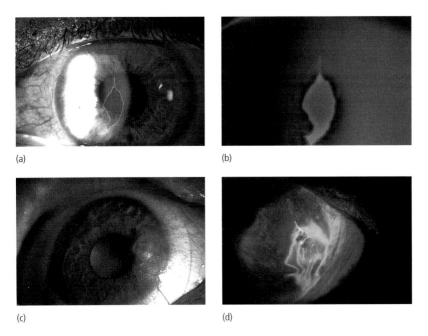

Figure 3.15 (a) A corneal abrasion (the corneal epithelial layer has been damaged); (b) fluorescein uniformly stains the area of damage. (c) A perforated cornea leaking aqueous (the leak is protected here with a soft contact lens); (d) (after removing the contact lens) the fluorescein fluoresces as it is diluted by the leaking aqueous.

Examination without a slit lamp

Without a slit lamp, the eye can still be meaningfully examined with a suitable light such as a penlight or ophthalmoscope. Comment can be made on:

- *The conjunctiva*: Is it injected (inflamed), is there a discharge, what is the distribution of redness, is a conjunctival haemorrhage present?
- *The cornea*: Is it clear, is there a bright reflection of light from the overlying tear film?
- *The anterior chamber*: Is it intact (if penetrating injury is suspected); is a hypopyon or a hyphema present (see Chapters 10 and 17)?
- *The iris and pupil*: Is the shape of the pupil normal?
- *The lens*: Is there an opacity in the red reflex observed with the ophthalmoscope?

Diagnostic use of fluorescein

Fluorescein dye (a phenolphthalein derivative) has the property of maximally absorbing light at 484 nm (blue light) and emitting light (i.e. fluorescing) at a different wavelength of 514 nm (green light). The instillation of fluorescein into the conjunctival sac can identify corneal abrasions (where the surface epithelial cells have been lost) and leakage of aqueous humour from the eye where the cornea has been penetrated or a wound is unsealed (Figure 3.15).

To examine an abrasion
- A weak, highly fluorescent solution of the dye is applied to the eye.
- The eye is examined with a blue light.
- The abrasion fluoresces bright green.

To determine if fluid is leaking from the eye (e.g. after penetrating corneal injury)
- A drop of 2% solution of fluorescein, which is poorly fluorescent, is applied to the eye.
- The eye is examined with a blue light.
- The dye, diluted by the leaking aqueous, becomes bright green at its junction with the dark, concentrated fluorescein (*Seidel test positive*).

Eversion of the upper lid

The underside of the upper lid is examined by everting it over a small blunt-ended object (e.g. a cotton bud) placed in the lid crease (Figure 3.16). This is an important technique to master, as foreign bodies may often lodge under the upper lid, causing considerable pain to the patient.

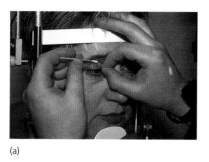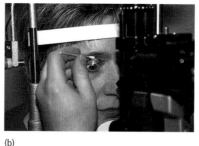

(a)   (b)

Figure 3.16 Lid eversion. (a) Placement of the cotton bud. (b) Eversion of the lid.

Retina

The retina is examined by:

- Direct ophthalmoscopy (the conventional ophthalmoscope) (Figure 3.17).
- Indirect ophthalmoscopy, which allows the extreme retinal periphery to be viewed. The examiner wears a head-mounted binocular microscope with a light source. A lens placed between the examiner and the eye of the subject is used to produce an inverted image of the retina.
- Special lenses (e.g. 90 dioptre and 3 mirror) are also used at the slit lamp.

The latter two techniques are reserved for specialists; the technique that must be mastered by the non-specialist is direct ophthalmoscopy.

The direct ophthalmoscope provides:

- an image of the *red reflex* – a red glow in the pupil zone due to light scattered from the vascular choroid;
- a magnified view of the optic nerve head, macula, retinal blood vessels and the retina to the equator.

It comprises:

- a light source, the size and colour of which can be changed;
- a system of lenses which permits the refractive error of both observer and patient to be corrected.

Confident use of the ophthalmoscope comes with practice. The best results are obtained if the pupil is first dilated with *tropicamide,* a mydriatic with a short duration of action.

The patient and examiner must be comfortable; the patient looks straight ahead at a distant object. The examiner's right eye is used to examine the patient's right eye, and the left eye to examine the left eye.

The examiner views the red reflex through the pupil at a distance of about 30 cm from the eye. Corneal or

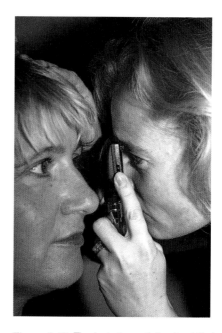

Figure 3.17 The technique of direct ophthalmoscopy. Note that the left eye of the observer is used to examine the left eye of the subject. The closer the observer is to the patient, the larger the field of view.

lens opacities appear as dark silhouettes against the red reflex, brought into focus by ratcheting down the ophthalmoscope from a high to a low hypermetropic (plus) correction, typically setting the lens to +4 (this technique is called distant direct ophthalmoscopy). The eye is then approached to within a couple of centimeters and the power of the lenses is adjusted in the myopic (minus) direction, to achieve focus on the retina.

The examiner may find it helpful to place a steadying hand on the subject's forehead, which can also be used to hold the upper lid open. The retina should now be in view. It is important to try and examine the retina in a logical sequence so that nothing is overlooked.

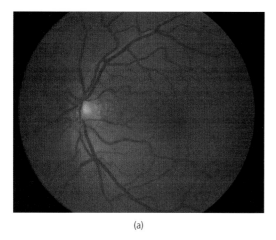
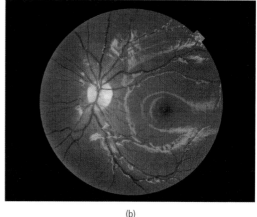

(a) (b)

Figure 3.18 (a) A normal left fundus from an adult. Note the optic disc with retinal veins and arteries passing from it to branch over the retina. The large temporal vessels form the *temporal arcades*. The macula lies temporal to the disc with the fovea at its centre. (b) This fundus picture is taken from a young subject, note the sheen from the retina, which is a normal appearance.

- First find the optic disc (Figure 3.18). With the eye looking straight ahead, approach the eye at an angle of 15° temporal to the line of gaze to avoid light reflection from the cornea. If blood vessels are seen, trace the vessels in the direction where they converge on the optic disc. Assess the margins of the optic disc, are they indistinct – as in papilloedema? Assess the colour of the disc, is it pale – as in optic atrophy? Assess the optic cup – is it enlarged, as it chronic glaucoma (see Chapter 11).
- Direct the ophthalmoscope slightly temporally and examine the macula. Is there a normal foveal reflex? In youth, the foveal pit appears as a bright pinpoint of light in the centre of the retina. Are there any abnormal lesions such as haemorrhages, exudates or cotton–wool spots?

- Return to the optic disc and follow each major vessel branch of the vasculature out to the periphery. Are the vessels of normal diameter? Do the arteries nip the veins where they cross (*A/V nipping* – in hypertension)? Are there any emboli in the arterioles? Also examine the surrounding retina for abnormalities.
- Examine the peripheral retina systematically, in a 360° sweep.

Special examination techniques

Diagnostic lenses

Ophthalmologists employ special lenses that can be used in conjunction with the slit lamp to examine particular ocular structures.

A *gonioscopy* lens is a diagnostic contact lens with a built-in mirror that permits examination of the iridocorneal angle. A larger lens with three mirrors allows the peripheral retina to be seen with the pupil dilated. Both are applied to the anaesthetized cornea, some requiring a lubricating drop. Other lenses can be used to obtain a stereoscopic view of the retina.

Retinoscopy

The technique of retinoscopy allows the refractive state of the eye to be measured (i.e. the required strength of a corrective spectacle lens). A streak of light from the retinoscope is directed into the eye. The reflection from the retina is observed through the retinoscope. By gently moving the retinoscope from side to side, the reflected

---

Direct ophthalmoscopy

Best performed in dim background illumination.

- Use an ophthalmoscope with a good illumination.
- Before examining the patient, set the ophthalmoscope power to a low plus, allowing you to focus through from the front to the back of the eye.
- Retinal examination requires that the examiner is close to the subject. An inadequate view will result if the examiner is too far away.
- Practice, practice, practice.

image is seen to move. The direction in which this image moves depends on the refractive error of the eye. By placing trial lenses of increasing or decreasing power in front of the eye, the direction in which the reflected image moves is seen to reverse. When this point is reached, the refractive error has been determined.

Investigative techniques

Ultrasound

The ultrasound B-scan (typical frequency 10 MHz) is used extensively in ophthalmology to provide information about the vitreous, retina and posterior coats of the eye (see Figure 3.19), particularly when they cannot be clearly visualized (if, for example, there is a dense cataract or vitreous haemorrhage). The ultrasound A-scan is used to measure the length of the eyeball prior to cataract surgery, to calculate the power of the artificial lens that is to be implanted in the eye (see Chapter 9).

High-frequency ultrasound (50 MHz) is used to visualize the anterior structures of the eye in detail, for example cornea, lens, ciliary body, anterior retina and anterior vitreous. This technique is referred to as ultrasound biomicroscopy.

Keratometry

The shape of the cornea (the radius of curvature) can be measured from the image of a target reflected from its surface. This is important in contact lens assessment (Chapter 4), refractive surgery (Chapter 4) and in calculating the power of an artificial lens implant in cataract surgery (Chapter 9). The technique of photo-keratometry (corneal topography) allows a very accurate contour map of the cornea to be produced (Figure 3.20). These techniques can be used to detect aberrations of shape such as a conical cornea (*keratoconus*).

Synoptophore

This machine permits the assessment of binocular single vision, the ability of the two eyes to work together to produce a single image. It can also assess the range over which the eyes can *diverge from* or *converge towards* each other, while maintaining a single picture (to measure the range of fusion).

Exophthalmometer

This device measures ocular protrusion (*proptosis*).

Electrophysiological tests

The electrical activity of the retina and visual cortex in response to specific visual stimuli, for example a flashing light, can be used to assess the functioning of the retina (*electroretinogram* or *ERG*), retinal pigment epithelium (*electrooculogram*) and the visual pathway (*visually evoked response* or *potential*).

Radiological imaging techniques

Computed tomography (CT) and magnetic resonance imaging (MRI) scans have largely replaced skull and orbital radiographs in the imaging of the orbit and visual pathway. The newer diagnostic techniques have enhanced the diagnosis of orbital disease (e.g. optic nerve sheath meningioma) and visual pathway lesions such as pituitary tumours. They have also become the first-line investigation in orbital trauma.

Fluorescein angiography

This technique (Figure 3.21) provides detailed information about the retinal circulation. Fluorescein dye is injected into the antecubital vein. A *fundus camera* is used to take photographs of the retina. A blue light is directed into the eye to 'excite' the fluorescein in the retinal circulation. The emitted green

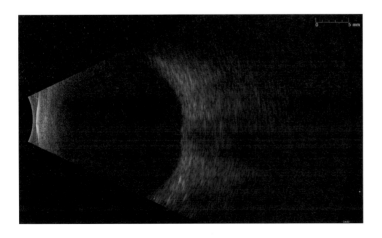

Figure 3.19 B-Scan ultrasound of a normal eye. Note the optic nerve shadow on the right in the centre.

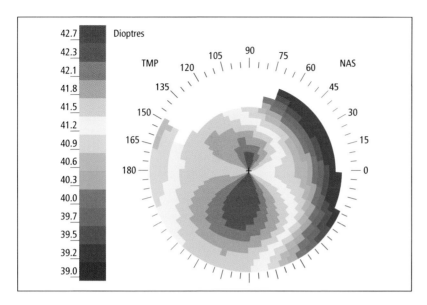

Figure 3.20 A contour map of the cornea obtained with a photokeratoscope. The colours represent areas of different corneal curvature and hence different refractive power. Red represents a lower radius of curvature and hence a higher refractive power.

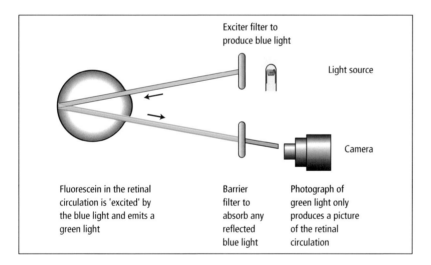

Figure 3.21 The technique of fluorescein angiography.

light is then photographed through a yellow barrier filter which absorbs any reflected blue light and allows the fluorescent image to be seen at high contrast.

In this way, a fluorescent picture of the retinal circulation is obtained (Figure 3.22). The dye leaks from abnormal blood vessels (e.g. the new vessels sometimes seen in diabetic eye disease). Areas of ischaemia, due to retinal capillary closure, fail to demonstrate the normal passage of dye (e.g. in a central retinal vein occlusion). The technique is useful both in diagnosis and in planning and following treatment.

Indocyanin green angiography (ICG) allows the choroidal vasculature to be imaged more accurately in a similar way.

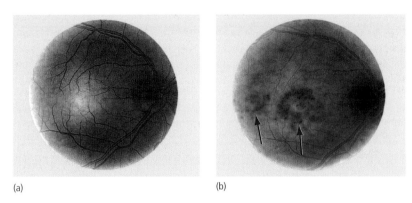

(a)

(b)

Figure 3.22 A fluorescein angiogram. (a) A photograph of the early phase, taken shortly after fluorescein has entered the eye: It can be seen in the choroidal circulation as background fluorescence, the retinal vessels being filled with the dye. (b) In the late phase, some minutes after injection of the dye, areas of hyperfluorescence (the dark areas, arrowed) can be seen around the macula. There has been leakage from abnormal blood vessels into the extravascular tissue space in the macular region (macular oedema).

OS, IR 30° + OCT 30° (8.6 mm) ART (9) Q: 30 [HS]

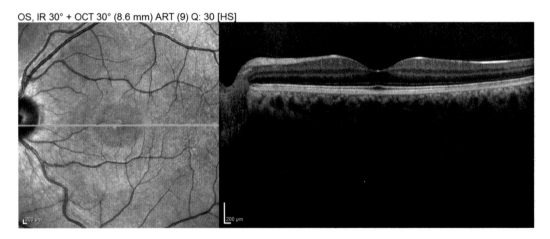

Figure 3.23 OCT scan of the macular region of retina. The scan represents the retina underneath the green line on the fundus picture. Note the depression at the fovea. The scan allows the layers of the retina to be seen.

Digital imaging and laser scanning techniques

New techniques of retinal imaging, such as confocal microscopy, have been developed to improve the quality of retinal and optic disc pictures and to permit quantitative assessment of features such as the area of the optic disc and optic disc cup (Chapter 11) and the size of retinal lesions (Chapter 12). These help in the assessment of patients with chronic diseases such as glaucoma, diabetes and macular degeneration, where the management requires an accurate assessment of any change over time.

Optical coherence tomography (OCT) (Figure 3.23) utilizes interferometry to create an *in vivo* cross-sectional map of the retina at a resolution of 10–15 μm. Sufficient media clarity is needed to obtain OCT scans. It is the technique of choice in the assessment and management

of age-related macular degeneration, diabetic macular disease and other retinal disorders.

KEY POINTS

- The eye is often affected by systemic disease. Always keep the possibility in mind when taking an ophthalmic history. It is always important to take a full medical history.

- A good ophthalmic history can initiate a differential diagnosis and influence subsequent clinical examination.

- It is possible to examine in detail every part of the eye with appropriate equipment. A simple penlight can however yield important clues to the diagnosis.

Assessment questions True or False

1. A red eye may be caused by:

a Acute glaucoma.

b Ocular infection.

c Iritis.

d Trauma.

e Retinal detachment.

2. Painful sudden loss or disturbance of vision may be caused by:

a Angle closure glaucoma.

b Endophthalmitis following cataract surgery.

c Giant cell arteritis.

d Raised intracranial pressure.

e Vitreous haemorrhage.

3. Visual acuity can be measured with:

a LogMAR chart.

b Perimeter.

c Snellen chart.

d Teller cards.

e Tonometer.

4. Physiological testing of the eye.

a A perimeter maps the field of vision.

b The Snellen chart is positioned at 4 m from the patient.

c The Cardiff acuity test relies on preferential looking.

d An isoptre on a visual field chart represents the eye's ability to see a point of light of given size and brightness.

e Intraocular pressure is measured with a perimeter.

5. Intraocular pressure:

a Is measured with a tonometer.

b Is measured with a pachymeter.

c Measurement is affected by the thickness of the cornea.

d Use of the Goldmann tonometer requires the cornea to be anaesthetized.

6. When examining the pupils:

a A pathologically small pupil is more apparent in dim light.

b A pathologically large pupil is more apparent in dim light.

c Healthy individuals may show asymmetry in pupil size.

d Iritis may cause irregularity of the pupil.

7. Pupils

a The term miosis means a constricted pupil.

b Anisocoria means that the pupils differ in size.

c Damage to oculomotor parasympathetic fibres causes miosis.

d A relative afferent pupillary defect indicates optic nerve disease.

e Normal pupils dilate during convergence.

8. Ptosis may be caused by:

a An inturned lower lid.

b Age-related dehiscence of the levator tendon from the tarsal plate.

c Myathenia gravis.

d Sixth nerve palsy.

e Third nerve palsy.

9. Lids

a When the lid margin is turned away from the eye, this is ectropion.

b When the lid margin is turned into the eye, this is entropion.

c Horner syndrome causes ptosis.

d In myasthenia, repeated lid blinking increases any ptosis.

10. Fluorescein

a Is excited by green light and emits in the blue wave band.

b Will stain a corneal abrasion.

c To detect its fluorescence, the eye must be examined with a blue light.

d Can be used to demonstrate a leak of aqueous from the anterior chamber.

e Is used to examine the vasculature of the retina.

11. The direct ophthalmoscope

a Produces a magnified image of the retina.

b Contains lenses which increase the magnification.

c Can be used to examine the red reflex.

d The retina can be seen by holding the instrument at a distance of 30 cm from the eye.

e The illumination can be altered.

12. Instruments

a Keratometry allows the protrusion of the eye to be measured.

b The synoptophore measures convergence and divergence.

c The exophthalmometer measures corneal shape.

d Retinoscopy is used to assess refractive error.

Answers

1. A red eye may be caused by:

a True. The conjunctiva is injected, the pupil dilated and the cornea cloudy.

b True. All ocular infections may present with a red eye.

c True. Typically, iritis presents with circumlimbal injection.

d True. Trauma may cause both conjunctival injection and a subconjunctival haemorrhage.

e False. A retinal detachment does not usually present with a red eye. There is a loss of vision.

2. Painful sudden loss or disturbance of vision may be caused by:

a True. The raised pressure causes the cornea to become oedematous and cloudy.

b True. The inflammation associated with the intraocular infection causes the vision to reduce.

c True. The patient may have a headache and pain in the jaw on eating (jaw claudication). The ischaemia of the optic nerve causes visual loss.

d False. Visual obscurations may occur, particularly on postural change, but these are not painful. The patient may however also have a headache associated with the raised intracranial pressure.

e False. Vitreous haemorrhage would not usually be associated with a painful eye.

3. Visual acuity can be measured with:

a True. This is particularly useful and provides more accurate measurement in patients with poorer vision.

b False. This is used to plot the field of vision.

c True. This is the conventional way to measure visual acuity.

d True. These are used in young children.

e False. This is used to measure intraocular pressure.

4. Physiological testing of the eye

a True. This is the conventional test of visual acuity.

b False. The chart is positioned at 6 m unless mirrors are used.

c True.

d True. This allows a map of the visual field to be created, linking the points perceived with similar size and brightness, similar to the contour lines of a map.

e False. A perimeter measures the visual field. A tonometer measures intraocular pressure.

5. Intraocular pressure:

a True. The Goldmann tonometer is the conventional instrument used to measure intraocular pressure.

b False. This is used to measure the thickness of the cornea.

c True. Intraocular pressure may be overestimated in patients with thicker corneas.

d True. The tip of the instrument touches the sensitive cornea.

6. When examining the pupils:

a True. The dim light causes the normal pupil to dilate.

b False. A pathologically large pupil is more apparent in bright light.

c True. There may be a small variation in pupillary size in normal people.

d True. The iris may become stuck to the lens and appear irregular.

7. Pupils

a True. Mydriasis refers to a dilated pupil.

b True. For causes, see Chapter 14.

c False. Blockade of these parasympathetic fibres results in mydriasis, because of the continued sympathetic dilator activity.

d True. This is an important test of optic nerve function, see page 45.

e False. They will constrict.

8. Ptosis may be caused by:

a False. This is an entropion.

b True. This is one of the commonest causes of ptosis.

c True. Myathenia gravis may cause a fatiguable ptosis.

d False. The sixth nerve innervates only the lateral rectus muscle palsy.

e True. Third nerve palsy may cause a severe ptosis.

9. Lids

a True. See Chapter 6.

b True. See Chapter 6.

c True. The third nerve carries nerve fibres to the levator muscle. See Chapter 16 for a full description.

d True. The muscle fatigues with the repeated effort of blinking.

10. Fluorescein

a False. Fluorescein is excited by blue light and emits green light.

b True. This is a ready way to demonstrate abnormalities of the corneal epithelium.

c True. The blue light excites the fluorescein causing it to emit green light.

d True. The dye, diluted by the leaking aqueous, becomes bright green at its junction with the dark, concentrated solution.

e True. This is called fluorescein angiography.

11. The direct ophthalmoscope

a True. The image is magnified some 16 times.

b False. The lenses allow the refractive error of patient and examiner to be corrected.

c True. This is an important part of the examination.

d False. To see the retina, the observer must be close to the eye.

e True. The size and colour of the illumination can be altered.

12. Instruments

a False. Keratometry involves the measurement of corneal shape.

b True.

c False. This allows the protrusion of the eye to be measured.

d True.

Reference

Anderson D.R. *et al.* (1982) *Testing the Field of Vision.* Mosby. ISBN 10: 0801602076 /ISBN 13: 9780801602078.

4

Clinical optics

Learning objectives

To understand:

✔ The different refractive states of the eye, accommodation and presbyopia.
✔ The means of correcting refractive error by cataract surgery.
✔ The correction of refractive errors with contact lenses, spectacles and refractive surgery.
✔ Preventing the development of myopia.

Introduction

Light can be defined as that part of the electromagnetic spectrum to which the retina is sensitive. The visible part of the spectrum lies between the wavebands 390 and 760 nm. For the eye to generate accurate visual information, light must be correctly refracted to be sharply focused on the retina. The focus must be adjustable to allow equally clear vision of near and distant objects. The cornea, or actually the air/tear interface, is the first refractive element of the eye, responsible for two-thirds of its focusing power; the crystalline lens provides the other third. These two refracting elements in the eye converge the rays of light because:

- The refracting surfaces of the cornea and lens are spherically convex.
- The cornea has a higher refractive index than air; the lens has a higher refractive index than the aqueous and vitreous humour. The velocity of light is reduced in a dense medium so that light is refracted towards the normal. Therefore, when passing from the air to the cornea, or from the aqueous to the lens, the light rays converge.

Refractive error (ametropia)

The single most common cause of poor vision on a global scale is uncorrected refractive error. The optically perfect eye requires no correction for distance, because, when no effort of focusing is made, parallel rays of light entering the eye from a distant object are brought to a point focus on the retina (see Figure 4.1). Such an individual can see sharply in the distance without accommodation. Any deviation from this state, with the point of focus shifted away from the retina with the eye at rest (without accommodation), is termed refractive error (or *ametropia*) and results in blurred uncorrected vision.

Ametropia may be divided into:

- *Myopia* (*short-sight*): Considering the upper diagram in Figure 4.2, you can see that the parallel rays of light entering the eye are brought to a point of focus *in front of* the retina. Therefore, at the retinal plane the image is blurred. This state is called *myopia*. This can occur because the eye is too long (*axial myopia*), or because the optical power of the eye (due to the cornea and lens) is too great (*refractive myopia*).

Ophthalmology: Lecture Notes, Thirteenth Edition. Bruce James, Anthony Bron, and Manoj V. Parulekar.
© 2024 John Wiley & Sons Ltd. Published 2024 by John Wiley & Sons Ltd.
Companion website: www.wiley.com/go/ophthalmology13e

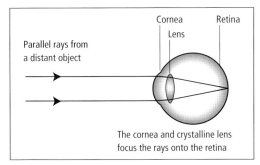

Figure 4.1 The rays of light in an emmetropic eye are focused on the retina.

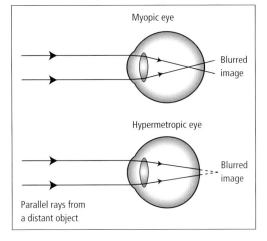

Figure 4.2 Myopia and hypermetropia.

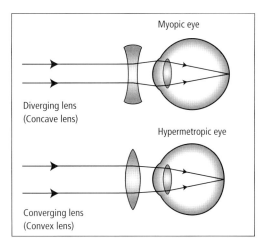

Figure 4.3 Correction of ametropia with spectacle lenses.

In either case, the ametropia can be corrected by placing a concave lens before the eye (Figure 4.3). A myopic eye is commonly described as *short-sighted*. This is because light diverging from an object close to a myopic eye is refracted to be focused sharply on the retina without the need for accommodation (see below). Shortsighted eyes can therefore see close objects clearly, and distant objects are blurred (hence shortsighted).

- *Hypermetropia* (*long-sight*): Now, considering the lower diagram in Figure 4.2, you can see that the parallel rays of light entering the eye are brought to a point of focus *beyond* the retina. Therefore, at the retinal plane the image is blurred. This state is called *hypermetropia*. This may occur because the eye is too short (*axial hypermetropia*), or because the optical power of the eye (due to the cornea and lens) is too weak (called *refractive hypermetropia*). This type of ametropia can be corrected by placing a convex lens before the eye (Figure 4.3). A hypermetropic eye is commonly described as *longsighted*. This is because parallel rays of light arising from distant objects and incident on the cornea can only be brought into focus on the retina by an accommodative effort, which increases the optical power of the lens. Since light arising from a near object diverges to reach the eye, even more accommodative effort is required to bring a near object into sharp focus. Hypermetropic eyes therefore see distant objects more clearly than close objects (hence longsighted).

- *Astigmatism:* Consider the two mirrors shown in Figure 4.4. The upper image in Figure 4.4 has a round spherical surface, and if you were to draw a line across the diameter of the mirror, no matter in which orientation (or *meridian*) you chose to draw your line, the curvature would be the same. Lenses with this same property are called *spherical* lenses.

- Now consider the ovoid mirror in Figure 4.4. You will notice that the curvature in one axis is different to the curvature of the mirror along the diameter at 90° to this. If you draw a line along a diameter of this mirror, the curvature changes as you rotate around the different *meridia* of the mirror. Lenses with this property are called *astigmatic* lenses.

Astigmatism, then, is the variation of surface curvature in different meridia of a lens. Consider Figure 4.5. You will see that light entering the eye in different meridia are focused differently depending on the curvature *in that meridian*. This means that the light entering the eye cannot be brought to a single point of focus. *Astigmatism* means literally 'without a point': 'stigma' meaning a 'mark' or 'point' in Greek.

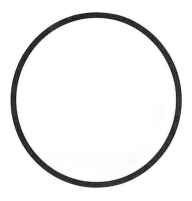

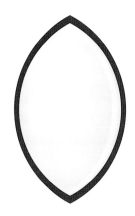

Figure 4.4 Curved surfaces of two mirrors: upper image a spherical mirror; lower image an ovoid mirror with an astigmatic curvature.

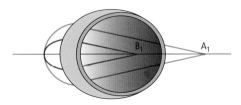

Figure 4.5 Astigmatism. (a) Light in the less steeply curved vertical meridian is focused to a point behind the retina in this example, at point A$_1$. (b) Light in the more steeply curved horizontal meridian is focused to a point in front of the retina, at point B$_1$.

All three types of ametropia can be corrected in one of three ways: spectacle lenses (Figure 4.3), contact lenses or refractive surgery. These diverge the

More globular shape of lens attained with accommodation

Figure 4.6 The curvature of the lens increases with accommodation (dotted line).

rays in myopia, converge the rays in hypermetropia and correct for the non-spherical (astigmatic) shape of the cornea in astigmatism. It should be noted that in hypermetropia, accommodative effort will bring distant objects into focus by increasing the power of the lens. This will use up the accommodative reserve for near objects.

Accommodation and presbyopia

As the object of regard is brought towards the eyes, the eyes converge to maintain fixation while focus is maintained by an increase in the power of the lens. This change in focus is brought about by the ciliary muscle contraction, which relaxes zonular tension on the lens equator and allows the lens to take up a more spherical shape. This is called *accommodation* (Figure 4.6).

The lens continues to grow throughout life. This increase in lens size and stiffness leads to a decrease in the elasticity of the lens with age. As a result, the ability to accommodate decreases with age, reaching a critical point at about 40-plus years, when the subject experiences difficulty with near vision (*presbyopia*). This occurs earlier in hypermetropes than in myopes. The problem is overcome with convex reading lenses, which provide the converging power no longer supplied by the lens of the eye.

Correction of refractive errors

Spectacles

Spectacles are available to correct most refractive errors. Lenses can be made to correct long- and short-sight and astigmatism. They are simple and safe to use but may be lost or damaged. Some people find them cosmetically unacceptable and prefer to wear contact lenses. The correction of presbyopia requires additional lens power to overcome the eye's reduced accommodation for near focus. This can be achieved with:

- separate pairs of glasses for distance and near vision;
- a pair of bifocal lenses, where the near correction is added to the lower segment of the distance lens;
- varifocal lenses, where the power of the lens gradually changes from the distance correction (in the upper part) to the near correction (in the lower part). This provides sharper middle-distance vision. Some people find these difficult to adapt to however.

People with particular needs, such as musicians, may also need glasses for middle distance.

Contact lenses

Contact lenses are slim lenses that rest upon the surface of the cornea, taking its place as the first refractive element of the eye. They are available to correct all forms of refractive error and provide a cosmetically attractive alternative to spectacles. Additionally, they can provide a means of correcting a refractive error, where the corneal surface is disturbed or optically irregular and does not allow spectacle correction. Occasionally, soft contact lenses without refractive power are used as therapeutic lenses, not to improve vision, but to relieve pain caused by ocular surface disease, for example a persistent epithelial defect. Modern contact lenses are very comfortable to wear, but any contact lens carries a small potential risk of infection.

Contact lenses are made either from rigid gas-permeable or from soft hydrophilic materials. All contact lenses retard the diffusion of oxygen to the cornea, but rigid gas-permeable lenses are relatively more permeable than soft lenses. Although soft lenses are better tolerated physically, gas-permeable lenses have certain advantages:

- Their greater oxygen permeability reduces the risk of corneal damage from hypoxia.
- Their rigidity allows easier cleaning and offers less risk of infection.
- Their rigidity permits an effective correction of astigmatism.
- Proteinaceous debris is less likely to adhere to the lens and cause an allergic conjunctivitis.

Daily disposable contact lenses are available which are discarded on the day of use, and therefore do not require cleaning, reducing the risk of infection.

Multifocal contact lenses, similar to varifocal spectacles, provide a focus for distance, intermediate and close viewing in a single lens. They are thus suitable for older patients with presbyopia. In one form, the lens powers required for the various viewing distances are incorporated in a series of concentric circles within the lens.

Optical correction after cataract extraction

The lens provides one-third of the refractive power of the eye, so that after cataract extraction (removal of an opaque lens) the eye is rendered highly hypermetropic. Without its lens, the eye is termed *aphakic*. Aphakic hypermetropia can be corrected by:

- the insertion of an intraocular lens (IOL) at the time of surgery – the preferred option.
- contact lenses, following surgery – where insertion of an IOL is not feasible.
- aphakic spectacles following surgery.

Intraocular lenses give the best optical results and are routinely used in the developed world and increasingly, in the developing world. These are placed at the site of the natural lens and mimic its performance. As they are unable to change shape, the eye cannot accommodate. An eye with an IOL is said to be *pseudophakic*.

Multifocal IOLs, which combine a distance and near correction, are also available. These may not suit everybody because of the optical side effects (reduced contrast and glare), so it is important to counsel patients pre-operatively. Multifocal lenses may allow patients to be independent of spectacles for both distance and near vision. Toric intraocular lenses have an astigmatic surface, and can be used for the correction of corneal astigmatism.

Contact lenses are worn at the surface of the cornea and produce slight increase of the retinal image size (110%) in an aphakic eye; this is not of visual significance, and so, where an IOL is not present, can be successfully used after unilateral or bilateral surgery, allowing balance between a phakic and aphakic eye. Insertion, removal and cleaning can be difficult for elderly patients or those with physical disability (e.g. arthritis).

Aphakic spectacles are corrective spectacles which are provided when no IOL has been used and a contact lens cannot be worn or provided. They have a number of disadvantages:

- They are powerful positive lenses which increase the retinal image to about 133% of normal, causing the patient to misjudge distances. They cannot be used to correct one eye alone if the other eye is *phakic* (the natural lens is *in situ*) or pseudophakic, because of the disparity in image size between the two corrected eyes (*aniseikonia*). This causes symptoms of dizziness and diplopia.
- Aphakic lenses induce many optical aberrations, including distortion of the image due to the thickness of the lens.

Aphakic lenses also restrict the usable field of vision due to their optical properties.

Low-vision aids

Patients with poor vision can be helped by advice on lighting conditions and low-vision aids (see also Chapter 20). Clinics specializing in low vision are available in most eye units. Devices used include:

- magnifiers for near vision (Figure 4.7);
- telescopes for distance vision;

- closed-circuit television to provide magnification and improve contrast;
- large-print books and tablet computers;
- talking clocks and watches;
- a variety of gadgets to help the patient manage household tasks.
- computer software allowing magnification of images and text may also be helpful.

Refractive surgery

Although refractive errors are most commonly corrected by spectacles or contact lenses, laser surgical correction has gained popularity. These techniques are aimed at reshaping the cornea to alter its refractive power, and are performed after the eye has stopped growing. Myopia is corrected by flattening the surface curvature of the cornea and hypermetropia by steepening it. Astigmatism can also be corrected. Various lasers are used including excimer (ultraviolet) and femtosecond (infrared) laser.

The excimer laser is used to precisely ablate a superficial layer of stromal tissue from the cornea to modify its shape In photorefractive keratectomy (PRK), the laser is applied to the corneal surface after removing the epithelium, which regrows in a few days. The laser

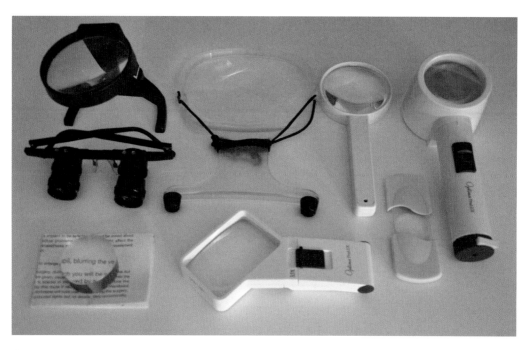

Figure 4.7 Some examples of low-vision aids. Most aid near tasks such as reading. Two monocular telescopes, to help with distance vision, are shown at the top.

can also be directly applied to the corneal stroma without removing epithelium. This can be achieved by creating a hinged, partial-thickness flap of corneal stroma in LASIK (laser-assisted *in situ* keratomileusis) or just an epithelial flap, leaving a thicker stroma for laser reshaping, in LASEK (Laser-assisted sub-epithelial keratomileusis). This may be important in those with a thin cornea. Laser is then applied to the stromal bed to alter its contour, and the flap is then restored to its original position.

Unlike PRK, LASIK provides a near instantaneous improvement in vision with minimal discomfort. The LASEK flap takes longer to heal than a LASIK flap. Serious complications during flap creation occur rarely.

Patients experience discomfort for a few days after PRK, although the level of pain can be reduced by provision of a bandage contact lens and treatment with topical or systemic non-steroidal anti-inflammatory drugs (NSAIDs). Some patients may develop dry-eye symptoms following refractive surgery.

The SMILE procedure involves cutting out a lenticule of central corneal stroma through a smile-shaped partial thickness corneal incision made with femtosecond laser. No flaps are raised, and healing is swift.

Intraocular lenses can also be placed in a phakic eye to correct severe myopic refractive error, but this carries all the risks of intraocular surgery including cataract formation. Alternatively, clear-lens extraction may be performed and an IOL placed in the eye, as with cataract surgery. A multifocal lens may overcome the effects of presbyopia by providing good vision for distance and near without the need for glasses. All intraocular surgery entails the risk of complications resulting in worse vision.

Prevention of myopia progression

As the incidence of myopia (shortsightedness) increases worldwide, there have been recent developments in preventing myopia progression. Treatment is started at the ages of 6–12 years old when progression is greatest. The principal of treatment is to defocus the rays of light reaching the mid-peripheral retina (which drives the excess growth of the eye). Low-dose Atropine 0.01% eye drops, and spectacle lenses or contact lenses with concentric rings of defocus are all being used with moderate success.

 KEY POINTS

- In myopia light focuses in front of the retina, in hypermetropia light focuses behind the retina.
- In astigmatism light cannot be brought to a single point of focus because of the variation in surface curvature and thus the refractive power, of the cornea.
- Patients with poor vision may be helped with low visual aids.

Assessment questions True or False

1. Clinical optics

a   The visible spectrum extends from 390 to 760 nm.

b   Emmetropia means that parallel rays of light are brought to a focus on the retina when accommodation is relaxed.

c   In myopia, the rays are focused in front of the retina, in hypermetropia, they are focused behind the retina.

d   Astigmatism suggests that the cornea is perfectly round.

e   Presbyopia refers to the loss of accommodation with age.

2. Correction of ametropia

a   A concave lens causes divergence of parallel rays and is used to correct myopia.

b   A convex lens causes convergence of parallel rays and is used to correct hypermetropia.

c   The natural lens provides 50% of the refractive power of the eye.

d   Aphakic spectacles magnify the retinal image.

e   The power of the crystalline lens decreases with accommodation.

Answers

1. Clinical optics

a   True. This is the part of the spectrum to which the retina is sensitive.

b   True. See Figure 4.1 for an explanation and diagram.

c   True. See Figure 4.2.

d   False. It suggests that the shape of the cornea is similar to a rugby ball.

e   True. The lens is unable to change shape sufficiently and the ability to accommodate is reduced.

2. Correction of ametropia

a   True. See Figure 4.3.

b   True. See Figure 4.3.

c   False. It produces about 33% of the refractive power of the eye.

d   True. This magnification effect creates optical problems for patients wearing aphakic spectacles.

e   False. The power of the lens increases with accommodation.

5

The orbit

Learning objective

✔ To understand the symptoms, signs, causes and investigation of orbital disease.

Introduction

The orbit provides:

- protection to the globe;
- attachments which stabilize the ocular movements;
- foramina for the transmission of nerves and vessels.

Despite the number of different tissues present in the orbit, the expression of diseases due to different pathologies is often similar.

Clinical features

Proptosis

Proptosis, or *exophthalmos,* is a forward displacement of the eye, which widens the palpebral aperture so that the upper and lower lid margins no longer overlap the corneal periphery above and below; a rim of white sclera may be exposed. The degree of protrusion can be measured with an *exophthalmometer.* A simple clinical test to detect *unilateral* proptosis is to stand behind the seated patient and tilt his head back slowly, observing as the eyes appear beyond the brow – if there is proptosis, the proptosed eye will appear before the normal eye.

Unilateral proptosis is diagnosed if there is a difference of more than 2 mm between the two eyes. Bilateral proptosis is present if the absolute value for either eye, measured with the exophthalmometer, exceeds

approximately 20 mm. Various other features may give a clue to the pathological process involved (Figure 5.1).

- If the eye is displaced directly forward (axial proptosis), it suggests a space-occupying lesion lying within the extraocular muscle cone, formed by the four rectus muscles (an *intra-conal lesion*). An example would be an optic nerve sheath meningioma.
- If the eye is displaced forward and to one side (nonaxial proptosis), a lesion outside the muscle cone is likely (an *extra-conal lesion*). For example, a tumour of the lacrimal gland displaces the globe to the nasal side.
- The presence of orbital varices can be demonstrated by asking the patient to perform a Valsalva manouvre. The increase in intracranial venous pressure, transmitted to the orbital veins, transiently displaces the globe forwards. Pulsatile proptosis may occur with arterial vascular lesions (carotid-cavernous sinus fistula).
- The speed of onset of proptosis may also give clues to the aetiology. A slow onset suggests a benign, space-occupying tumour, for example a dermoid cyst, whereas rapid onset occurs in inflammatory disorders, malignant tumours and carotid-cavernous sinus fistula.
- The presence of pain may suggest infection (e.g. orbital cellulitis).

Enophthalmos

Enophthalmos is a backward displacement of the globe, suggested by a narrowing of the palpebral fissure when the eyes are viewed from the front. It is a feature of an

Ophthalmology: Lecture Notes, Thirteenth Edition. Bruce James, Anthony Bron, and Manoj V. Parulekar.
© 2024 John Wiley & Sons Ltd. Published 2024 by John Wiley & Sons Ltd.
Companion website: www.wiley.com/go/ophthalmology13e

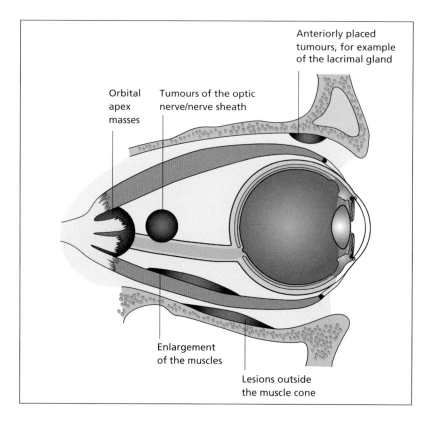

Anteriorly placed tumours, for example of the lacrimal gland

Orbital apex masses

Tumours of the optic nerve/nerve sheath

Enlargement of the muscles

Lesions outside the muscle cone

Figure 5.1 Sites of orbital disease.

orbital 'blowout fracture', when blunt injury to the globe and orbit fractures a thin orbital wall and displaces some of the orbital contents into an adjacent sinus. It was also said to occur in Horner syndrome, but this is really a pseudo-enophthalmos due to ptosis (a drooping of the upper lid), which narrows the palpebral aperture (see Chapter 14). It should be differentiated from *microphthalmos*, where the eyeball is smaller in size.

Pain

Inflammatory conditions, infective disorders and rapidly progressing tumours cause pain. This is not usually present with benign tumours.

Eyelid and conjunctival changes

Conjunctival injection and swelling suggest an inflammatory or infective process. Associated signs are important to determine. Infection affecting the anterior orbital structures, i.e. the lids only (*preseptal cellulitis*) causes protrusion of the lids but not of the globe, and therefore no proptosis, and eye movements and vision are unaffected. If infection involves the orbit behind the orbital septum (*orbital cellulitis*),

eye movements are reduced, vision may be reduced and there is significant proptosis. Both conditions are extremely painful, but this is a very much more serious condition.

Florid engorgement of the conjunctival vessels suggests a *carotid-cavernous sinus fistula* (see below).

Binocular diplopia

Binocular diplopia occurs when the eyes are not aligned, so that only one of the two eyes is directed at the object of interest. Thus, the image in the second eye does not fall upon the fovea and two images of the visual scene are perceived. This is due to the mechanical effects of an orbital space occupying lesion (for example a tumour) or enlargement of the muscles in *myositis* and *dysthyroid eye disease* (Graves disease). Eye movements may be restricted in a direction *away* from the field of action of the affected muscle (e.g. if the inferior rectus is thickened in thyroid eye disease, there will be restriction of upgaze).

Visual acuity

This may be reduced by:

- exposure keratopathy from severe proptosis, when the cornea is no longer protected by the lids and tear film. The corneal surface is uneven and its transparency is reduced;
- optic nerve involvement by compression or inflammation;
- distortion of the macula due to compression of the globe by a posterior, space-occupying lesion.

Investigation of orbital disease

Ultrasound, CT and MRI scans have greatly helped in the diagnosis of orbital disease – localizing the site of the lesion, demonstrating enlarged extraocular muscles in dysthyroid eye disease and myositis, or demonstrating fractures to the orbit. Additional systemic tests will be dictated by the differential diagnosis (e.g. tests to determine the primary site of a secondary tumour).

Differential diagnosis of orbital disease

Traumatic orbital disease is discussed in Chapter 17.

Disorders of the extraocular muscles

Dysthyroid eye disease and *ocular myositis* present with symptoms and signs of orbital disease. These are described in Chapter 16.

In children, a rapidly developing proptosis may be caused by a rare malignant tumour *rhabdomyosarcoma* (see Section 'Orbital tumours').

Infective disorders

Orbital cellulitis is a serious condition which can cause blindness and may spread to cause a brain abscess (Figure 5.2). The infection often arises from an adjacent ethmoid sinus, reflecting that the medial wall of the orbit is extremely thin. The commonest causative organisms are *Staphylococcus* and *Streptococcus*. The patient presents with:

- a painful, proptosed eye;
- conjunctival injection;
- periorbital inflammation and swelling;
- reduced eye movements;
- possible visual loss;
- systemic illness and pyrexia.

An MRI or a CT scan is helpful in diagnosis and in planning treatment. The condition usually responds to intravenous broad-spectrum antibiotics, but it may be necessary to drain an abscess or decompress the orbit, particularly if the optic nerve is compromised. Optic nerve function must be watched closely, checking acuity, monitoring colour vision and testing for a relative afferent pupillary defect. Orbital decompression is usually performed with the help of an ear, nose and throat (ENT) specialist.

Preseptal cellulitis involves lid structures alone (Figure 5.3). It presents with periorbital inflammation and swelling but not the other ocular features of orbital cellulitis. Eye movement is not impaired, and there is no risk to vision.

An orbital mucocoele arises from accumulated secretions within any of the paranasal sinuses when

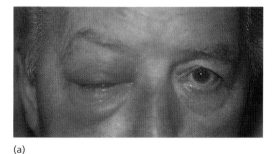

(a)

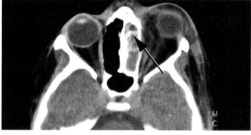

(b)

Figure 5.2 (a) The clinical appearance of a patient with right orbital cellulitis. (b) A CT scan showing a left opaque ethmoid sinus and subperiosteal orbital abscess.

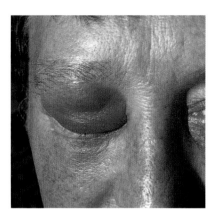

Figure 5.3 The appearance of a patient with preseptal cellulitis.

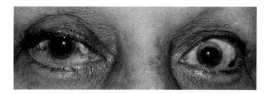

Figure 5.4 The ocular signs of a carotid-cavernous sinus fistula. Contrast the dilated vessels on the right to the normal appearance on the left.

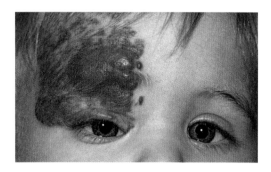

Figure 5.5 The appearance of a capillary haemangioma.

natural drainage of the sinus is blocked. Surgical excision may be required.

Inflammatory disease

The orbit may be involved in various inflammatory disorders, including sarcoidosis and inflammatory pseudotumour (or nonspecific orbital inflammation), a lymphofibroblastic disorder. Diagnosis of such conditions is difficult. The presence of other systemic signs of sarcoidosis may be helpful. High-resolution CT scans may be helpful in imaging an orbital pseudotumour. It may be necessary to biopsy the tissue to differentiate the lesion from a lymphoma but this can be difficult. The mainstay of treatment is systemic corticosteroid (and steroid-sparing agents in chronic cases).

Vascular abnormalities

An arteriovenous fistula may develop between the internal carotid artery or a dural artery in the cavernous sinus, and the cavernous sinus itself (*carotid-cavernous sinus fistula*) (Figure 5.4). As a result, the orbital veins are exposed to a high intravascular pressure, the eye is proptosed and the conjunctival veins are dilated and engorged. The patient may complain of a pulsatile tinnitus, and a bruit may be heard with a stethoscope placed over the closed eye, synchronous with the radial pulse. Extraocular muscle engorgement reduces eye movements, and increased pressure in the veins draining the eye causes increased intraocular pressure. Interventional radiological techniques can be used to close the fistula by embolizing and thrombosing the affected vascular segment.

The orbital veins may become dilated (*orbital varix*), causing intermittent proptosis when venous pressure is raised.

In infants, a capillary haemangioma may present as an extensive lesion of the orbit, affecting the skin of the lid (Figure 5.5). Swelling of the upper lid may cause sufficient ptosis to cause amblyopia. Fortunately, most undergo spontaneous resolution in the first 5 years of life. Treatment is indicated, if size or position obstructs the visual axis and risks the development of amblyopia (see Chapter 16). Although local injections of long-acting steroids have been the mainstay of treatment in past decades, they have been replaced by oral propranolol, an adrenergic beta-blocker, which is very effective in shrinking the haemangioma, with few adverse effects (Figure 5.6).

Orbital tumours

The following tumours may produce signs of orbital disease:

- lacrimal gland tumours;
- optic nerve gliomas;
- meningiomas;
- lymphomas;

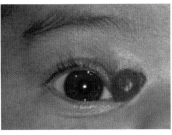

(a)

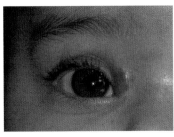

(b)

Figure 5.6 Before (a) and after (b) treatment of a capillary haemangioma with oral propranolol.

- rhabdomyosarcomas;
- metastasis from other systemic cancers (neuroblastomas in children, the breast, lung, prostate or gastrointestinal tract in adults).

A CT or MRI scan will help with the diagnosis (Figure 5.7). Again, systemic investigation, for example to determine the site of a primary tumour, may be required.

Malignant *lacrimal gland tumours* carry a poor prognosis. Benign tumours still require complete excision to prevent malignant transformation, which, in a proportion of cases but not all, may lead to dry eye. Optic nerve *gliomas* may be associated with *neurofibromatosis type 1 (NF1)*. Sporadic gliomas grow rapidly and need treatment (chemotherapy or surgery) while NF1-related gliomas tend to be indolent and can be observed in many cases. Meningiomas of the optic nerve are a rare association and may also be difficult to excise. Again, they can be monitored over time and some may benefit from treatment with radiotherapy. Meningiomas arising from the middle cranial fossa may spread through the optic canal into the orbit.

The treatment of *lymphoma* requires a full systemic investigation to determine whether the lesion is indicative of widespread disease or whether it is localized to the orbit. In the former case, the patient is

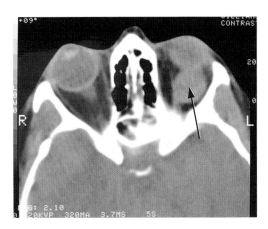

Figure 5.7 A CT scan showing a left-sided orbital metastasis.

treated with chemotherapy, in the latter, with localized radiotherapy.

In children, the commonest orbital tumour is a *rhabdomyosarcoma,* a rapidly growing, malignant tumour of embryonic tissues with features of striated muscle. Chemotherapy ± radiotherapy is effective if the disease is localized to the orbit.

Dermoid cysts

These congenital cystic lesions are caused by the continued growth of ectodermal tissue beneath the surface, which may present in the medial or lateral aspect of the superior orbit (Figure 5.8). Excision is usually performed for cosmetic reasons and to avoid traumatic rupture, which may cause scarring. Some may be attached to the underlying bone, or extend into or through the bone and a CT scan may be necessary before surgery to identify this. Dermoids can also occur at the corneoscleral junction (limbus). Here, they are solid rather than cystic.

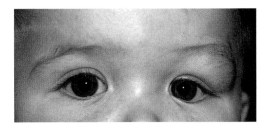

Figure 5.8 A left dermoid cyst.

KEY POINTS

- A full careful history and clinical examination will often reveal the cause of proptosis.
- Suspect orbital cellulitis in a patient with proptosis and periorbital and conjunctival inflammation, particularly when there is severe pain and the patient is systemically unwell.
- The commonest cause of bilateral proptosis is dysthyroid disease.
- The commonest cause of unilateral proptosis is also dysthyroid disease!
- Dysthyroid disease may be associated with the serious complications of exposure keratopathy and optic nerve compression.

Assessment questions True or False

1. **A 56-year-old female patient presents with a proptosed eye, deviated nasally.**
a   An eye displaced to one side of the orbit suggests an extra-conal lesion.
b   Rapid onset of proptosis might suggest a malignant tumour.
c   The patient may have dysthyroid eye (Graves) disease.
d   The patient may have a rhabdomyosarcoma of the extraocular muscles.
e   Diplopia is a common presenting feature of orbital disease.

2. **A 16-year-old boy presents with swollen eyelids, a red eye, proptosis, severe eye pain and tenderness and a pyrexia. The vision has become very blurred and colour vision is reduced.**
a   Orbital cellulitis is the most likely diagnosis.
b   A relative afferent pupillary defect may be present.
c   No investigations are necessary.
d   Urgent orbital decompression is indicated.

3. **A 70-year-old woman with a history of previous head trauma presents with sudden onset of a red, proptosed eye. Eye movements are reduced in all directions. Vision is intact. Intraocular pressure is increased. The most likely diagnosis is:**
a   Dysthyroid eye (Graves) disease.
b   A carotid-cavernous sinus fistula.

c   An orbital varix.
d   A dermoid cyst.

Answers

1. **A 56-year-old female patient presents with a proptosed eye, deviated nasally.**
a   True. It is likely that the lesion is outside the muscle cone causing an asymmetric deviation of the eye.
b   True. A rapid onset of proptosis is also seen in inflammatory disorders and carotid-cavernous sinus fistula.
c   True. See Chapter 16.
d   False. This is seen in much younger patients.
e   True. This may result from direct involvement of the muscle or its nerve supply.

2. **A 16-year-old boy presents with swollen eyelids, a red eye, proptosis, severe eye pain and tenderness and a pyrexia. The vision has become very blurred and colour vision is reduced.**
a   True. These are the classic symptoms.
b   True. The reduced acuity and colour vision suggests that the optic nerve is compromised, so that a relative afferent pupillary defect is expected.
c   False. An urgent CT of the orbit should be undertaken to confirm the diagnosis. Blood cultures may also be helpful.
d   True. Successful decompression may save optic nerve function.

3. **A 70-year-old woman with a history of previous head trauma presents with sudden onset of a red, proptosed eye. Eye movements are reduced in all directions. Vision is intact. Intraocular pressure is increased. The most likely diagnosis is:**
a   False. While possible, it is not the most likely diagnosis.
b   True. These are the classic features, including the history of trauma.
c   False. A varix causes an intermittent proptosis, worsened by an elevated venous pressure, as may occur with a Valsalva manoeuvre.
d   False. Dermoid cysts occur in a much younger age group. They do not cause proptosis and usually present as a swelling at the medial or lateral aspect of the orbit.

6

The eyelids

Learning objectives

To understand the symptoms, signs and causes of:

✔ Abnormal lid position.
✔ Anterior and posterior blepharitis.
✔ Lid swellings.

Introduction

The eyelids are important both in providing physical protection to the eyes and in ensuring a normal tear film and tear drainage. Diseases of the eyelids can be divided into those associated with:

- abnormal lid position;
- inflammation;
- lid swellings;
- abnormalities of the lashes.

Abnormalities of lid position

Ptosis

This is an abnormally low position of the upper eyelid (Figure 6.1).

Pathogenesis

It may be caused by the following factors:

Mechanical
a   A large lid lump pulling the lid down.
b   Lid oedema, increasing the volume and weight of the lid.

c   Downward tethering of the lid by conjunctival scarring.
d   Structural abnormalities, including a disinsertion of the aponeurosis of the levator muscle, usually in elderly patients.

Neurological
a   Third nerve palsy (see Chapter 16).
b   Horner syndrome, due to a sympathetic nerve lesion (see Chapter 14).
c   Marcus Gunn jaw-winking syndrome. Here, congenital ptosis is due to a developmental miswiring of the nerve supply to the pterygoid muscle of the jaw (cranial nerve V) and the levator of the eyelid (cranial nerve III) so that the eyelid moves in conjunction with chewing movements.

Myogenic
a   Myasthenia gravis (see also Chapter 16).
b   Some forms of muscular dystrophy.
c   Chronic progressive external ophthalmoplegia.

Symptoms

Patients present because:

- they object to the cosmetic effect;
- vision may be impaired when the lid crosses the visual axis;
- there are symptoms and signs associated with the underlying cause.

Ophthalmology: Lecture Notes, Thirteenth Edition. Bruce James, Anthony Bron, and Manoj V. Parulekar.
© 2024 John Wiley & Sons Ltd. Published 2024 by John Wiley & Sons Ltd.
Companion website: www.wiley.com/go/ophthalmology13e

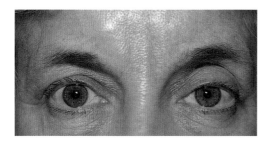

Figure 6.1 A mild left ptosis.

Signs

There is a reduction in size of the palpebral aperture. The upper lid margin, which usually overlaps the upper limbus by 1–2 mm, may partially cover the pupil or the eye may be completely closed. The function of the levator muscle can be tested by measuring the maximum travel of the upper lid from full downgaze to full upgaze (normally 15–18 mm). It is common for the eyebrows to be elevated in the presence of ptosis, as a compensatory event which offsets the ptosis. To remove this contribution to lid elevation, pressure is applied to the brow to prevent frontalis muscle action during the test (Figure 3.14).

Other signs may be present, such as a small pupil on the side of the ptosis in Horner syndrome or a large pupil, diplopia and reduced eye movements in third nerve palsy.

Myasthenia gravis

Myasthenia gravis is an autoimmune disease of the voluntary muscles in which fluctuating weakness is triggered by periods of muscle activity and relieved by rest. It is usually due to circulating antibodies that block the action of acetylcholine at postsynaptic, nicotinic, neuromuscular junctions. Muscles that control the ocular and eyelid movements, facial expression, chewing, talking and swallowing are often, but not always, involved. Involvement of respiratory muscles may be life threatening. Ocular involvement may occur on its own with few systemic features.

Four diagnostic tests may assist in the diagnosis of *ocular myasthenia*.

1 Repeated upgaze and downgaze movements result in fatigue and increased ptosis.
2 Ask the patient to look down for 15 seconds and then look up at an elevated target. The lid overshoots and then falls slightly after the period of rest (Cogan *twitch test*).

3 Ice applied to the lid for 2 minutes, through a rubber glove, significantly reduces a myasthenic ptosis.
4 Weakness of eyelid closure (orbicularis weakness).

Management

In the absence of a medically treatable disease such as myasthenia gravis, ptosis may require surgical correction. In very young children, this is usually deferred, unless the visual axis is covered and threatens to induce amblyopia.

Entropion

This is an inturning of the lid margin and lashes, usually of the lower lid, towards the globe (Figure 6.2). It may occur if the patient looks downwards or may be induced when the eyes are tightly closed. It is seen most commonly in elderly patients where the orbicularis muscle overrides the tarsal plate due to weak lower lid retractors (*involutional entropion*) or it may also be caused by conjunctival scarring, which draws the lid margin inwards (*cicatricial entropion*).

Abrasion of the lower cornea by the inturned lashes causes marked irritation and may be detected as *punctate fluorescein staining*. The bulbar conjunctiva may be red. Short-term treatment includes taping of the lower lid to turn the lashes away from the globe and the application of lubricants to soothe the eye. The condition can be alleviated for a period by the injection of *botulinum toxin* to paralyse the palpebral part of the orbicularis muscle of the lower lid, or cured permanently by surgery.

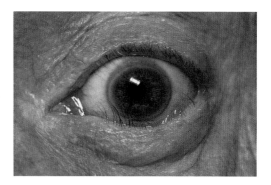

Figure 6.2 Entropion. The lid margin is rolled inwards and the lashes are touching the globe.

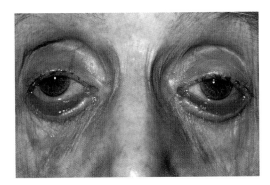

Figure 6.3 Ectropion. The lower lid is everted and the tarsal conjunctiva exposed.

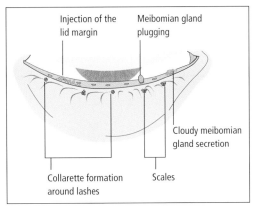

(a)

Ectropion

Here, there is an eversion of the lid away from the globe (Figure 6.3). Common causes include:

- age-related orbicularis muscle laxity;
- scarring of the periorbital skin;
- seventh nerve palsy.

The malposition of the lids everts the puncta and prevents drainage of the tears, leading to epiphora. It also exposes the conjunctiva and lower globe to drying (see Chapter 7). Ectropion causes an irritable eye. Surgical treatment is, again, effective.

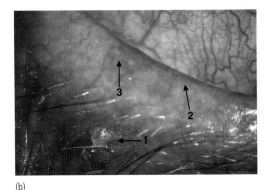

(b)

Figure 6.4 Blepharitis. (a) A diagram showing the signs. (b) The clinical appearance of the lid margin. Note (1) the scales on the lashes, (2) dilated blood vessels on the lid margin and (3) plugging of the meibomian glands.

Inflammation of the eyelids

Blepharitis

This is a common, symptomatic, chronic, inflammation of the lid margins (Figure 6.4). There are two forms, which can occur independently or may coexist in the same lids.

In *anterior blepharitis*, inflammation is concentrated anteriorly along the lash line of the lid margin and accompanied by squamous debris, which sometimes form collarettes at the lash bases. The conjunctiva becomes injected and there may be involvement of the cornea (*blepharokeratitis*). There is a strong association with skin diseases such as seborrhoeic dermatitis, atopic eczema and rosacea. Anterior blepharitis is often accompanied by a staphylococcal overgrowth and in some individuals, small infiltrates or ulcers may form in the peripheral cornea (*marginal keratitis*) due to an immune complex response to staphylococcal exotoxins. These are usually very responsive to a short course of topical steroid drops.

Posterior blepharitis is usually caused by *meibomian gland dysfunction,* often referred to as MGD. In MGD, the terminal ducts of the meibomian glands are obstructed by squamous debris and the lipid product of the glands, usually a clear oil, becomes viscous. It appears cloudy and opaque when expressed from the glands by pressure applied through the lid, and this is a simple and excellent diagnostic test for the condition.

Symptoms of blepharitis

These include:

- tired, itchy, sore eyes, worse in the morning;
- crusting of the lid margins in anterior blepharitis and redness in both.

Signs

In anterior blepharitis there may be:

- Redness and scaling of the lid margins; some lash bases may be ulcerated – a sign of staphylococcal infection.
- Debris in the form of collarettes around the eyelashes (cylindrical dandruff). This may indicate an infestation of the lash roots by *Demodex folliculorum*.
- A reduction in the number of eyelashes.

  In MGD, there may be:

- obstruction and plugging of the meibomian orifices;
- thickened, cloudy, expressed meibomian secretions;
- injection of the lid margin and conjunctiva;
- tear film abnormalities and punctate keratitis.

In scarring conditions of the conjunctiva, such as trachoma and pemphigoid, the meibomian orifices may be dragged backwards into the tarsal conjunctiva.

Both forms of blepharitis are strongly associated with seborrhoeic dermatitis, atopic eczema and rosacea. In rosacea, there is hyperaemia and telangiectasia of the facial skin and a rhinophyma may occur. This is a bulbous, red, irregular swelling of the nose with hypertrophy of the sebaceous glands.

Treatment

This is often difficult and must be long term for these chronic conditions.

For anterior blepharitis, lid scrubs with a cotton bud wetted with bicarbonate solution or lid wipes helps to remove squamous debris from the lash line. Commercial products are also available. Topical steroids can reduce inflammation but must be used infrequently, to avoid steroid complications such as raised intraocular pressure (glaucoma). Staphylococcal lid disease may also require therapy with topical antibiotics (e.g. fusidic acid gel), and occasionally with systemic antibiotics. *Demodex* infestation responds to the application of 'tea tree oil' but its aetiological role is controversial because infestation with the mite is extremely common in asymptomatic individuals.

For MGD, abnormal secretions can be expressed by lid massage after heating the glands through the closed lids with a hot, moist flannel or using one of a number of commercial heating appliances. Massage is applied through the lid skin, with a gentle force to the tarsal plate applied with a firm rod from the attached border of the lid to the lid margin. Alternatively, an in-office treatment is available which directs heat to the inner surface of the lids while applying a rhythmic compression along their full extent. This is claimed to offer prolonged relief from symptoms but is a costly procedure. If this treatment fails, then there may be a place for topical azithromycin drops or, occasionally, for a short course of an oral tetracycline such as doxycycline or minocycline.

Where meibomian gland obstruction is extensive, the absence of an oily layer on the tear film can induce an evaporative dry eye, which requires treatment with artificial tears, lipid-containing drops or moisturising sprays (see Chapter 7).

Prognosis

Although symptoms may be ameliorated by treatment, blepharitis may remain a chronic problem.

Benign lid lumps and bumps

Chalazion

This is a common, painless condition in which an obstructed meibomian gland causes a granuloma within the tarsal plate (Figure 6.5). It is more common in children. Symptoms are of an unsightly lid swelling which usually resolves within 6 months. If the lesion persists, it can be incised and the gelatinous contents curetted away.

An abscess (*internal hordeolum*) may also form within the meibomian gland and, unlike a chalazion,

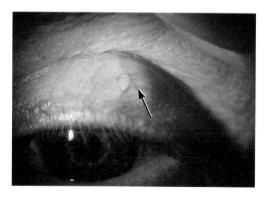

Figure 6.5 Chalazion.

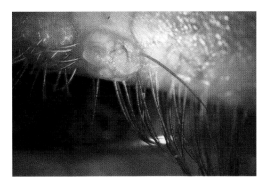

Figure 6.6 Molluscum contagiosum.

this is painful. It may respond to topical antibiotics but usually incision is necessary.

A stye (*external hordeolum*) is an exquisitely painful abscess within an eyelash follicle. Treatment requires the removal of the associated eyelash and application of hot compresses. Most cases are self-limiting, but occasionally systemic antibiotics are required.

Molluscum contagiosum

This umbilicated lesion found on the lid margin is caused by a pox virus (Figure 6.6). It causes irritation of the eye by shedding virus into the eye. The eye is red, and small elevations of lymphoid tissue are found on the tarsal conjunctiva (*follicular conjunctivitis*). Treatment requires excision of the lid lesion.

Cysts

Various cysts may form on the eyelids. Sebaceous cysts are opaque. They rarely cause symptoms. They can be excised for cosmetic reasons. A cyst of Moll is a small translucent cyst on the lid margin caused by obstruction of a sweat gland. A cyst of Zeis is an opaque cyst on the eyelid margin caused by blockage of an accessory sebaceous gland. These too can be excised for cosmetic reasons.

Squamous cell papilloma

This is a common, frond-like lid lesion with a fibrovascular core and thickened squamous epithelium (Figure 6.7a). It is usually asymptomatic but can be excised for cosmetic reasons with cautery to the base.

Xanthelasmas

These are lipid-containing bilateral lesions which may in youth be associated with hypercholesterolaemia (Figure 6.7b). It is worth checking the blood cholesterol. They are excised for cosmetic reasons.

Keratoacanthoma

This is a brownish pink, fast-growing lesion with a central crater filled with keratin (Figure 6.7c). Treatment is by excision. Careful histology must be performed as some may have the malignant features of a squamous cell carcinoma (see below).

Naevus (mole)

These lesions are derived from naevus cells (altered melanocytes) and can be pigmented or non-pigmented. No treatment is necessary.

Malignant tumours

Basal cell carcinoma (BCC)

This is the most common form of malignant tumour (Figure 6.8). Ten percent of cases occur in the eyelids and account for 90% of eyelid malignancies. The tumour is:

- slow growing;
- locally invasive;
- non-metastasizing.

Patients present with a painless lesion on the eyelid which may be nodular, sclerosing or ulcerative (the so-called *rodent ulcer*). Typically, it has a *pale, pearly margin*. A high index of suspicion is required. Treatment is by:

- Excision biopsy with a margin of normal tissue surrounding the lesion. For large lesions threatening important tissues, excision may be controlled with frozen sections and serial sections used to determine the need for additional tissue removal (Mohs surgery). This minimizes destruction of normal tissue.
- Cryotherapy.
- Radiotherapy.

The prognosis is usually very good, but deep invasion of the tumour can be difficult to treat.

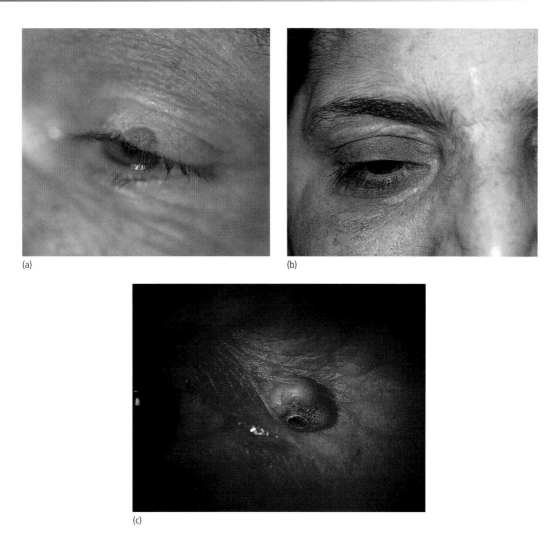

Figure 6.7 (a) A squamous cell papilloma. (b) Xanthelasma. (c) Keratoacanthoma.

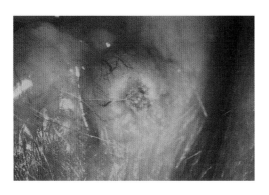

Figure 6.8 A basal cell carcinoma.

Squamous cell carcinoma

This is a less common but more malignant tumour which can metastasize to the lymph nodes. It can arise *de novo* or from pre-malignant lesions. It may present as a hard nodule or a scaly patch. Treatment is by excisional biopsy with a margin of healthy tissue.

When a squamous cell carcinoma is suspected, it is essential to check for the presence of affected cervical lymph nodes.

Ultraviolet (UV) exposure is an important risk factor for both basal cell and squamous cell carcinoma.

Abnormalities of the lashes

Trichiasis

This is a common condition in which aberrant eyelashes are directed backwards towards the globe. It is distinct from entropion since the lid margin remains normally apposed to the globe. The lashes rub against the cornea and cause irritation and abrasion. It may result from any cicatricial process. In developing countries, trachoma (see Chapter 18) is an important cause and trichiasis is an important basis for the associated blindness. Localized (short segment) trichiasis with only a few misdirected eyelashes can be treated with epilation of the offending lashes, electrolysis delivered to the lash base, or cryotherapy applied through the lid. Long segment trichiasis, affecting most eyelashes, is treated surgically with the lid split operation and everting sutures.

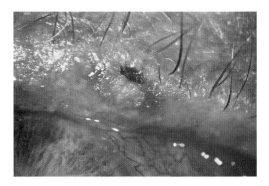

Figure 6.9 The clinical appearance of the eye referred to in Question 3.

 KEY POINTS

- Blepharitis is a common cause of sore 'tired' irritable eyes.
- Abnormalities of eyelid position can cause corneal disease.
- A red eye with a follicular conjunctivitis may be due to a small, umbilicated, molluscum contagiosum on the lid.
- Measure serum cholesterol levels in young patients with xanthelasma.
- Always consider the possibility of malignancy in lid lesions.

2. **Meibomian gland dysfunction is associated with**

a Cloudy expressed meibomian secretions.
b Injection of the lid margin.
c Marginal keratitis.
d An inturned eyelid.
e Squamous debris around the base of an eyelash.

3. **A 70-year-old patient presents with the single lesion shown in Figure 6.9. It is slowly increasing in size. The most likely diagnosis is**

a Keratoacanthoma.
b Basal cell carcinoma.
c Squamous cell carcinoma.
d Molluscum contagiosum.
e Xanthelasma.

Assessment questions True or False

1. **A 55-year-old woman presents with a small ptosis, and miosis on the same side. She is a smoker. The likely diagnosis is**

a Myasthenia gravis.
b Marcus Gunn syndrome.
c Horner syndrome.
d Third nerve palsy.
e Conjunctival scarring.

Answers

1. **A 55-year-old woman presents with a small ptosis, and miosis on the same side. She is a smoker.**

a False. This may cause a ptosis but does not cause miosis.
b False. The eyelid moves in conjunction with jaw movements, again there is no miosis.
c True. There is an interruption of the sympathetic supply to the iris dilator and to the smooth muscle of the upper lid. In this patient, this may be caused by a tumour of the lung.
d False. There would be a ptosis but the pupil would be *dilated*.
e False. Once again this would not affect the size of the pupil.

2. Meibomian gland dysfunction is associated with

a   True. Expressed secretions may be cloudy or opaque and as thick as toothpaste.

b   True. Injection of the lid margin occurs in both forms of blepharitis.

c   False. Marginal keratitis is more likely to be associated with anterior blepharitis.

d   False. There is no association with an inturned eyelid.

e   False. Squamous debris around the base of a lash is a feature of anterior blepharitis.

3. A 70-year-old patient presents with the single lesion shown in Figure 6.9. It is slowly increasing in size.

a   False. There is no central crater filled with keratin.

b   True. Slow growth is usual, the shape is typical and the pearly margin is also characteristic.

c   False. The appearance differs and the condition is less common. It can however metastasize and must be considered in the differential diagnosis.

d   False. These lesions are usually umbilicated and may be associated with a red eye and tarsal follicles.

e   False. These lipid-laden lesions, usually bilateral, are not ulcerated.

7

The lacrimal system

Learning objectives

To understand the symptoms, signs, causes and treatment of:

✔ dry eyes.
✔ watery eyes.

Introduction

Disorders of the lacrimal system are common and may produce chronic symptoms with a significant morbidity. In a quiet environment, the lacrimal glands normally secrete about 1.5 µl of tears per minute. Some tears are lost by evaporation, while the remainder drain via the nasolacrimal system into the nose. The tear film is re-formed with each blink.

Abnormalities are found in:

- tear secretion and evaporation;
- tear drainage.

Abnormalities in tear secretion and evaporation – Dry eye

Dry eye disease (DED) is a condition of the ocular surface caused by either a *deficiency of tear secretion* or *excessive evaporation*. The resulting tear *hyperosmolarity* leads to ocular surface damage and inflammation and chronic symptoms of ocular discomfort with visual loss. Tear hyperosmolarity, which can be measured simply at the bedside (Figure 7.1), is a key diagnostic feature. It is envisaged that damage to the ocular surface increases tear instability, amplifies tear hyperosmolarity and results in a self-perpetuating *vicious circle* of disease. An alternative term for DED is *keratoconjunctivitis sicca* (*KCS*). Its prevalence in adult populations ranges between 5% and 50%.

There is currently a greater understanding of the contribution of personal behaviour and environment to DED. Any circumstance that increases tear evaporation may trigger its onset or exacerbate its severity, including conditions of low relative humidity, high air flow and raised ambient temperature such as that imposed by air-conditioning. This may be encountered in the home, in hotels, and during air travel, and in commercial offices where workers spend prolonged periods working at computers. Digital display users experience slow blink rates, incomplete eye closure and increased width of the palpebral aperture, which contribute to drying of the ocular surface; the act of reading may also slow the blink rate. Younger patients are more symptomatic than the old because of a greater sensory integrity. Important risk factors for DED include the frequent, long-term use of eye drops containing preservatives and the chronic use, particularly in the elderly, of systemic medications which suppress tear production, such as antihypertensive agents and antidepressants.

Two major forms of DED exist, aqueous-deficient and evaporative.

Aqueous-deficient dry eye

Aqueous-deficient dry eye (ADDE) is due to inflammatory damage to the lacrimal glands by invading lymphocytes, causing a deficiency of

Ophthalmology: Lecture Notes, Thirteenth Edition. Bruce James, Anthony Bron, and Manoj V. Parulekar.
© 2024 John Wiley & Sons Ltd. Published 2024 by John Wiley & Sons Ltd.
Companion website: www.wiley.com/go/ophthalmology13e

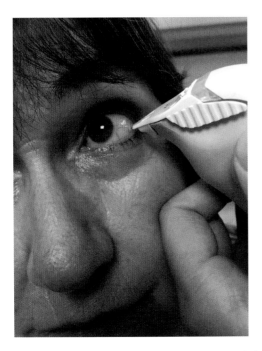

Figure 7.1 Tear lab device for measuring the osmolarity of the tear film.

lacrimal secretion. It is more common in women than in men and its prevalence increases with age. Less commonly, ADDE may occur as a congenital lacrimal deficiency, result from a lymphomatous or sarcoid infiltration of the lacrimal gland or from obstruction to lacrimal secretion by conjunctival scarring in trachoma, Stevens Johnson syndrome or mucous membrane pemphigoid.

Sjögren syndrome

Aqueous-deficient DED may occur in combination with a dry mouth, in the debilitating autoimmune condition of *primary Sjögren Syndrome*, usually with other mucous membranes and organ systems affected. Inflammatory damage is caused by activated T-cells that target the glands. An accompanying MGD frequently adds an evaporative component to the DED and increases its severity. When Sjögren syndrome occurs in association with a specific autoimmune connective tissue disorder, the condition is called *secondary Sjögren syndrome*. Rheumatoid arthritis is the commonest cause and others include systemic lupus erythematosis, primary biliary cirrhosis and scleroderma. Sjögren syndrome is nine times as common in women than men and has an earlier onset than age-related dry eye. Genetic makeup is important and there may be hormonal and infective triggers. Diagnosis of Sjögren syndrome is confirmed by the finding of reduced lacrimal and salivary function, the presence of raised titres of *anti-Rho* and *anti-La* antibodies and the demonstration of T-cell infiltration in minor salivary gland biopsy.

Evaporative dry eye – Meibomian gland dysfunction

Evaporative dry eye (EDE) is due to an excessive evaporative loss from the ocular surface in the presence of normal lacrimal secretory function. The commonest cause is Meibomian gland dysfunction (MGD), itself a common condition in the adult population, in which delivery of Meibomian oil to the tear film is obstructed by changes in the terminal ducts of the glands and by an increase in viscosity of the delivered lipid. This leads to tear film instability and increased water loss. Meibomian gland dysfunction is a feature of certain dermatoses such as rosacea, seborrheic and atopic dermatitis and Meibomian gland obstruction also occurs as a toxic response to the use of 13 cis-retinoic acid in the treatment of acne vulgaris. Disorders of lid congruity, aperture and dynamics can also cause EDE, so that it is a possible complication of proptosis, ectropion and Parkinson disease – where blink rate is reduced.

Symptoms of dry eye disease

Patients with dry eye have symptoms of grittiness, burning, photophobia, lid heaviness and ocular fatigue, which are worse in the evening because the eyes dry progressively during the day. Symptoms can be graded and the score used in diagnosis. Vision is unstable, and in more severe cases, visual acuity may be reduced by corneal damage.

Signs

Tear film *instability* is a feature of both aqueous-deficient and evaporative dry eye which can be revealed by fluorescein instillation. In normal subjects, the stained tear film can remain intact for an extended period in the absence of blinking, whereas in DED, the tear film shows dark spots of *early tear film break-up* occur during blink suppression, diagnostically, <5 seconds after the last blink (Figure 7.2). At the same time, fluorescein uptake into damaged epithelial cells can be demonstrated in a characteristic pattern of fluorescent dots over the exposed corneal and conjunctival surface (Figure 7.3). This can be graded to provide a severity score (Figure 7.4).

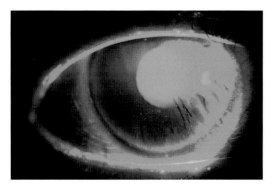

Figure 7.2 Tear breakup following the instillation of fluorescein dye. Note hypofluoescent streaks and also punctate staining.

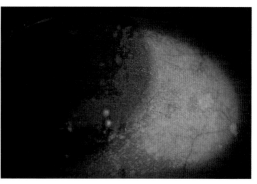

Figure 7.3 Fluorescein staining demonstrating corneal and conjunctival punctate lesions in a severe dry eye.

GRADING OF CORNEAL AND CONJUNCTIVAL STAINING

OXFORD SCHEME

PANEL	GRADE	VERBAL DESCRIPTOR
A 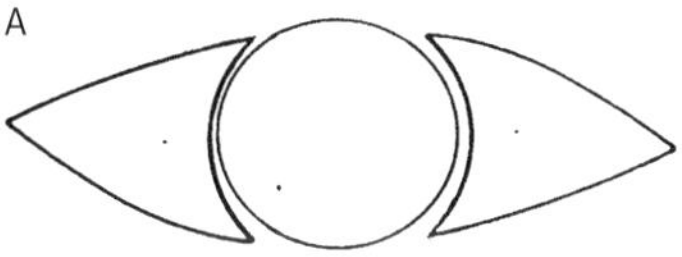	0	Absent
B 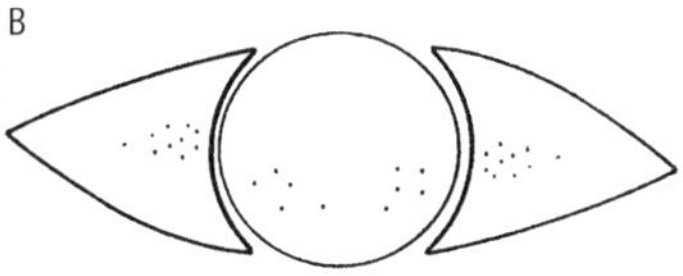	I	Minimal
C 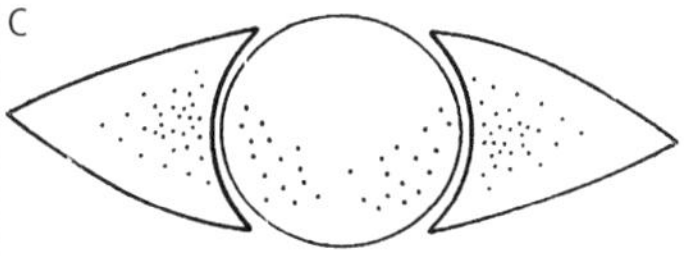	II	Mild
D 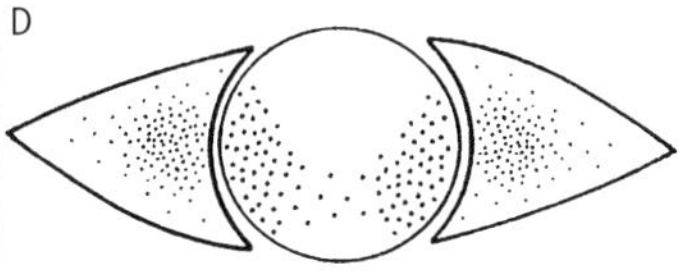	III	Moderate
E 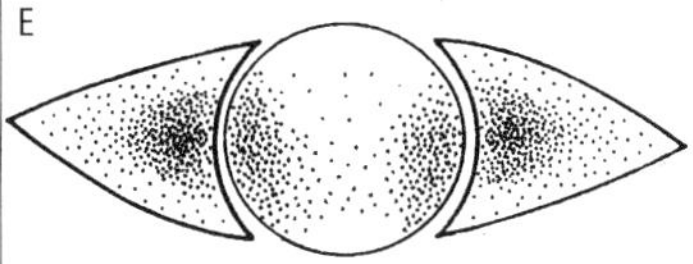	IV	Marked
>E	V	Severe

Figure 7.4 The Oxford grading scale. Note increasing severity of interpalpebral staining with increasing severity of dry eye.

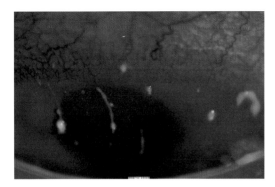

Figure 7.5 Fluorescein staining of filamentary keratitis.

In severe cases, tags of abnormal mucus may attach to the corneal surface (Figure 7.5) (*filamentary keratitis*), causing pain due to tugging during blinking.

In ADDE, a reduction in reflex tear secretion can be demonstrated by the Schirmer test, in which the length of wetting of a standard filter paper strip, hooked over the lateral third of the lid margin, provides a criterion of lacrimal deficiency. A diagnostic value would be <10 mm wetting in 5 minutes. Occasionally, reflex overproduction of tears due to ocular irritation may confuse the diagnosis.

Treatment

Treatment of ADDE involves topical therapy, built up in a step-wise fashion according to the severity of the condition, often starting with inexpensive, low-viscosity cellulose polymers which prolong the residence time of a moisturizing drop and allow inflammatory mediators to be flushed from the ocular surface. Other agents are available which are directed towards lubrication, water retention, protection from hyperosmolar damage (*osmoprotection*), stabilization of the tear film lipid layer and promotion of epithelial cell viability.

Tear substitutes should be instilled regularly throughout the day and not simply as-needed for symptomatic relief and the use of substitutes containing preservatives should be avoided or severely limited since these may exacerbate the condition. A mild steroid preparation to suppress inflammatory signs may be used for a limited period, while monitoring for complications such as raised ocular pressure (glaucoma). Where inflammatory features are not major or have been suppressed, preparations containing *hyaluronic acid* are of particular value. Their non-Newtonian property (less viscous when moving, more viscous when stationary) allows them to be formulated at relatively high viscosity, which extends their retention time, while they 'shear thin' during the blink or saccade, avoiding intolerance due to frictional drag.

In ADDE, when tear flow is greatly reduced, it may be necessary to occlude the puncta with plugs, or more permanently with surgery, to conserve the tears. This is preceded by a short period of topical steroid therapy to prevent the build-up of inflammatory mediators in the tears when drainage is blocked. Agents such as topical cyclosporin A, tacrolimus and lifitegrast, which inhibit the migration of activated lymphocytes to the ocular surface, are used in longer term anti-inflammatory therapy. A role for oral *n*-omega-3 fatty acids (such as *n*-3 eicosapentaenoic (EPA) and docosahexaenoic (DHA) acids), is not established.

Where MGD contributes to the DED, the main goal should be to reduce lid margin inflammation and restore the Meibomian contribution to the tear film lipid layer. Treatment is designed to achieve a more efficient control of the tear film stability, applying heat and massage to the lids, antibiotic drops or ointment and systemic antibiotics where necessary (Chapter 6).

Other forms of evaporative dry eye

Malposition of the globe or lid margins

If the lids are not adequately apposed to the eye (*ectropion*), or there is incomplete lid closure (*lagophthalmos* – for example, in a seventh nerve palsy), or if the eye protrudes (*proptosis*) as in dysthyroid eye disease, the preocular tear film will not form adequately and an evaporative form of dry eye will result. It also occurs in conditions of infrequent blinking, such as Parkinson disease.

Correction of the lid deformity is required for ectropion. In other instances, if the defect is temporary, artificial tears and lubricants can be applied. If lid closure is inadequate, a temporary ptosis can be induced with a local injection of botulinum toxin into the levator muscle to effect a short-term paralysis and lowering of the upper lid. A more permanent result can be obtained by suturing together part of the apposed margins of the upper and lower lids to reduce the palpebral aperture (e.g. *lateral tarsorrhaphy*; Figure 7.6), or the use of gold/platinum weights inserted into the lids to assist closure.

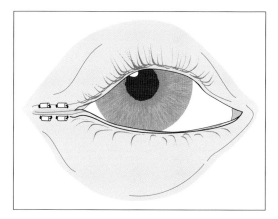

Cicatricial conjunctival disorders

Loss of goblet cells occurs in most forms of dry eye, but particularly in cicatricial conjunctival disorders such as erythema multiforme (Stevens–Johnson syndrome). In this, there is an acute episode of inflammation causing macular 'target' lesions on the skin and discharging lesions on the eye, mouth and vulva. In the eye, this is followed by conjunctival shrinkage, with adhesions forming between the globe and the conjunctiva (*symblepharon*). There may be both an aqueous, a meibomian and a mucin deficiency, and problems due to lid deformity and trichiasis. Mucous membrane pemphigoid, chemical burns of the eye, and trachoma (chronic inflammation of the conjunctiva caused by chlamydial infection; see Chapters 8 and 18) may have a similar end result.

The symptoms are similar to those seen with an aqueous deficiency. Examination may reveal scarred, abnormal conjunctiva and areas of fluorescein staining on the cornea and conjunctiva. Treatment requires the application of artificial lubricants and anti-inflammatory agents and may require reconstructive surgery in severe cases.

Vitamin A deficiency (*xerophthalmia*) is a condition causing childhood blindness on a worldwide scale. It is associated with generalized malnutrition in countries such as India and Pakistan. Goblet cells are lost from the conjunctiva and the ocular surface becomes keratinized (*xerosis*). An aqueous deficiency may also occur. A characteristic corneal melting and perforation which occurs in this condition (*keratomalacia*) may be prevented by early treatment with vitamin A (see Chapter 18 for a more detailed description).

Disorders of tear drainage

When tear production exceeds the capacity of the drainage system, excess tears overflow onto the cheeks leading to a watering eye. It may be caused by:

- reflex tearing, due to irritation of the ocular surface, for example by a corneal foreign body, infection or blepharitis,
- obstruction of any part of the drainage system (when the tearing is termed *epiphora*).

Obstruction of tear drainage (infantile)

The nasolacrimal system develops as a solid cord which subsequently canalizes and is patent just before term. Congenital obstruction of the duct is common, when the distal end of the nasolacrimal duct remains imperforate, causing a watering eye. If the canaliculi also become partially obstructed, the non-draining pool of fluid in the sac may become infected and accumulate within the sac as a *mucocoele,* or cause *dacryocystitis*. Diagnostically, the discharge may be expressed from the puncta by pressure over the lacrimal sac. The conjunctiva, however, *is not* inflamed and the eye is white. Most obstructions resolve spontaneously in the first year of life. If epiphora persists beyond this time, patency can be achieved by passing a probe via the punctum through the nasolacrimal duct to perforate the occluding membrane (*probing*). A general anaesthetic is required.

Obstruction of tear drainage (adult)

The tear drainage system may become blocked at any point, such as the puncta or canaliculi, but the most common site is the nasolacrimal duct. Causes include infections or direct trauma to the nasolacrimal system and, occasionally, topically applied drugs.

History

The patient complains of a watering eye, sometimes associated with stickiness. The eye is white. Symptoms may be worse in the wind or in cold weather. There may be a history of previous trauma or infection.

Signs

A stenosed punctum may be apparent on slit lamp examination. Epiphora is unusual if one punctum continues to function. Acquired obstruction beyond

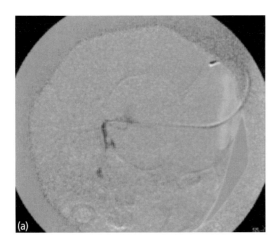

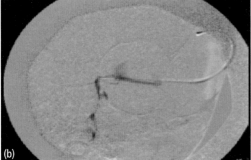

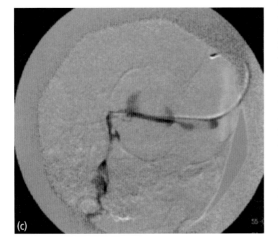

Figure 7.7 The phases of a dacryocystogram. The cannula is inserted into the lower canaliculus and the dye injected into the nasolacrimal system. (a) The dye has just entered the lacrimal sac. (b) The dye has started to outline the nasolacrimal duct. (c) The dye has passed into the nose. (*Source:* Courtesy of Dr Timothy Taylor.)

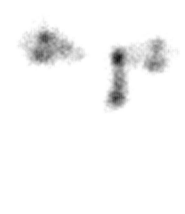

RT ANTERIOR LT

Figure 7.8 A dacryoscintigram. This picture was taken 25 minutes after instillation of the technetium. The dye has passed through to the nasolacrimal duct and the nose on the left hand side. On the right it has entered the lacrimal sac but not the nasolacrimal duct, indicating an obstruction to flow here.

the punctum is diagnosed by syringing the nasolacrimal system with saline, using a fine cannula inserted via the punctum, into a canaliculus. A patent system is indicated when the patient tastes the saline as it reaches the pharynx. If there is an obstruction of the nasolacrimal duct, then fluid will regurgitate from the non-cannulated punctum. Another useful test is the fluorescein dye disappearance test where a drop of fluorescein sodium is instilled into the conjunctival sac, and dye clearance observed 5 minutes later. Complete or near-complete clearance of the dye would be expected in the presence of a patent and functioning lacrimal drainage system. The exact location of the obstruction can be confirmed by injecting a radio-opaque dye into the nasolacrimal system (*dacryocystogram*). X-rays are then used to follow the passage of the dye through the system (Figure 7.7). A more physiological test follows the passage of a drop of technetium isotope instilled into the lateral conjunctival sac, through the drainage system, using a gamma camera (*dacryoscintigram*) (Figure 7.8).

Treatment

It is important to exclude other ocular disease that may contribute to watering, such as blepharitis. Repair of the occluded nasolacrimal duct requires

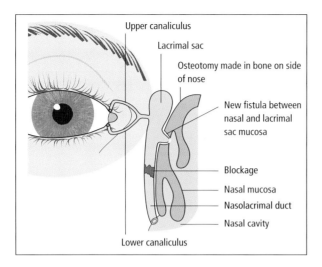

Figure 7.9 The principle of a DCR (dacryocystorhinostomy).

surgery to connect the mucosal surface of the intact lacrimal sac to the nasal mucosa by removing the intervening bone (*dacryocystorhinostomy* or DCR; Figure 7.9). The operation can be performed through an incision on the side of the nose but it may also be performed endoscopically through the nasal passages, thus avoiding a scar at the root of the nose.

Infections of the nasolacrimal system

Closed obstruction of the drainage system predisposes to infection of the sac *(dacryocystitis;* Figure 7.10).

The organism involved is usually *Staphylococcus or Streptococcus.* Patients present with a painful swelling on the medial side of the orbit, overlying the enlarged, infected sac. Treatment is with systemic antibiotics. A *mucocoele* results from a collection of mucus in an obstructed sac; it is not grossly infected and is often painless and non-tender. In either case a DCR may be necessary to remove its contents and achieve a patent nasolacrimal system.

 KEY POINTS

- Dry eyes can cause significant ocular symptoms and signs.
- A watery eye in a newborn child is commonly due to non-patency of the nasolacrimal duct. Most spontaneously resolve within the first year of life.
- In an adult, increased lacrimation may be due to disease of the ocular surface, including a foreign body or blockage of the tear drainage system.

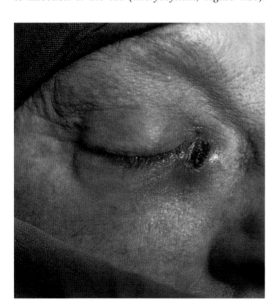

Figure 7.10 Dacryocystitis pointing through the skin.

Assessment questions True or False

1. **Sjögren syndrome is associated with**
   a   Keratoconjunctivitis sicca (KCS – dry eye).
   b   Rheumatoid arthritis.
   c   Dryness of the mouth.
   d   Staining of the cornea with fluorescein.

2. **A 60-year-old man presents with painless watering of the eye, worse when outside in the wind. Sometimes there is a sticky discharge. The white of the eye is never inflamed. No abnormal masses are palpable, but pressure over the lacrimal sac causes a mucopurulent discharge to be expressed from the lower punctum.**

a The most likely diagnosis is an ectropion.
b The most likely diagnosis is a blocked nasolacrimal duct.
c The site of a nasolacrimal obstruction can be confirmed with a dacrocystogram.
d The most likely diagnosis is blepharitis.
e The most likely diagnosis is dacryocystitis.

Answers

1. **Sjögren syndrome**
a True. There is a deficiency of lacrimal secretion.
b True. The association with connective tissue disease is called secondary Sjögren syndrome.
c True. Dry eye and dry mouth are key features of Sjögren syndrome.
d True. Dry eye damages the corneal (and conjunctival) epithelium.

2. **A 60-year-old man presents with painless watering of the eye, worse when outside in the wind.**
a False. This may cause epiphora, but there would not usually be a discharge, nor would there be a mucopurulent discharge expressed from the lower punctum.
b True. The symptoms and signs are typical of the condition.
c True. The radio-opaque dye outlines the nasolacrimal system.
d False. Although blepharitis can cause epiphora, no mucopurulent discharge would be expressible from the lower punctum.
e False. There is no inflammatory swelling over the lacrimal sac.

8

Conjunctiva, cornea and sclera

Learning objectives

To understand:

✔ The symptoms, signs, causes and treatment of conjunctival disease.

✔ The symptoms, signs, causes and treatment of corneal disease.

✔ The difference between episcleritis and scleritis.

Introduction

Disorders of the conjunctiva and cornea are a common cause of ocular symptoms. The surface of the eye is regularly exposed to the external environment and subject to trauma, infection and allergic reactions. These account for the majority of diseases in these tissues. Degenerative and structural abnormalities account for a minority of problems.

Symptoms

Patients may complain of the following:

1 Pain and irritation. Conjunctivitis alone is seldom associated with anything more than mild discomfort. Pain signifies something more serious such as corneal injury or infection. This symptom helps differentiate conjunctivitis alone from corneal disease.
2 Redness. Due to dilatation of conjunctival vessels. In conjunctivitis, the entire conjunctival surface including that covering the tarsal plates is involved. If the redness is localized to the episclera, near the limbus *(a ciliary flush)*, the following should be considered:
   a keratitis (an inflammation of the cornea);
   b uveitis (see Chapter 10);
   c acute glaucoma (see Chapter 11).
3 Discharge. Purulent discharge suggests a bacterial conjunctivitis. Viral conjunctivitis is associated with a more watery discharge. Blurring of vision caused by a discharge is cleared by blinking.
4 Visual loss that is not cleared by blinking. This occurs only when the central cornea is affected. Loss of vision that is not transient is thus an important symptom requiring urgent action.
5 Patients with corneal disease may also complain of photophobia.

Signs

The following features may be seen in conjunctival disease:

• Papillae. These are raised lesions on the upper tarsal conjunctiva, about 1 mm or more in diameter with a central vascular core. They are *a non-specific sign* of chronic inflammation. They result from

Ophthalmology: Lecture Notes, Thirteenth Edition. Bruce James, Anthony Bron, and Manoj V. Parulekar.
© 2024 John Wiley & Sons Ltd. Published 2024 by John Wiley & Sons Ltd.
Companion website: www.wiley.com/go/ophthalmology13e

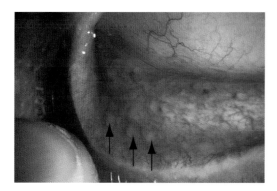

Figure 8.1 The clinical appearance of follicles.

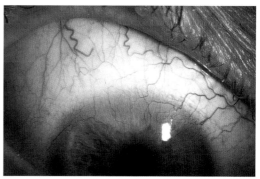

Figure 8.2 Pannus.

inflammatory infiltrates within the conjunctiva, constrained by the presence of multiple, tiny fibrous septa. *Giant papillae*, several mm in diameter, are typical of allergic eye disease and are formed by the coalescence of papillae (see Figure 8.4). They are also seen as a reaction to contact lens wear.

- Follicles (Figure 8.1). These are raised, gelatinous, oval lesions about 1 mm in diameter, found usually in the lower tarsal conjunctiva and upper tarsal border, and occasionally at the limbus. Each follicle represents a lymphoid collection with its own germinal centre. Unlike papillae, the causes of follicles are more specific, implying e.g. viral or chlamydial infections, or sometimes toxic reaction to topical medication.
- Dilation of the conjunctival vasculature also termed 'injection'.
- Subconjunctival haemorrhage, often *bright red* in colour because blood is fully oxygenated by the ambient air, diffusing through the conjunctiva.

The features of corneal disease are different, and include the following:

- Focal or diffuse *epithelial oedema,* giving rise to a superficial corneal haze.
- *Stromal oedema,* giving rise to increased corneal thickness and loss of stromal transparency. There may be an accompanying epithelial oedema.
- Focal, white, *cellular infiltrates* in the stroma, which may attract new blood vessels. Slit-lamp examination at high magnification reveals invading polymorphs, migrating from the vascular limbus.
- Deposits of inflammatory cells on the corneal endothelium (termed *keratic precipitates* or *KPs*). Neutrophils are responsible for fine KPs and lymphocytes or macrophages for coarse, or *'mutton fat'* KPs (see Chapter 10).
- Chronic keratitis may stimulate the peripheral ingrowth of subepithelial blood vessels (*pannus*; Figure 8.2). In acute keratitis, new blood vessels

may invade the stroma at any level. Stromal oedema, which causes swelling and separates the collagen lamellae, facilitates blood vessel invasion.

- *Punctate keratitis* is a common feature of many corneal diseases. It is best detected using fluorescein dye, which is taken up into dead or dying surface epithelial cells, which fluoresce a bright green under a blue light, enhanced when viewed through a yellow filter. Staining may be isolated, scattered or confluent and the pattern may give a clue to the cause of the disease. The term punctate epithelial erosion (PEE) is also used to describe the same phenomenon, but there is no evidence that the dots of stain occupy the space left by a desquamated cell and so the term is a misnomer. Punctate staining can also be shown on the bulbar conjunctiva using the stain lissamine green, which in this case provides better contrast than fluorescein.
- More extensive epithelial loss, due to chemical or physical trauma, is referred to as an *abrasion*. Abrasions are very painful.

Conjunctiva

Inflammatory diseases of the conjunctiva

Bacterial conjunctivitis

Patients present with:

- bilateral redness of the eyes;
- a sticky, purulent discharge;
- ocular irritation.

The commonest causative organisms are *Staphylococcus, Streptococcus, Pneumococcus* and *Haemophilus*. The condition is usually self-limiting, although a broad-spectrum antibiotic eye drop is often used to hasten resolution. Conjunctival swabs for culture are indicated in severe disease or if the condition fails to resolve.

Antibiotics

Some of the antibiotics available for topical ophthalmic use are as follows (see Appendix 2):

- Azithromycin.
- Ceftazidime.
- Cefuroxime.
- Chloramphenicol.
- Ciprofloxacin.
- Fusidic acid.
- Gentamicin.
- Neomycin.
- Ofloxacin.

Chloramphenicol is an effective broad-spectrum agent. An unproven risk of bone marrow aplasia following topical therapy has restricted its use in some countries and, where it is available, as a matter of caution, its long-term use is not recommended.

Ophthalmia neonatorum

Ophthalmia neonatorum (ON) refers to any conjunctivitis that occurs in the first 30 days of neonatal life and requires urgent treatment. Infection is acquired during vaginal delivery. *Urgent swabs for gram stain and culture are mandatory*. Examination may be difficult because of a profuse purulent discharge, but corneal examination is essential to exclude ulceration.

The frequency of ON varies geographically depending on socio-economic factors and the standard of health care but the commonest causes are as follows:

- Bacteria, including *Streptococcus, Staphylococcus, Haemophylus, Pseudomonas* and *Neisseria* species.
- Of these, *Neisseria gonorrhoeae* is the most severe and threatens both sight and health. It usually develops within the first 5 days of birth and progresses rapidly. Corneal perforation may occur. Systemic complications include rhinitis, stomatitis, arthritis, meningitis and septicaemia. Patients should be managed with the help of a paediatrician. Due to increasing resistance to penicillin, a systemic, third-generation cephalosporin (ceftriaxone (or cefotaxime) given im or iv) is used to treat

the condition. The eye must be kept clean with 0.9% saline irrigation. Topical bacitracin ointment can also be given but systemic treatment is the most important. Parents should be referred to a sexually transmitted diseases (STD) clinic.

- *Chlamydia.* This is more common and may be responsible for a chronic conjunctivitis and sight-threatening corneal scarring. The onset is usually between 5 and 14 days of birth but may be later. The discharge may be serosanguinous, later becoming mucopurulent. The infection may be complicated by the development of pneumonia. First-line treatment for local and systemic disease is erythromycin and azithromycin can also be used. Topical preparations have a role in prophylaxis. It is important to refer parents to an STD clinic.
- *Herpes simplex*, which can cause corneal scarring. While HSV type 1 is the usual cause in the adult, HSV type 2 may be responsible in the neonate. A history of maternal genital infection must be sought. There may be skin vesicles, oedema of the eyelids and a hazy cornea on the affected side as well as conjunctival injection and discharge. Topical and systemic antivirals are used to treat the condition. Systemic antiviral treatment is given because of the risk of infection to other organs including the central nervous system. Recurrence is common.

Viral conjunctivitis

This is distinguished from bacterial conjunctivitis by the following:

- A watery discharge with limited purulent features.
- The presence of conjunctival follicles (hence *follicular conjunctivitis*). Preauricular lymph nodes are also enlarged.
- There may also be lid oedema and excessive lacrimation.

The commonest causative agent is adenovirus, and to a much lesser extent Coxsackie and picornavirus. *Adenovirus conjunctivitis* is self-limiting but *highly contagious* and frequently occurs in epidemics. There is a risk of hospital-acquired infection, which can arise where there is failure to hand wash and disinfect equipment when managing patients with a red eye and conjunctivitis. Certain adenovirus serotypes can cause a troublesome and painful *keratoconjunctivitis* with a coarse, scattered, superficial punctate keratitis, in which vision is affected. This may have long-term visual sequelae. Adenoviruses can also cause a conjunctivitis associated with the formation of a pseudomembrane across the conjunctiva. Patients must be given hygiene instruction to minimize the spread of infection In the home (e.g. frequent hand washing; using separate towels). Treatment of keratoconjunctivitis is controversial. No effective commercial antiviral is available. Antibacterial therapy is not indicated unless there is a secondary bacterial infection. The judicious use of topical steroids damps down symptoms and causes corneal opacities to resolve, but rebound inflammation is common and steroids must be weaned slowly to limit the reappearance of corneal opacities.

Chlamydial infections

Different serotypes of the obligate intracellular organism *Chlamydia trachomatis* are responsible for two forms of ocular infections.

Adult inclusion keratoconjunctivitis

This STD is caused by chlamydial serotypes D–K and may take a chronic course (up to 18 months), unless adequately treated. Patients present with a mucopurulent follicular conjunctivitis and develop a *micropannus* (superficial peripheral corneal vascularization) associated with subepithelial scarring. Urethritis or cervicitis is common. Diagnosis is confirmed by detection of chlamydial antigens, using immunofluorescence (ELISA test), or by identification of typical inclusion bodies by Giemsa staining in conjunctival swab or scrape specimens; this is of low sensitivity however.

Inclusion conjunctivitis is treated with systemic tetracycline because of the likelihood of genital tract infection. Other systemic agents in use include doxycycline and erythromycin, and azithromycin may be given as a single dose. The patient should be referred to an STD clinic.

Trachoma

Trachoma is caused by chlamydial serotypes A–C and is the commonest infective cause of blindness in the world, although it is uncommon in developed countries (more details will be found in Chapter 18). It predominantly affects children. Houseflies clustering about the face and eyes act as a vector, and the disease is encouraged by poor hygiene and overcrowding in a dry, hot climate. The hallmark of the disease is subconjunctival fibrosis caused by frequent re-infections associated with the unhygienic conditions. Blindness may occur due to corneal scarring from recurrent keratitis and trichiasis (Figure 8.3).

Trachoma is treated with oral or topical tetracycline or erythromycin. Azithromycin, an alternative, requires only a single oral dose. Entropion and trichiasis require surgical correction.

Allergic conjunctivitis

This may be divided into acute and chronic forms:

1 Hayfever or seasonal allergic conjunctivitis is an acute IgE-mediated reaction to airborne allergens (usually pollens, for example ragweed, and mite allergens) which interact with IgE-primed conjunctival mast cells. This leads to mast cell degranulation with the release of preformed histamine, responsible for the acute phase response. In the late-phase response, synthesis and release of prostaglandins and leukotrienes amplifies conjunctival hyperaemia, oedema, increased vascular permeability, discharge of goblet cell mucin and inflammatory cell infiltration. Symptoms and signs include:
   a   itchiness;
   b   conjunctival injection and swelling (chemosis);
   c   lacrimation, including a mucous discharge;
   d   allergic rhinitis.

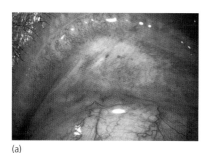
(a)

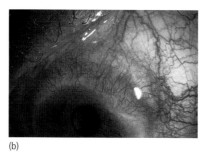
(b)

Figure 8.3 Trachoma: scarring of (a) the upper lid (everted) and (b) the cornea.

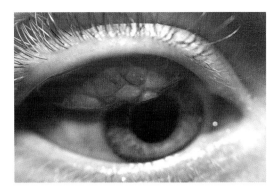

Figure 8.4 The appearance of giant (cobblestone) papillae in vernal conjunctivitis.

2 Vernal keratoconjunctivitis (VKC or spring catarrh) is also mediated by IgE. It often affects male children with a history of atopy. It is usually seasonal but may be present all year long (perennial) and may become a chronic and intractable disease. Symptoms and signs include:

a itchiness;

b photophobia;

c lacrimation;

d papillary conjunctivitis on the upper tarsal plate (papillae may coalesce to form giant cobblestones; Figure 8.4);

e limbal follicles and white spots;

f punctate epithelial keratitis;

g an opaque, oval plaque which in severe disease replaces an upper zone of the corneal epithelium (shield ulcer).

Initial therapy is with mast cell stabilizers (e.g. sodium cromoglycate, nedocromil, lodoxamide) and antihistamines (e.g. levocabastine), or with agents combining mast cell stabilizing and antihistamine properties (e.g. olopatidine). Topical steroids are required in severe cases but long-term use is avoided if possible because of the risks of steroid-induced glaucoma or cataract. In such cases, topical cyclosporine or tacrolimus may be used. Mucolytics (acetylcysteine) may be required to help dissolve the corneal plaque but surgical removal may be necessary.

Contact lens wearers may develop a reaction to their lenses, leading to a *giant papillary conjunctivitis* (GPC) with a mucoid discharge. This is more a mechanical irritation than a true allergic reaction. While this may respond to topical treatment with mast cell stabilizers, it is often necessary to stop lens wear for a period, or even permanently if symptoms recur.

Conjunctival degenerations

Cysts are common in the conjunctiva but rarely cause symptoms. If necessary, they can be removed. *Pingueculae* are small, yellowish, paralimbal lesions in the horizontal meridian that are unassociated with irritation and never impinge on the cornea (Figure 8.5a).

Pterygia are wing-shaped elevations of the interpalpebral conjunctiva, usually bilateral, and located nasally. The apex of the pterygium is directed towards the cornea, onto which it progressively extends with time (Figure 8.5b). Pterygia cause redness and discomfort and if extensive, they may encroach onto the visual axis to cause visual loss. They result from excessive exposure to scattered or direct ultraviolet radiation, and are thus more common in outdoor workers, particularly in countries with a high sunlight exposure. Histologically, collagen structure is altered. Lubrication drops may help with symptoms of ocular irritation in a limited way. Surgical excision may be indicated, particularly when vision is threatened; a risk of recurrence is reduced by the use of antimitotic therapy at the time of surgery.

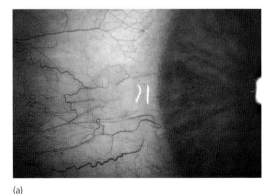
(a)

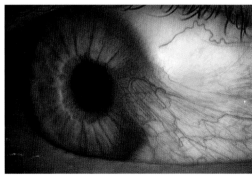
(b)

Figure 8.5 The clinical appearance of (a) a pinguecula and (b) a pterygium.

Conjunctival tumours

These are rare. They include:

- Squamous cell carcinoma. An irregular raised area of conjunctiva which may invade the deeper tissues. They may be treated with topical chemotherapeutic drugs or by excision.
- Malignant melanoma. The differential diagnosis from benign pigmented lesions (e.g. a naevus or melanosis) may be difficult. Review is necessary to assess whether the lesion is increasing in size. Excision biopsy, to achieve a definitive diagnosis, may be required. Management is with surgical excision, cryotherapy and adjuvant chemotherapy. Immunotherapy may also become a possible option for metastatic disease.

Cornea

Infective corneal lesions

Herpes simplex keratitis

Type 1 herpes simplex virus (HSV1) is a common and important cause of ocular disease. Type 2, which causes genital disease, may occasionally cause keratitis and infantile chorioretinitis. Primary infection by HSV1 is usually acquired early in life by close contact such as kissing. It may be asymptomatic, but otherwise is accompanied by:

- fever;
- vesicular lid lesions;
- follicular conjunctivitis;
- preauricular lymphadenopathy.

Primary infection may cause a conjunctivitis, with or without punctate keratitis. It is followed by resolution and latency of the virus in the trigeminal ganglion. 'Recurrent' infection involves reactivation of the latent virus, which travels centrifugally to nerve terminals in the corneal epithelium to cause an epithelial keratitis. There may be no past clinical history. The risk of reactivation is increased if the patient is debilitated (e.g. systemic illness, immunosuppression). The pathognomonic appearance is of a *dendritic ulcer* (Figure 8.6). These linear, branching, epithelial ulcers may heal without a scar but they may progress to a stromal keratitis, associated with an inflammatory infiltration and oedema, and ultimately a loss of corneal transparency and permanent scarring. This stage of the disease represents an immunogenic response to the viral antigen.

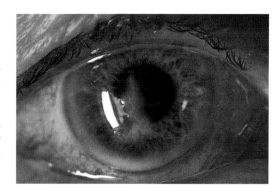

Figure 8.6 A dendritic ulcer seen in herpes simplex infection.

If corneal scarring is severe, a corneal graft may be required to restore vision. Uveitis and glaucoma may accompany the disease. *Disciform keratitis* is another immunogenic reaction to herpes antigen in the stroma and presents as disc- or ring-shaped stromal oedema and clouding without ulceration, often associated with iritis.

Treatment is with topical antiviral agents such as aciclovir. Topical steroids must not be given to patients with a dendritic ulcer, since they may exacerbate the disease and cause extensive corneal ulceration. In patients with stromal involvement (keratitis), steroids are used deliberately but cautiously, under ophthalmic supervision and with antiviral cover, to suppress the immunogenic response. Patients undergoing corneal graft surgery for past HSV keratitis commonly receive an extended course of prophylactic, oral antiviral cover to minimize recurrence.

Antivirals

Dendritic lesions are treated with topical antivirals and typically heal within 2 weeks. Some of those available are:

- aciclovir;
- ganciclovir;
- vidarabine;
- trifluorothymidine.

Herpes zoster ophthalmicus (ophthalmic shingles)

This is caused by the *varicella zoster virus* that is responsible for chickenpox (Figure 8.7). The ophthalmic division of the trigeminal nerve is affected.

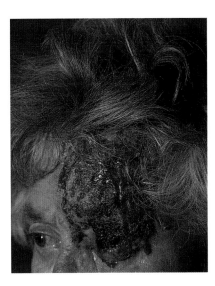

Figure 8.7 The clinical appearance of herpes zoster ophthalmicus.

Unlike herpes simplex infection, there is usually a prodromal period with the patient systemically unwell. Ocular manifestations are usually preceded by pain and the appearance of vesicles in the distribution of the ophthalmic division of the trigeminal nerve. Ocular problems are more likely if the *nasociliary branch* of the nerve is involved (signalled by vesicles at the root of the nose). Signs include:

- lid swelling (which may be bilateral);
- keratitis;
- iritis;
- secondary glaucoma.

Reactivation of the disease is often linked to unrelated systemic illness. Oral antiviral treatment given for seven days (e.g. aciclovir, famciclovir) is effective in reducing post-infective neuralgia (a severe chronic pain in the area of the rash) *if given within 3 days of the eruption of skin vesicles*. Ocular disease may require antibacterials to prevent secondary infection. Steroid use is controversial.

The prognosis of herpetic eye disease has improved since antiviral treatment became available. Both simplex and zoster cause anaesthesia of the cornea, termed *neurotrophic keratitis*, leading to non-healing indolent corneal ulcers. These are difficult to treat.

Vaccination against herpes zoster is available. It lasts for about 8 years and is usually recommended to people over 60 or those with a compromised immune system.

Bacterial keratitis

Bacteria

Some of the bacteria responsible for corneal infection:

- *Staphylococcus epidermidis*.
- *Staphylococcus aureus*.
- *Streptococcus pneumoniae*.
- *Coliforms*.
- *Pseudomonas*.
- *Haemophilus*.

Pathogenesis

A host of bacteria may infect the cornea. Some are found on the lid margin as part of the normal flora, but the conjunctiva and cornea are normally protected against infection by:

- blinking;
- washing away of debris by the flow of tears;
- entrapment of foreign particles by mucus;
- the antibacterial properties of the tears;
- the barrier function of the corneal epithelium (*Neisseria gonorrhoeae* is the only organism that can penetrate the intact epithelium).

Predisposing causes of bacterial keratitis include:

- keratoconjunctivitis sicca (dry eye);
- a breach in the corneal epithelium (e.g. following surgery or trauma);
- contact lens wear;
- prolonged use of topical steroids.

Symptoms and signs

These include:

- *pain,* usually severe unless the cornea is anaesthetic;
- purulent discharge;
- ciliary injection;
- visual loss (severe if the visual axis is involved);
- hypopyon – sometimes (a mass of white cells collected in the anterior chamber; see Chapter 10);
- a white corneal opacity identifies the site of polymorphonuclear infiltration of the stroma and is often visible with the naked eye (Figure 8.8).

Treatment

Scrapes are taken from the base of the ulcer under topical anaesthesia, for Gram staining and culture. The patient is then treated with intensive topical anti-

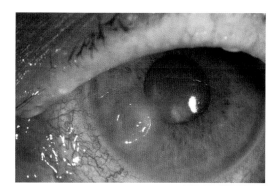

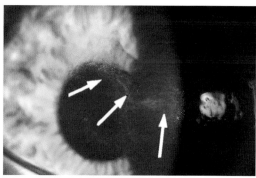

Figure 8.8 Clinical appearance of a bacterial corneal ulcer.

Figure 8.9 The clinical appearance of acanthamoeba keratitis. Arrows indicate keratoneuritis.

biotics, often with dual therapy using concentrated, combined preparations to cover most organisms (e.g. cefuroxime against Gram-positive bacteria with gentamicin for Gram-negative bacteria). Such preparations are usually formulated locally and because they are unlicensed, they are used on a physician's responsibility basis. The use of commercial fluoroquinolones such as ciprofloxacin and ofloxacin, as a monotherapy, is gaining popularity.

Drops are given hourly, day and night, for the first couple of days and are then reduced in frequency with clinical improvement. In severe or unresponsive keratitis, the cornea may perforate. This can be treated initially with tissue adhesives to seal the wound (cyanoacrylate glue) and later, when inflammation has settled, by a corneal transplant. A persistent scar may also require a corneal graft to restore vision.

Acanthamoeba keratitis

This freshwater amoeba can cause an extremely painful infective keratitis (Figure 8.9). It became more common with the increasing use of soft contact lenses. The risk is reduced with disposable daily wear lenses and increased by swimming when wearing contact lenses. The keratitis may be accompanied by prominent, infiltrated, corneal nerves and when advanced may spread into the sclera. Diagnosis may be made non-invasively using *in vivo* confocal microscopy to reveal amoebic cysts, or the amoeba can be isolated from a corneal scrape and from the contact lens case, using selected stains on potassium hydroxide (KOH) wet mounts. It can also be cultured on special plates coated with *Escherichia coli* (an *E coli* lawn), to identify strains, but molecular techniques such as PCR are faster and becoming increasingly specific and efficient.

Topical chlorhexidine, polyhexamethylene biguanide (PHMB) and propamidine are used to treat the condition. Prolonged treatment over a period of several months is often needed.

Fungal keratitis

This is unusual in the United Kingdom but more common in warmer climates such as India and the southern United States. In India, it accounts for 30–50% of infective keratitis. It should be considered in:

- corneal ulcers unresponsive to antibacterial therapy;
- cases of trauma with vegetable matter e.g. a tree branch;
- cases associated with the prolonged use of steroids.

The whitish inflammatory stromal infiltrate of fungal keratitis may be difficult to distinguish from that of bacterial keratitis, but the presence of satellite lesions outside the main lesion may be an important clue to diagnosis. Liquid and solid Sabouraud media are used to grow the fungi, often requiring prolonged incubation. Treatment requires topical antifungal drops such as natamycin, voriconazole and amphotericin.

Interstitial keratitis

This term is used for any vascular keratitis that affects the corneal stroma without epithelial involvement. In the past, the most common cause was congenital syphilis, leaving a midstromal scar interlaced with the empty ('ghost') blood vessels. Corneal grafting may be required when the opacity is marked and visual acuity reduced.

Corneal dystrophies

These are rare inherited corneal disorders often with a striking and characteristic appearance. They affect different layers of the cornea and often affect corneal transparency (Figure 8.10). They may be divided into the following:

- Anterior dystrophies involving the epithelium. These may present with painful attacks as in inherited recurrent corneal erosion. In Meesmann dystrophy, tiny microcysts are scattered throughout the epithelium. Both are dominantly inherited.
- Stromal dystrophies presenting with visual loss. If very anterior, they may also cause corneal erosion and pain. Examples are granular corneal dystrophy (dominant trait) (Figure 8.10) and macular dystrophy (recessive trait).
- Posterior dystrophies which affect the endothelium occur in congenital and adult forms. Loss of endothelial pumping results in corneal oedema which leads to a gradual loss of vision. An example is Fuchs dystrophy, which may present in middle to late adult life. It may be a sporadic condition or be inherited as a dominant trait. An X-linked form of endothelial dystrophy exists. The clinical features of Fuchs dystrophy are identical to those seen in other forms of endothelial failure (see below).

Disorders of shape

Keratoconus

Keratoconus is a painless disorder, usually sporadic but sometimes inherited, in which progressive central corneal thinning leads to an ectatic conical shape and marked myopia and astigmatism (Figure 8.11a). With time, stromal corneal scarring occurs, which

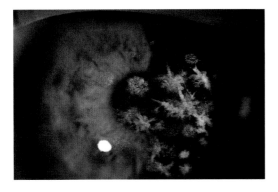

Figure 8.10 Granular dystrophy – a dominant stromal dystrophy.

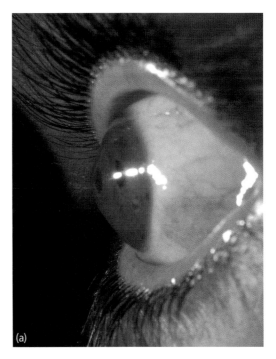

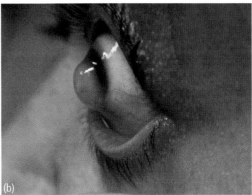

Figure 8.11 (a) Keratoconus note the prominent cone shape of the cornea on this lateral view. (b) Sudden rupture of Descemet membrane and endothelium may cause acute corneal oedema (hydrops).
(*Source:* Courtesy of Tom Butler.)

may further reduce vision. Onset is in youth, with a typical history of myopia which, with the development of irregular astigmatism, becomes uncorrectable by spectacle lenses. When suspected, it can be diagnosed from the presence of a distorted red reflex during ophthalmoscopy or at an earlier stage with instruments that record surface corneal topography. The condition is due to a failure of cohesion between the stromal collagen fibrils and lamellae of unknown cause, causing them to slip over one another and unravel. This leads to stromal thinning and ectasia. Thinning may be pronounced (Figure 8.11b) but rarely leads to perforation.

The optical impact of keratoconus is readily treated in its early stages with rigid contact lenses which arch over the irregularly shaped cornea and restore the optics of the eye. When contact lenses cannot be worn, or if, with time, they cannot correct the acuity, surgical intervention is required. In the past, this has consisted of a penetrating keratoplasty involving the replacement of the central cornea with a full thickness corneal allograft. Because the keratoconus cornea is avascular, visual results were good with a low risk of graft rejection. More recently, using lamellar techniques, it has been possible to replace the corneal stroma alone, leaving the healthy endothelium intact. Since graft rejection involves, in particular, an immune attack on the grafted endothelium, this approach has further reduced the risk of rejection.

A recent advance, which is far less invasive and may even slow progression of the disorder, is cross-linking of the anterior stromal collagen. This is achieved by exposing the riboflavin-soaked anterior stroma to UVA radiation; the generation of free radicals results in cross-linking of the collagen and inhibits progression of the disease. It is not suitable for advanced cases with thin corneas.

Corneal degenerations

Endothelial failure – Bullous keratopathy

The function of the corneal endothelium (Figure 8.12a) is to transfer water from the corneal stroma to the anterior chamber and thus maintain a minimum corneal thickness. This ensures the regular order and separation of the stromal collagen fibrils that is necessary for corneal transparency. Endothelial cell loss, from whatever cause, is repaired by cell spreading, which entails an enlargement of cells and a fall in cell density. When cell density falls below a critical level, a loss of barrier and pumping functions occurs which leads to stromal oedema and clouding as the regular packing of the collagen fibres is disrupted. This may be detected at an early stage as an increase in corneal thickness, or inferred by the presence of punctate excrescences in Descemet layer of the cornea (*corneal guttae*), which are collections of abnormal basal laminar material synthesized by the sick endothelial cells (Figure 8.12b).

As the condition advances, oedema spreads to affect the corneal epithelium and may result in

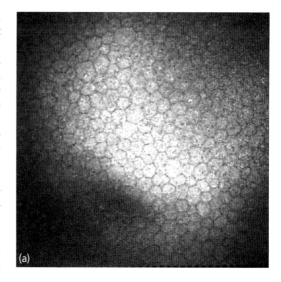

(a)

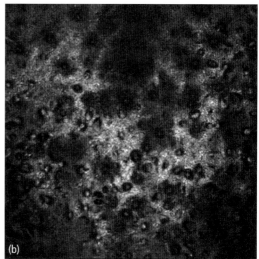

(b)

Figure 8.12 The corneal endothelium viewed by confocal microscopy. (a) The normal, hexagonal mosaic. (b) Endothelial failure. The normal mosaic is no longer visible and the endothelium is studded with drop-like excrescences (guttae) located in Descemet layer. (*Source:* Courtesy of Paula Hedges.)

epithelial bullae, which accounts for the name, bullous keratopathy. These bullae can rupture and give rise to painful erosions. Causes of endothelial cell damage include uveitis, cataract surgery, corneal graft failure and, as noted earlier, inherited endothelial disease (Fuchs dystrophy). Endothelial failure is the commonest indication for corneal graft surgery and, increasingly, is treated by endothelial keratoplasty (see below).

Band-shaped keratopathy

Band-shaped keratopathy is the subepithelial deposition of calcium phosphate in the exposed part of the cornea where CO_2 loss and the consequent raised pH favour its deposition (Figure 8.13). It is seen in eyes with chronic uveitis or glaucoma, and may cause visual loss or discomfort if epithelial erosions occur over the band. If symptomatic, it can be scraped off surgically, aided by a chelating agent such as sodium edetate to remove the calcium at the time of surgery. The excimer laser can also be effective in treating these patients by ablating the deposits. Band keratopathy can also be a sign of systemic hypercalcaemia, as in hyperparathyroidism or renal failure. The lesion is then more likely to occupy the 3 o'clock and 9 o'clock positions of the paralimbal cornea.

Lipid arcus

This is an asymptomatic, peripheral white ring-shaped lipid deposit, separated from the limbus by a clear interval. It is often seen in normal, elderly people (*arcus senilis*), but in younger patients, under 50 years, it may be a sign of hyperlipoproteinaemia. It does not affect vision and no treatment is required.

Corneal thinning

A rare cause of painful peripheral corneal thinning is *Mooren ulcer*, a condition of progressive corneal melting with an immune basis, which starts near the limbus and spreads relentlessly across the cornea. Corneal melting can also be seen in collagen diseases such as rheumatoid arthritis and Wegener granulomatosis. Treatment can be difficult, and both sets of disorders require systemic and topical immunosuppression and antiproteases. Where there is an associated dry eye, it is important to ensure adequate corneal wetting and corneal protection (see Chapter 7).

Corneal grafting – transplantation

Full thickness keratoplasty

Human donor corneal tissue from one individual can be grafted into the host cornea of another individual to restore corneal clarity or repair a perforation (Figure 8.14). This is termed a corneal allograft, and the classical approach of *penetrating keratoplasty* involves replacement of a full thickness disc of cornea with a donor disc, which is sutured in place.

Donor corneas obtained from enucleated cadaver eyes can be banked, so that corneal grafts can be performed as a planned (elective) procedure. Up to 90% of such first-time keratoplasties in avascular corneas succeed without HLA cross-matching and with only the use of topical corticosteroid drops to prevent rejection. By contrast, other forms of solid organ grafts such as kidney or liver transplants require both HLA-matching and systemic immunosuppression. The reason for this difference is that the cornea is the site of an *immune privilege* which protects the graft from rejection. The normal, avascular cornea lacks lymphatics and in the absence of these, the transfer of foreign alloantigens to the draining lymph nodes is restricted. This limits the opportunity to activate lymph node T-cells which would otherwise threaten graft survival. Protection is reinforced by the production of factors that inhibit lymphangiogenesis or lead to the deletion of activated T-cells following keratoplasty. Additionally, the delivery of graft alloantigens into the anterior chamber initiates the generation of antigen-specific, regulatory T-cells (T-regs) which suppress the immune response. This process, referred to as Anterior Chamber-Associated Immune Deviation (ACAID), involves the release of the cytokine IFN-γ.

Graft survival is much lower when the host cornea is heavily vascularized, probably in part because the cornea is also richly provided with lymphatics which

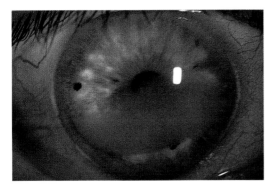

Figure 8.13 Band-shaped keratopathy.

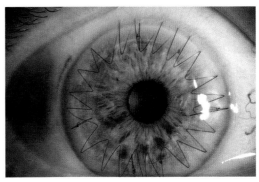

Figure 8.14 A full thickness corneal graft. Note the interrupted and the continuous 10/0 nylon sutures at the interface between graft and host.

undermine the graft's immune privilege. Although tissue can be HLA-matched for the grafting of vascularized corneas at high risk of rejection, the value of this is still uncertain.

The patient is treated with steroid eye drops for some time after surgery to prevent graft rejection. Complications such as astigmatism can be dealt with surgically or by suture adjustment. Increasingly, methods are being used to transplant only the damaged part of the cornea, for example the endothelial layer when disease of this layer results in corneal oedema or the stroma when there is a corneal opacity or it is grossly thinned as in keratoconus.

Newer techniques of lamellar keratoplasty

The various layers of the cornea can be replaced individually. For patients with endothelial disease, it is possible to selectively replace the endothelial layer with donor endothelial tissue. These include DSEK (Descemet stripping endothelial keratoplasty) and DMEK (Descemet Membrane Endothelial Keratoplasty). Since no sutures are required, there are no risks of suture-related complications such as induced astigmatism, and visual recovery is faster. The graft used in DSEK incorporates a thin layer of the donor stroma, DMEK allows an even thinner graft to be used with no stroma. DALK (Deep Anterior Lamellar Keratoplasty) involves replacing the corneal epithelium and stroma without disturbance of the endothelium, minimizing the risk of rejection.

Graft rejection

Any patient who has had a corneal graft and who complains of redness, pain or visual loss must be seen urgently by an eye specialist, as this may indicate graft rejection. Examination shows graft oedema, iritis and a line of activated T-cells attacking the graft endothelium. Intensive topical steroid application in the early stages can restore graft clarity.

Sclera

Episcleritis

This inflammation at the surface of the sclera causes a patch of redness and mild or no discomfort. This distinguishes it from scleritis and it is rarely associated with systemic disease. It is usually self-limiting but, as symptoms may be tiresome, topical anti-inflammatory treatment can be given. In rare, severe diseases, systemic non-steroidal anti-inflammatory treatment may be helpful.

Scleritis

This is a sight-threatening condition, usually accompanied by deep and severe ocular pain. A systemic cause should be sought since it is associated with collagen vascular disease in almost 50% of cases, most commonly rheumatoid arthritis, but also granulomatous polyangiitis (Wegener granulomatosis), polyarteritis nodosa and systemic lupus erythematosis. Both inflammatory and ischaemic scleral lesions occur, usually anteriorly but sometimes posteriorly. Anteriorly, the sclera may show *diffuse* or *nodular* swelling (Figure 8.15), but less commonly a *necrotizing* form occurs with full thickness tissue loss, uveal exposure and the risk of perforation. The following may complicate the condition:

- *Scleromalacia perforans*: a diffuse scleral thinning seen in rheumatoid arthritis.
- *Keratitis*: usually peripheral and sometimes with *persistent ulceration*.

- Uveitis.
- Cataract formation.
- Glaucoma.

The condition is due to an immune complex-dependent microangiopathy and treatment requires anti-inflammatory treatment with or without systemic immunosuppression. Non-steroidal anti-inflammatory agents may suffice in diffuse or nodular scleritis but treatment may require high doses of systemic steroids, combined with cytotoxic therapy in severe disease. Newer immunomodulatory agents such as monoclonal antibodies (e.g. iadalimumab) and tumour necrosis factor (TNF) alpha inhibitors (e.g. mycophenolate) may be of benefit in refractory non-infectious cases. Scleral grafting may be required to prevent perforation of the globe.

Scleritis affecting the posterior part of the globe may cause choroidal effusions, or may simulate a tumour.

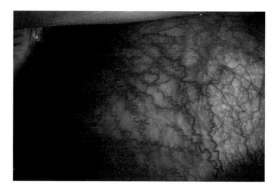

Figure 8.15 The appearance of scleritis.

KEY POINTS

- Avoid the unsupervised use of topical steroids in treating ophthalmic conditions, since complications may be serious.
- In contact lens wearers, a painful red eye is serious; it may imply an infective keratitis.
- Redness, pain and reduced vision in a patient with corneal graft suggest rejection, which is an ophthalmic emergency.
- Good hygiene and hand washing is vital if contact with an adenoviral conjunctivitis is suspected, to prevent spread.

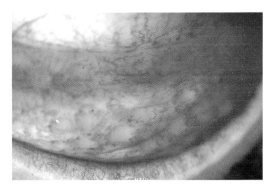

Figure 8.16 The clinical appearance of the eye referred to in Question 1.

Assessment questions
True or False

1. **An 11-year-old child presents with a red watery eye and slightly blurred vision. Her sister had similar symptoms a week ago. The appearance of the lower lid is shown in Figure 8.16.**

   a The most likely diagnosis is uveitis.
   b The most likely diagnosis is viral conjunctivitis.
   c The most likely diagnosis is bacterial conjunctivitis.
   d The child should be treated with steroids.
   e Papillae are present.

2. **A 26-year-old patient presents with an itchy watery eye. She is photophobic and the vision has become blurred. She has a history of asthma. The appearance of the (a) upper tarsus and (b) eye is shown in Figure 8.17.**

   a The most likely diagnosis is uveitis.
   b The most likely diagnosis is epithelial herpes simplex keratitis.
   c The most likely diagnosis is an allergic conjunctivitis.
   d Treatment is with antihistamines, mast cell stabilizers and topical steroids.
   e Treatment is with aciclovir.

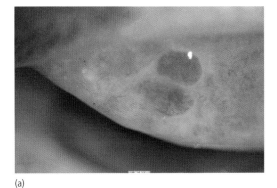

(a)

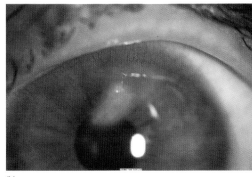

(b)

Figure 8.17 The clinical appearance of the eye referred to in Question 2. (a) The inverted upper lid. (b) The cornea stained with fluorescein.

3. A 67-year-old lady presents with pain on the right side of her forehead for 3 days. She has been feeling generally unwell. She has just noticed the appearance of vesicles on the skin.

a   The most likely diagnosis is herpes simplex.
b   The most likely diagnosis is herpes zoster.
c   The most likely diagnosis is acanthamoeba keratitis.
d   Ocular complications may include keratitis, iritis and secondary glaucoma.
e   The patient should be prescribed systemic aciclovir in high dosage.

4. A contact lens wearer presents with a red painful eye. There is a purulent discharge and vision is decreased. Figure 8.18 shows the appearance of the eye.

a   The most likely diagnosis is a bacterial corneal ulcer.
b   Acanthamoeba keratitis is another possibility in a contact lens wearer.
c   The most likely diagnosis is a corneal dystrophy.
d   The patient has band keratopathy.
e   Treatment with intensive topical antibiotics is necessary.

5. A 24-year-old lady presents with a red eye. There is no discharge. The redness is located in the temporal quadrant of the bulbar conjunctiva. There is slight discomfort; the vision is normal. There is no other medical history.

a   The most likely diagnosis is bacterial conjunctivitis.
b   The most likely diagnosis is keratoconus.
c   The most likely diagnosis is episcleritis.
d   The most likely diagnosis is scleritis.
e   Treatment is with a non-steroidal anti-inflammatory agent.

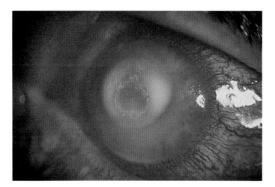

Figure 8.18 The clinical appearance of the eye referred to in Question 4.

6. Identify the conditions shown in Figure 8.19.

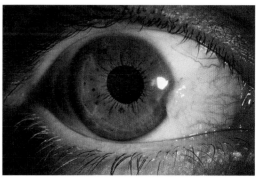

(a)

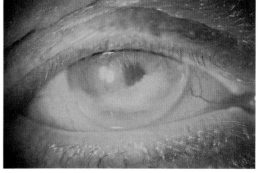

(b)

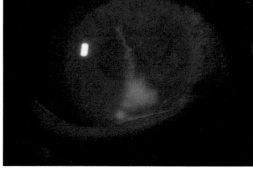

(c)

Figure 8.19 See Question 6. (a) the lesion on the right involving conjunctiva and cornea. (b) The corneal lesion and (c) the corneal lesion stained with fluorescein.

Answers

1. **An 11-year-old child presents with a red watery eye and slightly blurred vision.**

a   False. While the symptom of redness fits, the watering and similar symptoms experienced by her sister suggest that an infection is more likely.

b   True. The symptoms are typical of an adenovirus conjunctivitis, a condition which is highly contagious.

c   False. The discharge would be mucopurulent.

d   False. While steroids can help the corneal complications of adenovirus infection, they are difficult to wean. You would also wish to exclude a herpes simplex infection before considering their use.

e   False. These elevations are called 'follicles' and are composed of lymphoid cells.

2. **A 26-year-old patient presents with an itchy watery eye.**

a   False. The inflammation is not localized at the limbus, papillae are present and there is an opaque corneal plaque on the cornea.

b   False. The corneal lesion does not resemble a dendritic ulcer.

c   True. The redness, papillae and corneal lesion are typical of severe vernal keratoconjunctivitis.

d   True. This is a serious condition that may affect the long-term clarity of the cornea. Mucolytic drops are also given to remove or help dissolve the corneal plaque.

e   False. Aciclovir is an antiviral agent used in the treatment of herpes simplex keratitis.

3. **A 67-year-old lady presents with pain on the right side of her forehead.**

a   False. Vesicles would not be a feature of the disease in this age group.

b   True. This is a classical presentation.

c   False. The skin is not affected in acanthamoeba keratitis.

d   True. The effects on the eye can be widespread.

e   True. If this is given in the first 3 days of the disease, it can reduce symptoms and help reduce severe post-herpetic neuralgia.

4. **A contact lens wearer presents with a red painful eye.**

a   True. Contact lens wear is the commonest risk factor in the developed world. Other causes are trauma, prolonged steroid use, dry eye and an anaesthetic cornea (as seen in herpetic eye disease).

b   True. The eye is usually very painful.

c   False. These rarely cause a red painful eye.

d   False. Band keratopathy is caused by a deposition of calcium salts in the superficial cornea. It may sometimes cause a red painful eye, but the appearance differs.

e   True. This is an ophthalmic emergency.

5. **A 24-year-old lady presents with a red eye.**

a   False. There is no discharge and injection is not usually localized in conjunctivitis.

b   False. Keratoconus is a disorder of corneal shape and occurs in a white eye.

c   True. The symptoms and signs are very suggestive.

d   False. The diagnosis is possible but less likely than episcleritis. Scleritis causes a deep, boring pain.

e   True. Simple episcleritis is self-limiting. Nodular episcleritis may be helped by topical anti-inflammatory agents. If there is a lack of response, a systemic NSAID (e.g. flurbiprofen) may be used.

6. **Identify the conditions shown in Figure 8.19.**

a   Pterygium.

b   Band keratopathy.

c   Herpes simplex dendritic ulcer stained with fluorescein.

9

The lens and cataract

Introduction

Diseases of the lens may affect its transparency, shape or position.

Cataract

Definition and causes

Cataract is the name given to any *light-scattering opacity* within the lens. When it lies outside the pupillary zone, it may have little effect on vision. Small opacities within the visual axis (central) as well as diffuse lens opacities can result in visual loss. Cataract is the commonest cause of treatable blindness in the world. The majority of cataracts occur in older subjects and are referred to as *age-related*. They result from the effects of a cumulative exposure of the lens to environmental and other influences, such as diabetes, UV and ionizing radiation, corticosteroids and smoking. Age of onset is lower in countries with the highest prevalence of cataract, reflecting the interaction of special cataractogenic factors such as high UV exposure, poor diet and chronic disease. A smaller number of cataracts are associated with specific ocular or systemic diseases or defined physicochemical

mechanisms. Some congenital, infantile and even adult cataracts may be inherited.

Some ocular causes of cataract

- *Ocular trauma*: such as a penetrating injury, but also blunt trauma to the globe.
- *Uveitis*.
- High myopia.
- Topical medications (such as steroid eye drops).
- *Intraocular tumour*: ciliary body tumours may impinge physically on the lens.

Some systemic causes of cataract

- Diabetes.
- Other metabolic disorders (including galactosaemia and hypocalcaemia).
- Systemic drugs (particularly steroids, also chlorpromazine).
- X-radiation.
- Infection (congenital rubella).
- Atopy (accompanying atopic dermatitis).
- Inherited (congenital cataracts and some adult cataracts as in *myotonic dystrophy*).
- Syndromes (Down syndrome, Lowe syndrome).

Ophthalmology: Lecture Notes, Thirteenth Edition. Bruce James, Anthony Bron, and Manoj V. Parulekar.
© 2024 John Wiley & Sons Ltd. Published 2024 by John Wiley & Sons Ltd.
Companion website: www.wiley.com/go/ophthalmology13e

Symptoms

A cataract of sufficient degree causes:

- painless loss of vision;
- glare – due to light scattering;
- (Monocular diplopia or polyopia). The multiple images are due to the lens opacities bending the rays of light to differing degrees. The diplopia/polyopia persists on covering the fellow eye i.e. monocular in contrast to diplopia associated with a squint which is only present with both eyes open i.e. binocular.
- a change in refraction – for example, a myopic shift with nuclear cataract.

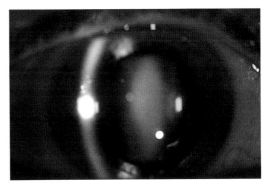

(a)

Cataracts occurring during critical stages of visual development i.e. early childhood, can deprive the retina of a formed image. This may result in amblyopia, a failure of visual maturation which may be profound and irreversible (see later).

Reduced visual acuity affects reading at all distances including reading a book, watching TV and the interpretation of road signs when driving. Driving at night may be a particular problem, because of the glare of oncoming headlights. In some patients the acuity, measured in a dark room, may seem satisfactory, but if the same test is carried out in bright light or sunlight, the acuity reduces as a result of glare and loss of contrast. Constriction of the pupils in bright light may also restrict light entry.

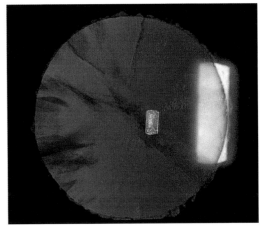

(b)

Signs

A cataract appears as a dark silhouette against the red reflex when the eye is examined with the direct ophthalmoscope (see Chapter 3). Slit-lamp examination allows the precise location, and morphology to be examined in detail. Age-related cataract may be *nuclear, cortical* or *subcapsular,* alone or in combination (Figures 9.1 and 9.2).

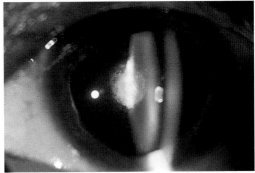

(c)

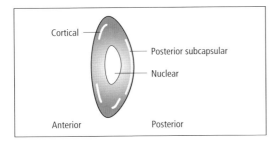

Figure 9.1 The location of different types of cataract.

Figure 9.2 The clinical appearance of cataract at the slit lamp. (a) A nuclear cataract (b) a cortical spoke cataract, silhouetted against the red reflex and (c) a posterior subcapsular cataract.

Nuclear cataract

The nucleus of the lens contains all those lens fibres that were laid down before birth. Like the deeper fibres of the lens cortex, they lack organelles and their proteins undergo little or no turnover with age. The proteins are therefore as old as the individual and with time, suffer progressive oxidative damage. A proportion of the crystallins, the major lens proteins, undergo cross-linking and the formation of molecular aggregates of sufficient size to scatter light. Furthermore, biochemical changes result in brown products, so, with ageing, the lens nucleus becomes cloudy, yellowish and then brown in colour. At some point, this may be of sufficient degree to be called *nuclear cataract*. Colour perception and contrast sensitivity may be altered but, initially, visual acuity may not be greatly affected. The hardness conferred to the lens nucleus by protein cross-linking may create problems when performing lens fragmentation during phacoemulsification surgery.

Cortical cataract

This form of cataract is due to a breakdown of groups of fibres in the lens cortex. Because these fibres are radially arranged in a pattern that relates to depth and clock position, the affected zones have a radial, spoke-like appearance and may be peripheral or extend more centrally. Peripheral spoke opacities have no effect on vision but those that encroach upon the visual axis will do so and may require action if symptomatic.

Posterior subcapsular cataract

This form of cataract lies immediately deep to the posterior lens capsule and therefore affects lens fibres that have been laid down most recently.

Posterior subcapsular cataract may arise acutely following blunt injury to the eye or after vitreous surgery (vitrectomy), or it may evolve slowly after X-radiation to the orbit and with steroid treatment.

Features suggesting an ocular cause of cataract include pigment deposition from previous inflammation, or damage to the iris, suggesting previous ocular trauma.

Investigation

A systemic cause for cataract should always be kept in mind, particularly in youth and in patients under the age of 60 years. A careful family history and a history of past diseases and medications can provide important clues. Unilateral cataract is likely to have a local cause. Congenital cataract can be detected by routine ocular screening at or near the time of birth.

Treatment

Although much effort has been directed towards slowing the progression of, or preventing cataract, management remains surgical. There is no need to wait for the cataract to 'ripen' and cause major visual loss. The test is whether or not the cataract produces sufficient visual symptoms to reduce the quality of life of an individual. Patients may have difficulty in recognizing faces, reading, carrying out their occupation or achieving the driving standard. Some patients may be greatly troubled by glare. Prior to surgery, patients must be informed of any coexisting eye disease which may influence the outcome of cataract surgery and the visual prognosis.

Cataract surgery

The operation (Figure 9.3) requires access to the lens across the anterior chamber via an opening in the anterior lens capsule, removal of most of the lens fibres and epithelial cells and insertion of a lens implant of appropriate optical power. The eye without a lens is termed *aphakic* and with a lens implant, *pseudophakic*. The implant is held in place within the 'capsular bag'. Surgery is usually performed under local rather than general anaesthesia. Local anaesthetic is infiltrated around the globe and lids or given topically. Usually the patient can attend as a day case, without admission to hospital, returning home shortly after surgery.

The following procedures are available:

- Emulsification of the lens, using an ultrasound probe introduced through a small incision at the limbus (*phacoemulsification* or '*phaco*') (Figure 9.3). Usually the wound does not require suturing. *This is now the preferred method in the developed world.* The use of the femtosecond laser to make incisions in the cornea and anterior capsule as well as to partially emulsify the lens is a developing field in cataract surgery.
- Alternatively, an extended incision at the limbus, or a smaller incision in the sclera, followed by *extracapsular cataract extraction* (ECCE) (see Chapter 18). Here, after opening the capsule, the bulk of the lens substance is expressed from the eye with gentle pressure and residual material is aspirated with a cannula. The incision must be sutured and the sutures removed postoperatively. In developing countries, a modification of this

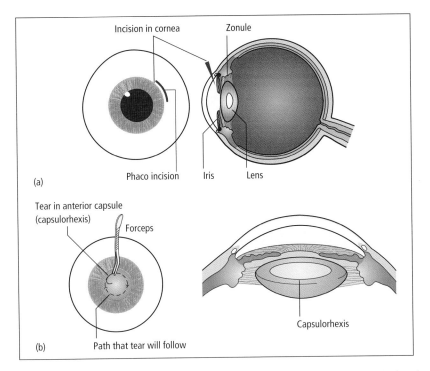

Figure 9.3 Stages in the removal of a cataract and the placement of an intraocular lens by phacoemulsification. (a) An incision is made in the cornea or anterior sclera, giving access to the anterior chamber. A small, stepped, self-sealing incision is made. (b) The capsule is pierced and torn in a circle leaving a strong smooth edge to the remaining anterior capsule. The circular disc of the anterior capsule so created is removed from the anterior chamber. A cannula is then placed under the anterior capsule and fluid injected to separate the lens nucleus from the cortex, allowing the nucleus to be rotated within the capsular bag. (c) The nucleus can be emulsified in situ. The phacoemulsification probe, introduced through the small corneal or scleral incision, shaves away the nucleus. (d) The remaining soft lens matter is aspirated, leaving only the posterior capsule and the peripheral part of the anterior capsule. (e) An intraocular lens is implanted into the capsular bag. To introduce the lens implant through the small phacoemulsification wound, the lens must be folded in half or injected through a special introducer into the eye. Once in the capsular bag, the lens unfolds like a butterfly opening its wings and settles into position, held in place by supporting loops. The incision usually does not require suturing.

technique requiring no sutures, is called small incision cataract surgery (SICS).

The optical power of the *lens implant* is calculated (*biometry*) prior to surgery by measuring the length of the eye *ultrasonically* and the curvature of the cornea (and thus its optical power) optically (*keratometry*). The power of the lens is generally calculated to provide good distance acuity without glasses (i.e. emmetropia). The choice of implant power is influenced by the refraction of the fellow eye and whether it too has a cataract that will require surgery. Where surgery on the fellow eye is likely to be delayed, it is important that the patient is not left with a major difference in the refractive state of the two eyes (*anisometropia*), since the difference in retinal image size (*aniseikonia*) may not be tolerated visually.

Postoperatively, the patient is given a short course of steroid and antibiotic drops. New glasses, if required, can be prescribed after a few weeks, once the incision has healed. Visual rehabilitation and the prescription of new glasses are much quicker after phacoemulsification. Since the patient cannot accommodate, a spectacle correction is usually required postoperatively for close work even if it is not needed for distance. Multifocal intraocular lenses, which provide good distance, intermediate and near vision without glasses, are now in use. There may be a reduction in contrast sensitivity with such lenses and some patients may

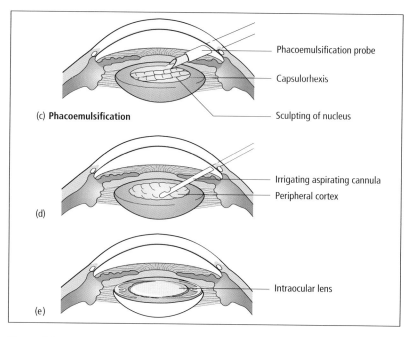

(c) **Phacoemulsification**

— Phacoemulsification probe

— Capsulorhexis

— Sculpting of nucleus

(d)

— Irrigating aspirating cannula
— Peripheral cortex

(e)

— Intraocular lens

Figure 9.3 (*Continued*)

experience glare. Astigmatism can be corrected with a toric intraocular lens. See Chapter 4 for more details on correcting refraction after cataract surgery.

Surgery may sometimes induce a degree of corneal astigmatism. Where sutures were used, their postoperative removal may reduce this. This is done prior to measuring the patient for new glasses but after the wound has healed and steroid drops have been stopped. Excessive corneal curvature can be induced in the line of a tight suture. Removal usually solves this problem and is easily accomplished in the clinic under local anaesthetic with the patient sitting at the slit lamp. Loose sutures must be removed to prevent infection but it may be necessary to re-suture the incision if healing is imperfect. Sutureless phacoemulsification through a smaller incision avoids these complications. Pre-existing astigmatism can be corrected with a modified entry site or relaxing incisions at the periphery of the cornea or a toric intraocular lens.

Complications of cataract surgery

1 *Vitreous loss:* If the posterior capsule is accidentally torn during the operation, the vitreous gel may prolapse forward into the anterior chamber, where it represents a risk for glaucoma by obstructing aqueous outflow via the trabecular meshwork. Prolapsed gel may also cause retinal traction and increase the risk of retinal detachment, and may interfere with placement of the lens implant. The gel requires careful aspiration and excision (*vitrectomy*) at the time of surgery. Placement of the intraocular lens usually follows during the same procedure, but may need to be deferred to a secondary procedure.

2 *Iris prolapse:* The iris may protrude through the surgical incision in the immediate postoperative period, appearing as a dark elevation at the incision site accompanied by pupil distortion. This requires prompt surgical repair.

3 *Endophthalmitis:* A serious but rare infective complication of cataract extraction (less than 0.1%). Patients usually present within a few days of surgery with:
   a   a painful red eye;
   b   reduced visual acuity;
   c   a collection of white cells in the anterior chamber (hypopyon).
   This is an extreme ophthalmic emergency. The patient requires urgent sampling of the aqueous and vitreous for microbiological analysis and intravitreal injection of a broad-spectrum antibiotic

at the time of sampling (e.g. vancomycin and ceftazidime) to provide immediate cover. Further management is dependent on the microbiological report and clinical response. The use of intravitreal corticosteroids in conjunction with the antimicrobials is debated.

4 *Cystoid macular oedema:* The macula may become oedematous following routine uncomplicated surgery. The risk is greater if surgery was accompanied by vitreous loss or inflammation. It may settle with time but can produce a severe and permanent reduction in acuity. The release of *prostaglandin* from inflamed intraocular tissues plays an important role and prompt treatment with topical NSAIDs and steroid can alleviate the oedema in a proportion of patients. It may be necessary to inject steroids into or around the eye in resistant cases.

5 *Retinal detachment:* Modern techniques of cataract extraction are associated with a low rate of detachment, but the risk is increased if there has been vitreous loss. The symptoms, signs and management are described in Chapter 12.

6 *Opacification of the posterior capsule* (Figure 9.4): Normally, the thin capsular layer that lies behind the implant is crystal clear. However, in approximately 20% of patients, clarity of the posterior capsule decreases in the months following surgery, when residual epithelial cells migrate across its surface to form an opaque scar. Vision then becomes blurred and there may be problems with glare. This is often referred to as an 'aftercataract'. The treatment is *YAG laser capsulotomy,* using a neodymium yttrium garnet (Nd-YAG) laser to create a small central opening in the capsule as an outpatient procedure. There is a small risk of cystoid macular oedema or retinal detachment following *YAG capsulotomy.* Research aimed at reducing capsule opacification has shown that the lens implant material, the shape of the lens edge and overlap of the intraocular lens by a small rim of anterior capsule are important factors in preventing this complication.

Congenital cataract

Infants with a family history of congenital cataract should be assessed by an ophthalmologist shortly after birth as a matter of urgency. The presence of congenital or infantile cataract is a threat to sight, not only because of the immediate obstruction to vision but also because of the disturbance to retinal image formation during the sensitive period of visual development (the first 5 years) that impairs visual maturation and leads to amblyopia (see Chapter 19). This in turn may trigger the onset of a squint (see Chapter 16). If bilateral cataract is present in early infancy and has a significant effect on retinal image formation in both eyes, this will cause bilateral amblyopia, squint and *nystagmus,* a horizontal oscillation of the eyes. In this case, both cataractous lenses require urgent surgery and the fitting of contact lenses to correct the aphakia. The management of contact lenses requires considerable input and motivation from the parents of the child.

The treatment of unilateral congenital cataract remains controversial. The results of surgery vary widely and visual improvement may be limited in many cases because amblyopia develops despite adequate optical correction with a contact lens. To maximize the chances of success, treatment must be performed within the first few weeks of life and be accompanied by a coordinated patching routine to

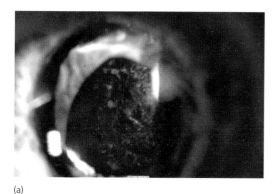
(a)

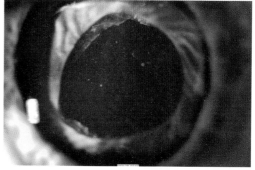
(b)

Figure 9.4 (a) An opacified posterior capsule. (b) The opacity is cleared by laser capsulotomy.

the fellow eye to stimulate visual maturation in the amblyopic eye and minimize the risk of squint. Intraocular lenses are routinely implanted in children over 2 years old. This age limit has lowered in recent years, and many surgeons routinely implant children over 6 months to 1 year. There is an inevitable myopic shift as the eye grows, making the choice of lens implant power difficult. There is also a significant risk of subsequent glaucoma in infants undergoing surgery for congenital cataract, particularly when this is performed prior to 6 months of age.

Disorders of lens shape

Abnormal lens shape is very unusual. In Alport syndrome, a recessively inherited condition accompanied by deafness and nephropathy, there may be a bilateral, conical anterior protrusion of the anterior lens surface (*anterior lenticonus*). It is caused by mutations influencing the structure of type IV collagen, a key component of basal laminae within the glomerulus, the Organ of Corti and the lens capsule. *Posterior lenticonus* may also occur, but is usually a non-syndromic, unilateral condition, which is rarely inherited.

An abnormally small lens may be associated with short stature and other skeletal abnormalities.

Disorders of lens position (ectopia lentis)

Weakness of the zonule causes lens displacement, which is termed *subluxation* if minor, or *dislocation* when more advanced. The lens takes up a more rounded form and the eye becomes more myopic, with considerable astigmatism. This may be seen:

- following ocular trauma;
- in inherited disorders:
  - *Homocystinuria* is a recessive disorder with ectopia lentis, learning disability, skeletal abnormalities and a risk of thrombotic complications. The lens is usually displaced downwards.
  - *Marfan syndrome is* a dominant disorder with skeletal and cardiac abnormalities and a risk of dissecting aortic aneurysm. The lens is usually displaced upwards. Here, there is a defect in the zonular protein due to a mutation in the *fibrillin* gene.

The irregular myopia and astigmatism of subluxation can be corrected optically, but if the lens is substantially displaced from the visual axis, an aphakic

correction may be required. Surgical removal may be indicated, particularly if the displaced lens has caused a secondary glaucoma or vision cannot be corrected optically. Surgery can be challenging in some cases, and involves removal of the entire lens in its capsular bag. Lens implantation may be possible using special techniques.

 KEY POINTS

- In adult cataract, extraction is indicated if the reduction in vision is interfering with the patient's quality of life.
- Pain, redness and reduced vision soon after intraocular surgery may indicate an intraocular infection (endophthalmitis) requiring urgent treatment.
- Gradual reduction in vision following cataract surgery may indicate that the remaining posterior lens capsule has become opacified (aftercataract); this can be easily treated with laser surgery.
- A dislocated lens may indicate that the patient has Homocystinuria or Marfan Syndrome.
- Timely treatment of childhood cataract is important to prevent irreversible amblyopia.

Assessment questions True or False

1. **Cataract causes:**
   a   A sudden loss of vision.
   b   A gradual loss of vision.
   c   Glare.
   d   Ocular pain
   e   A change in refractive error.

2. **Cataract may be caused by or associated with:**
   a   Trauma.
   b   Steroids.
   c   Diabetes.
   d   Myotonic dystrophy.
   e   Hypocalcaemia.

3. **Complications of cataract surgery include:**
   a   Recurrence of the cataract.
   b   Endophthalmitis.
   c   Astigmatism.

d   Glaucoma.

e   Cystoid macular oedema.

4.   A 60-year-old lady has just had a cataract operation. Three days later she presents to her general practitioner with a painful red eye. The vision, which was initially much improved, has become blurred and she is seeing lots of floaters.

a   The GP should reassure her that the eye is settling down.

b   The patient has endophthalmitis and needs to be referred to an eye unit immediately.

c   Treatment of the condition requires steroid drops only.

d   Treatment of the condition requires intravitreal antibiotics.

e   This is a rare complication of cataract surgery.

Answers

1.   Cataract causes:

a   False. The change in vision is gradual.

b   True. The patient may not be aware that a change in vision is occurring until they notice that particular visual tasks are becoming difficult.

c   True. This can be a particularly troubling symptom even in patients with good visual acuity.

d   False. Cataract is painless.

e   True. For example, in nuclear cataract an increase in the density of lens proteins at the centre of the lens causes a myopic shift.

2.   Cataract may be caused by or associated with:

a   True.

b   True.

c   True.

d   True.

e   True.

3.   Complications of cataract surgery include:

a   False. Most lens material is removed by surgery, the cataract does not recur but the posterior capsule may opacify later (aftercataract). Laser capsulotomy can restore vision by creating a hole in the capsule, on the visual axis.

b   True. This is the most feared complication. Patients with pain, redness of the eye and reducing vision following cataract surgery must be seen immediately.

c   True. The incision at the periphery of the cornea can change the shape of the cornea inducing astigmatism. This can sometimes be used to advantage, however, to reduce pre-existing astigmatism.

d   True. Modern phacoemulsification surgery may, however, actually reduce the pressure in the eye in the long term.

e   True. This accumulation of fluid at the macula may reduce visual acuity, usually temporarily, following cataract surgery.

4.   A 60-year-old lady just had a cataract operation.

a   False. The patient has endophthalmitis, a serious eye emergency, and must be referred immediately.

b   True. Immediate and urgent referral is essential to maximize the chance of successful treatment.

c   False. But these may form part of the treatment of endophthalmitis in conjunction with antibiotics.

d   True. This is the mainstay of treatment.

e   True. Fortunately, this is a rare complication but vigilance is nonetheless necessary both in its prevention and for early diagnosis.

10

Uveitis

Learning objectives

To understand:

✔ The definition of uveitis and the ocular structures involved.
✔ The symptoms, signs, causes and treatment of uveitis.

Introduction

Inflammation of the uveal tract (the iris, ciliary body and choroid) is termed *uveitis* (Figure 10.1). It is usual for structures adjacent to the inflamed uveal tissue to become involved in the inflammatory process. It may be classified anatomically:

- *Iritis* or *anterior uveitis* refers to inflammation of the iris.
- Inflammation of the ciliary body is termed *cyclitis,* of the pars plana is *pars planitis* and of the vitreous is *vitritis.* As a group, these are termed *intermediate uveitis.*
- Inflammation of the posterior uvea is termed *posterior uveitis* and may involve the choroid (*choroiditis*), the retina (*retinitis*) or both (*chorioretinitis*).
- *Panuveitis* refers to more extensive involvement of the uveal tract, with inflammatory changes affecting the anterior chamber, vitreous and retina and/or the choroid.
- Any form of uveitis is accompanied by increased vascular permeability (Figure 10.2). In anterior uveitis, white cells can be seen circulating in the aqueous humour of the anterior chamber with a slit lamp. Protein, which also leaks into the anterior chamber from the blood vessels, is picked out by its light-scattering properties in the beam of the slit lamp as *'flare'*. Similarly, cells and protein are seen in the vitreous in intermediate and posterior uveitis and termed vitritis and vitreous haze, respectively.

Epidemiology

The incidence of uveitis is about 37,714 per 100,000 people. About 75% of these are anterior uveitis.

About 50% of patients with uveitis have an associated systemic disease.

History

The patient may complain of:

- ocular pain;
- photophobia;
- blurring of vision;
- redness of the eye.

Isolated intermediate and posterior uveitis however are not painful. Although a significant number of cases of uveitis are isolated (without systemic involvement), the patient must be questioned about other relevant symptoms that may help determine the presence of associated systemic disease, these include:

- Respiratory symptoms such as shortness of breath, cough and the nature of any sputum produced (associated sarcoidosis or tuberculosis).
- Skin problems. Erythema nodosum (painful raised red lesions on the arms and shins) may be present in granulomatous diseases such as sarcoidosis and Behçet disease. Patients with Behçet may also have

Ophthalmology: Lecture Notes, Thirteenth Edition. Bruce James, Anthony Bron, and Manoj V. Parulekar.
© 2024 John Wiley & Sons Ltd. Published 2024 by John Wiley & Sons Ltd.
Companion website: www.wiley.com/go/ophthalmology13e

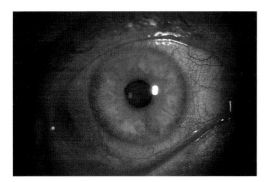

Figure 10.1 External ocular appearance in a patient with anterior uveitis. Note the inflammatory response at the limbus.

thrombophlebitis, dermatographia and oral and genital ulceration. Psoriasis (in association with arthritis) may be accompanied by uveitis.

- Joint disease. Back pain, due to ankylosing spondylitis, is associated with acute anterior uveitis. In children, juvenile chronic arthritis may be associated with uveitis. Reiter disease (classically urethritis, conjunctivitis and a seronegative arthritis) may also be associated with anterior uveitis.
- Bowel disease. Occasionally, uveitis may be associated with inflammatory bowel diseases such as ulcerative colitis, Crohn disease and Whipple disease.
- Infectious disease. Syphilis with its protean manifestations can cause uveitis (particularly posterior choroiditis). Herpetic disease (herpes simplex and zoster) may also cause uveitis. Cytomegalovirus (CMV) may cause uveitis, particularly in patients with AIDS. Fungal infections and metastatic infections may also cause uveitis, usually in immunocompromised patients.

Signs

On examination:

- The visual acuity may be reduced.
- The eye will be inflamed, mostly around the limbus (*ciliary injection* or *ciliary flush* Figure 10.1).

Anterior uveitis (Figure 10.2)

- Inflammatory cells may be visible clumped, together on the endothelium of the cornea, particularly inferiorly (*keratic precipitates* or *KPs*).
- Slit-lamp examination will reveal aqueous cells, and a flare due to exuded protein. If the inflammation is

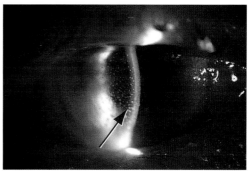

(a)

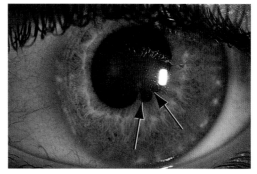

(b)

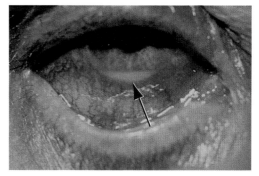

(c)

Figure 10.2 Signs of anterior uveitis: (a) keratic precipitates on the corneal endothelium; (b) posterior synechiae (adhesions between the lens and the iris) give the pupil an irregular appearance; (c) a hypopyon – white cells gravitated to form a fluid level in the inferior anterior chamber.

severe, there may be sufficient white cells to collect as a fluid level inferiorly (*hypopyon*).
- The vessels on the iris may be dilated.
- The iris may adhere to the lens and bind down the pupil (*posterior synechiae or PS*). *Peripheral anterior synechiae (PAS)* between the iris and the trabecular meshwork or cornea may occlude the drainage angle.

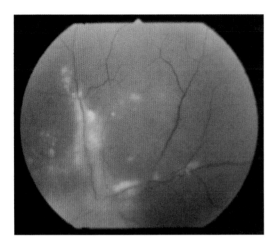

Figure 10.3 Retinitis in a patient with sarcoidosis.

- The intraocular pressure may be elevated by PAS or increased aqueous protein blocking the trabecular meshwork (drainage channels for aqueous).

Intermediate and posterior uveitis

- There may be cells in the vitreous.
- There may be retinal or choroidal foci of inflammation (Figure 10.3), which may be distributed along blood vessels (*perivascular sheathing*).
- Macular oedema may be present (see Chapter 12).

Investigations

These are aimed at determining a systemic association and are directed in part by the type of uveitis present. An anterior uveitis is more likely to be associated with ankylosing spondylitis, and these patients are usually human leucocyte antigen (HLA B27) positive. The presence of large KPs and inflammatory nodules on the iris may suggest sarcoidosis: a chest radiograph, serum calcium and 24 hour urinary calcium, and serum angiotensin-converting enzyme levels would be appropriate. In toxoplasma retinochoroiditis, the focus of inflammation often occurs at the margin of an old inflammatory choroidal scar. Posterior uveitis may have an infectious or systemic inflammatory cause. Some diseases such as CMV infections in HIV-positive patients have a characteristic appearance (Figure 10.7), and with an appropriate history may require no further diagnostic tests. Associated symptoms may also point towards a systemic disease (e.g. fever, diarrhoea, weight loss). Not all cases of anterior uveitis require investigation at first presentation unless associated systemic symptoms are present.

Treatment

This is aimed at:

- suppressing inflammation in the eye, and relieving symptoms in anterior uveitis;
- preventing damage to ocular structures, particularly to the macula and the optic nerve, which may lead to permanent visual loss.

Steroid therapy is the mainstay of treatment. In anterior uveitis, this is delivered by eye drops. However, topical steroids do not effectively penetrate to the posterior segment. Posterior uveitis is therefore treated with systemic steroids, or with steroids injected onto the orbital floor or into the sub-Tenon space (Figure 10.4), from whence they can diffuse into the eye across the ocular coat.

In anterior uveitis, dilating the pupil relieves the pain from ciliary spasm and prevents the formation of posterior synechiae by separating the iris from the anterior lens capsule. Synechiae, once established can interfere with normal dilation of the pupil, result in pupil-block glaucoma due to interruption of aqueous flow through the pupil, and may result in cataract formation. Dilation is achieved with mydriatics, for example cyclopentolate or atropine drops. Atropine has a prolonged action lasting several days to 1 week. An attempt to break any synechiae that have formed should be made with initial intensive treatment with short-acting cyclopentolate and phenylephrine drops. A subconjunctival injection of mydriatics may help to break resistant synechiae.

In posterior uveitis/retinitis, visual loss may occur either from direct destruction to the retina and choroid (e.g. in toxoplasmosis or CMV infection) or from fluid accumulation in the layers of the macula (macular oedema). Apart from systemic or injected steroids, specific antiviral or antibiotic medication may also be required. Some rare but severe forms of non-infectious uveitis, e.g. that associated with Behçet disease, may require treatment with other systemic immunosuppressant drugs. Antimetabolites (e.g. azathioprine, methotrexate and mycophenolate), calcineurin inhibitors (e.g. cyclosporine) and alkylating agents (e.g. cyclophosphamide) may be effective but require appropriate specialist supervision. Monoclonal

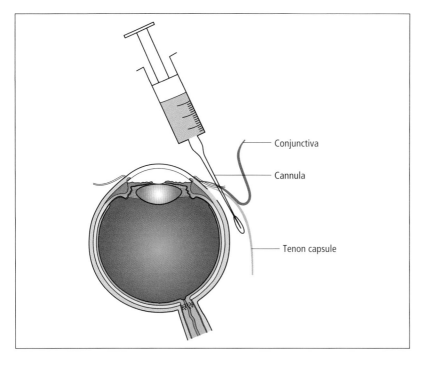

Conjunctiva

Cannula

Tenon capsule

Figure 10.4 The principle of a sub-Tenon injection. A cannula is placed in the potential space between the sclera and Tenon capsule. Injection of steroid separates the two layers and the steroid spreads to surround the eye.

antibodies may also have a role in refractory cases. Long-term treatment may be necessary.

Specific conditions associated with uveitis

There is a large number of systemic diseases associated with uveitis. A few of the more common ones are outlined in Table 10.1.

Ankylosing spondylitis

This is a seronegative (rheumatoid factor negative) spondyloarthropathy causing inflammation of the tendons, ligaments and joints of the spine. Untreated, the condition leads to a disabling, gross rigidity and flexion deformity of the spine with the head directed downwards. Genetic factors are involved in the disease. Ninety percent of patients with acute anterior uveitis have the tissue-type HLA B27, although the prevalence of uveitis in people with HLA B27 is only 1%. Approximately 20% of

Table 10.1 Some causes of uveitis (not an exhaustive list).

Infectious	Non-infectious ocular disease	Systemic disease-associated
Toxoplasmosis	Sympathetic ophthalmitis	Juvenile chronic arthritis
Herpes simplex Herpes zoster	Fuchs heterochromic cyclitis	Ankylosing spondylosis
CMV (AIDS)	Angle-closure glaucoma	Psoriatic arthritis
Tuberculosis	Retinal detachment	Sarcoidosis
Fungal	Intraocular tumours	Behçet disease
	Autoimmune reaction to advanced cataract. Phacogenic uveitis	Vogt–Koyanagi–Harada disease (VKH)
	Following ocular injury or surgery	Reiter disease Inflammatory bowel disease

patients with ankylosing spondylitis will develop acute anterior uveitis. Males are affected more frequently than females (3 : 1).

History

Recurrent anterior uveitis may be the presenting feature of this condition. Close enquiry will usually reveal an insidious history of low backache, typically worse on waking and relieved by exercise. Stiffness at rest is a useful symptom which helps differentiate the condition from disease of the intervertebral discs. The peripheral joints may be affected in a minority of patients.

Signs

These are typical of an anterior uveitis.

Investigation

The presence of symptoms and signs in an HLA B27-positive individual is indicative. Sacroiliac spinal MRI may detect early changes in the sacroiliac joints and radiographs or MRI scans may reveal the classical features of the disease (Figure 10.5).

Treatment

Treatment of the arthropathy is with painkillers, disease-modifying drugs, NSAIDs, physiotherapy and biologics such as etanercept and adalimumab which are directed against the action of tumour necrosis factor-α (TNF-α). Ocular treatment is as previously outlined. The patient will benefit from a rheumatological opinion and may require intermittent anti-inflammatory treatment and physiotherapy.

Prognosis

Patients may experience recurrent attacks. The outlook for vision is good if the acute attacks are treated early and vigorously.

Reiter disease

This condition predominantly affects males, nearly all of whom are HLA B27-positive. It comprises:

- urethritis;
- arthritis (typically of the large joints);
- conjunctivitis.

Some 40% of patients develop acute anterior uveitis.

Juvenile idiopathic arthritis-related uveitis

A seronegative arthritis (negative for rheumatoid factor) which presents in children, either as a systemic disease with fevers and lymphadenopathy, or as an oligoarticular (formerly pauciarticular) or polyarticular arthritis. The oligoarticular form has the higher risk of chronic anterior uveitis, particularly if the patient is positive for antinuclear antibodies.

Facet fusion

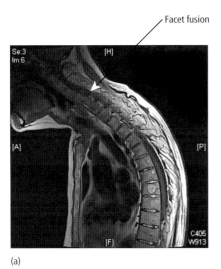

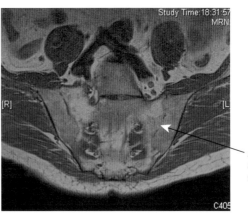

Ankylosis across the sacroiliac joint

(a) (b)

Figure 10.5 MRI appearance of (a) the spine and (b) the fused sacroiliac joints of a patient with ankylosing spondylitis. (*Source:* Courtesy of Tom Meagher.)

History

The anterior uveitis is chronic and usually asymptomatic. A profound visual defect may be discovered by chance if lens, glaucoma or retinal damage caused by chronic uveitis has developed slowly.

Signs

The eye is white (unusual for iritis), but other signs of an anterior uveitis are present. Because the uveitis is chronic, cataract may occur and patients may develop glaucoma, either as a result of the uveitis or as a result of the steroid drops used to treat the condition. Macular oedema may also occur. Approximately 70% of cases show bilateral involvement.

Investigation

Rheumatoid factor is negative but patients frequently have a positive antinuclear antibody.

Treatment

It is important to screen children with juvenile arthritis regularly for uveitis, since they may be asymptomatic at its earliest stages and only present when potentially blinding complications occur.

Ocular treatment is as previously outlined. Patients may be put on systemic treatment such as Methotrexate or an anti-TNF-α monoclonal antibody drug for the joint disease, or for the uveitis in resistant cases. Early control of the uveitis is the best way to prevent the ocular complications. Glaucoma can be very difficult to treat, and, if medical treatment fails to control pressure, it may require surgery.

Fuchs heterochromic uveitis

This is a rare, unilateral, chronic uveitis usually presenting in young adults. The cause is uncertain, it may be immune-mediated and there are no systemic associations.

History

The patient does not usually present with a typical history of iritis. Blurred vision and floaters may be the initial complaint.

Signs

A mild anterior uveitis is present, but without signs of conjunctival or ciliary injection, and there are no posterior synechiae. There are KPs distributed diffusely over the cornea and there is iris heterochromia, the iris colour of the affected eye being different from that of the fellow eye, due to a loss of epithelial pigment cells. The vitreous may be inflamed and condensations (the cause of the floaters) may be present. About 70% of patients develop cataract. Glaucoma occurs to a lesser extent.

Treatment

Steroids are not effective in controlling the inflammation and are thus not prescribed. Patients usually respond well to cataract surgery when it is required. The glaucoma is treated conventionally.

Toxoplasmosis

History

The infection may be congenital or acquired. Most ocular toxoplasmosis was thought to be congenital, with the resulting retinochoroiditis being reactivated in adult life. However, there is now evidence that it is often acquired during a glandular fever-like illness, caused by toxoplasmosis. The patient may complain of hazy vision and floaters, and the eye may be red and painful.

Signs

The retina is the principal structure involved, with secondary inflammation occurring in the choroid (*retinochoroiditis*). An active lesion is often located at the posterior pole, appearing as a creamy focus of inflammatory cells at the margin of an old chorioretinal scar (such scars are usually atrophic, with a pigmented edge) (Figure 10.6). Inflammatory cells cause a vitreous haze, and the anterior chamber may also show evidence of inflammation.

Investigation

The clinical appearance is usually diagnostic, but a positive anti-toxoplasma antibody test is suggestive. However, a high percentage of the population have positive IgG titres due to prior infection.

Treatment

Reactivated lesions will subside, but treatment is required if the macula or optic nerve is threatened or if the inflammatory response is very severe. Systemic steroids are administered with antiprotozoal drugs such as pyrimethamine (with folinic acid) and sulphadiazine, used in combination. A trimethoprim–sulfamethoxazole combination is also effective and may be better tolerated and more available.

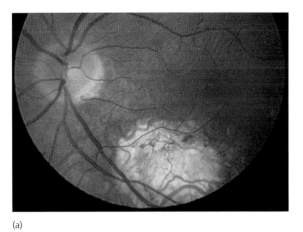
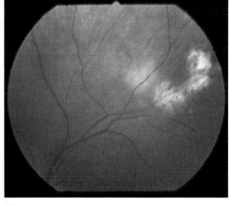

(a)   (b)

Figure 10.6 The appearance of (a) an inactive toxoplasma retinitis and (b) a reactivated lesion. The active lesion appears pale with indistinct edges; it lies adjacent to the inactive one.

Behçet and Vogt–Koyanagi–Harada diseases

There are two form of uveitis which are seen infrequently in western countries but make an important contribution to the prevalence of uveitis in the Middle East, Asia and also in Japan. The prevalence of the disease is these countries is in the order of 8 per 10,000 (42 per 10,000 in Turkey).

Behçet disease

Behçet disease is a condition that causes wide-ranging symptoms and signs including mouth ulcers, genital ulcers and an anterior uveitis with hypopyon. Additional central nervous system (CNS), genitourinary, gastrointestinal (GI) and skin problems and thrombosis also occur. The disease is due to a chronic vasculitis affecting small blood vessels. The protean nature of the disease may require the support of several different specialists. As it is most common in Mediterranean countries, Turkey, the Middle East, Japan and southeast Asia, it has sometimes been called the Silk Route disease, after the ancient trade routes that ran through these areas. The diagnosis is a clinical one. There is a strong association with HLA B51.

Treatment

Colchicine tablets are often prescribed for mouth or genital ulcers, and dapsone may also be effective. There are also treatments that can be applied locally to the ulcers.

Immunosuppressives are the usual treatment for moderate to severe Behçet syndrome, for example azathioprine, and also ciclosporin (cyclosporine/cyclosporin), tacrolimus and mycophenolate. These agents act as steroid-sparing drugs. Anti-TNF drugs and interferon alpha may be effective.

Vogt–Koyanagi–Harada disease

Vogt–Koyanagi–Harada disease (VKH) is a multisystem disorder presenting with a bilateral panuveitis with exudative retinal detachments and followed by neurological and cutaneous manifestations such as alopecia (focal baldness) and loss of lash and skin pigments (poliosis and vitiligo). It is a cell-mediated autoimmune disease probably directed against tyrosinase-related proteins, TRP1 and TRP2 contained in melanocytes. VKH is more common in females than males (2 : 1) and affects individuals aged 20–50 years, although it has been reported in children as young as 4 years. VKH disease occurs most commonly in patients with a genetic predisposition to the disease, including Asian, Middle Eastern, Hispanic, and Native American populations. Several HLA associations have been found in patients with VKH disease, including HLA-DR4, HLA-DR53 and HLA-DQ4.

A prodromal stage, with fever, headache, tinnitus and cerebrospinal fluid (CSF) pleocytosis, is followed after several days by a posterior uveitis leading to bilateral serous retinal detachments. There is also a vigorous granulomatous, anterior uveitis with mutton-fat (large, greasy-looking) KPs. After several weeks, the detachments subside and there is both depigmentation of the choroid and hyperpigmentation of the retina. Skin changes include vitiligo and poliosis of the lashes, eyebrows and hair, with the vitiligo distributed symmetrically over the head, eyelids and trunk. Treatment requires systemic steroids and immunosuppressive therapy.

AIDS and CMV retinitis

Ocular disease is a common manifestation of AIDS. Patients develop a variety of ocular conditions:

- microvascular occlusion causing retinal haemorrhages and cotton-wool spots (axonal swelling proximal to infarcted areas of the retinal nerve fibre layer);
- corneal endothelial deposits possibly associated with concurrent rifabutin treatment;
- neoplasms of the eye and orbit;
- neuro-ophthalmic disorders;
- opportunistic infections, of which the most common is CMV retinitis. This was previously seen in more than one-third of AIDS patients, but the population at risk has decreased significantly since the advent of *highly active antiretroviral therapy* (HAART) in the treatment of AIDS. It typically occurs in patients with a blood CD^{4+} cell count of less than 50/ml. Toxoplasmosis, herpes simplex and herpes zoster are among other infections that may be seen.

History

The patient may complain of blurred vision or floaters. A diagnosis of HIV disease has usually already been made and other AIDS-defining features may have presented.

Signs

CMV retinopathy comprises a whitish area of retina, associated with haemorrhage, which has been likened in appearance to 'cottage cheese and ketchup' or 'pizza pie' (Figure 10.7). The lesions may threaten the macula or the optic disc. There is usually an associated sparse inflammation of the vitreous.

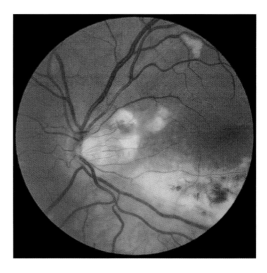

Figure 10.7 The retinal appearance in a patient with AIDS and CMV retinitis. Note the cotton-wool spot at the 1 o'clock position.

Treatment

Chronic antiviral therapy with ganciclovir and/or foscarnet given parenterally is the current mainstay of therapy; these drugs may also be given into the vitreous cavity. Cidofovir is available for intravenous administration. Ganciclovir and its prodrug valganciclovir are available orally which makes it easier to administer. Intraocular depot systems for the long-term delivery of anti-CMV agents into the vitreous are under active development, and an intraocular ganciclovir implant is available. Oral therapy is the preferred first-line treatment.

Prognosis

Prolonged treatment is required to prevent recurrence.

Sympathetic ophthalmitis

This is a devastating complication of ocular injury. A penetrating or surgical injury to one eye involving the retina may rarely excite a peculiar form of uveitis which involves not only the injured eye but also the fellow eye. This is termed sympathetic ophthalmitis. The uveitis may be so severe that in the worst cases sight may be lost from both eyes. This was a major problem in war injuries, with limited initial surgical repair. Fortunately, systemic steroids, initially given intravenously, and new immunosuppressive agents like ciclosporin, have greatly improved the chances of conserving vision. Sympathetic ophthalmitis usually develops within 3 months of the injury or last ocular operation but may occur at any time. The cause appears to be an immune response to retinal antigens, initiated at the time of injury. Enucleation (removal) of the traumatized eye shortly after the injury (within a week or so) and prior to the onset of signs in the fellow eye can reduce the risk to the fellow eye, and can be considered if the visual potential of the injured eye is very poor and there is major disorganization. The advent of newer immunosuppressive drugs has improved outcomes, and the role of surgical removal of the traumatized eye is less important in current management.

Symptoms

The patient may complain of pain and decreased vision in the uninjured fellow eye, but loss of accommodation can be the first sign.

Signs

The iris appears swollen, and yellow–white spots may be seen on the retina. There is a panuveitis.

Treatment

High-dose systemic and topical steroids, and also oral ciclosporin, are required to reduce the inflammation and prevent long-term visual loss. It is vital to warn patients with ocular trauma or multiple eye operations to attend an eye casualty department if they experience any problems with their normal eye.

Uveitis associated with other ocular disease

Uveitis may be associated with the following ocular diseases:

- Posterior scleritis
- Retinal detachment
- Angle closure glaucoma

 KEY POINTS

- Active treatment of uveitis is required to prevent long-term complications.
- Angle-closure glaucoma may cause an anterior uveitis and may present with similar symptoms. Look for a dilated pupil and check the intraocular pressure.
- Patients with a retinal detachment may occasionally present with an anterior uveitis. The retina should always be examined in patients with uveitis.
- Patients with uniocular injury should be warned of the symptoms of sympathetic ophthalmitis and the need for urgent rapid treatment.

Assessment questions
True or False

1. **Uveitis can be an inflammation of**
   a   The lens.
   b   The iris.
   c   The ciliary body.
   d   The choroid.
   e   The optic nerve.

2. **Uveitis**
   a   Is always associated with a red eye.
   b   May be complicated by macular oedema.
   c   Posterior synechiae may form between the iris and the lens.
   d   May cause oculomotor palsies.
   e   May be associated with retinitis.

3. **A 33-year-old West Indian patient presents with a red eye, without discharge, photophobia and blurred vision. The eye is uncomfortable. He has recently become short of breath and developed painful, raised, tender red lesions on his shins.**
   a   The patient has uveitis.
   b   The patient has ankylosing spondylitis.
   c   The patient probably has sarcoidosis.
   d   Treatment is with steroid eye drops and cycloplegics.
   e   Glaucoma and cataract are possible ocular complications of the condition or its treatment.

4. In acquired immunodeficiency syndrome

a   Haemorrhages and cotton-wool spots may be seen on the retina.

b   Opportunistic infection has increased since the development of highly active antiretroviral therapy (HAART).

c   CMV retinopathy causes focal white spots on the retina associated with haemorrhage.

d   Ganciclovir and foscarnet are used to treat CMV retinitis.

e   Oculomotor palsies may be seen in AIDS.

Answers

1. Uveitis can be an inflammation of

a   False. The lens is not inflamed in uveitis.

b   True. Inflammation of the iris results in the presence of anterior chamber cells.

c   True. Inflammation of the ciliary body results in cyclitis.

d   True. Inflammation of the choroid is termed choroiditis.

e   False. The optic nerve is not inflamed in uveitis.

2. Uveitis

a   False. The eye is usually white in choroiditis, heterochromic cyclitis and in children with uveitis associated with juvenile arthritis.

b   True. Posterior uveitis may be associated with the accumulation of fluid in the macula region of the retina.

c   True. Areas of adhesion between the iris and the lens are a complication of anterior uveitis.

d   False. The condition affects the eye alone. Associated systemic diseases may however cause neurological problems (e.g. sarcoidosis).

e   True. Retinitis refers to inflammation of the retina and will accompany a choroiditis.

3. A 33-year-old West Indian patient presents with a red eye, without discharge, and with photophobia and blurred vision.

a   True. The symptoms are classical.

b   False. Although kyphosis in ankylosing spondylitis may cause shortness of breath, this condition is not associated with erythema nodosum.

c   True. The uveitis, shortness of breath and erythema nodosum are suggestive.

d   True. His systemic disease also requires investigation and treatment.

e   True. Both anterior uveitis and prolonged treatment with topical steroids may cause cataract or open-angle glaucoma. Anterior uveitis may also cause closed-angle glaucoma.

4. In acquired immunodeficiency syndrome

a   True. Haemorrhages and cotton-wool spots may be a sign of AIDS.

b   False. There has been a reduction in opportunistic infections.

c   True. CMV retinopathy comprises a whitish area of retina associated with haemorrhages, likened to cottage cheese.

d   True. Ganciclovir and foscarnet are given parenterally and/or intravitreally.

e   True. Neuro-ophthalmic disorders may be seen.

11

Glaucoma

Learning objectives

To understand:

- ✔ The nature of glaucoma.
- ✔ The difference between primary and secondary glaucoma; open- and closed-angle glaucoma.
- ✔ The different symptoms and signs of open- and closed-angle glaucoma.
- ✔ The three major forms of glaucoma therapy.

Introduction

The glaucomas are a group of diseases causing damage to the optic nerve (*optic neuropathy*) by the effects of raised ocular pressure on the optic nerve head. Ischaemia of the optic nerve head independent of the level of intraocular pressure may also be important. Axon loss results in visual field defects and a loss of visual acuity if the central visual field is involved. In chronic glaucoma the visual loss is gradual, irreversible and initially may not be apparent to the patient, particularly as one eye is often more severely affected than the other. Glaucoma is thus known as a silent blinding disease.

Pathophysiology

The level of intraocular pressure is determined by a balance between production and removal of aqueous humour (Figure 11.1). Aqueous is actively secreted into the posterior chamber by the ciliary processes, by a combination of active transport and ultrafiltration. It then passes through the pupil into the anterior chamber and leaves the eye, predominantly via the trabecular meshwork, Schlemm canal and the episcleral veins, to reach the bloodstream (*the conventional pathway*). A small but important proportion of the aqueous (4%, but possibly more in younger people) drains across the ciliary body into the supra-choroidal space and is absorbed into the venous circulation (*the uveoscleral pathway*). The tone of the ciliary muscle affects the flow through this pathway.

Two theories have been advanced to explain how elevated intraocular pressure, acting at the nerve head, damages the optic nerve fibres:

1 Raised intraocular pressure causes mechanical damage to the axons.
2 Raised intraocular pressure causes ischaemia of the nerve axons by reducing blood flow at the nerve head.

The pathophysiology of glaucoma is probably multifactorial and both mechanisms are important.

Classification

The usual cause of raised intraocular pressure in glaucoma is an increased resistance to aqueous outflow at the trabecular meshwork. The mechanism by which this occurs provides a means to classify the primary glaucomas, based on the physical appearance of the drainage angle when it is viewed by *gonioscopy* (Figure 11.2 and see below).

Ophthalmology: Lecture Notes, Thirteenth Edition. Bruce James, Anthony Bron, and Manoj V. Parulekar.
© 2024 John Wiley & Sons Ltd. Published 2024 by John Wiley & Sons Ltd.
Companion website: www.wiley.com/go/ophthalmology13e

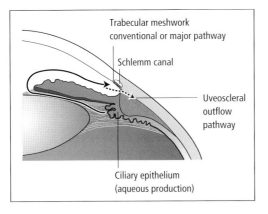

Figure 11.1 Diagram of the drainage angle, showing routes taken by aqueous from production to absorption.

Classification of the glaucomas

1. Primary glaucoma:
   - Open-angle glaucoma (POAG) and normal tension glaucoma (NTG).
   - Acute and chronic angle-closure glaucoma (PACG).
2. Childhood glaucoma:
   - Primary congenital glaucoma (PCG) typically presents in first few months of life.
   - Juvenile open-angle glaucoma (JOAG) 3–40 years old.
   - Secondary to acquired conditions (e.g. tumours, uveitis and trauma).
   - Secondary to inherited ocular disorders (e.g. aniridia – absence of the iris) or systemic abnormalities (e.g. Sturge–Weber syndrome – abnormal blood vessels on the face and in the eye and brain).
3. Secondary glaucoma, both open and closed angle:
   - Trauma.
   - Ocular surgery.
   - Associated with other ocular disease (e.g. uveitis).
   - Raised episcleral venous pressure.
   - Drug induced (e.g. steroids).

- Where the increased resistance occurs within the meshwork itself and the angle is not obstructed by peripheral iris, this is termed *open-angle glaucoma*.
- Where the increased resistance is due to the peripheral iris blocking the trabecular meshwork, this is termed, *angle-closure glaucoma*.

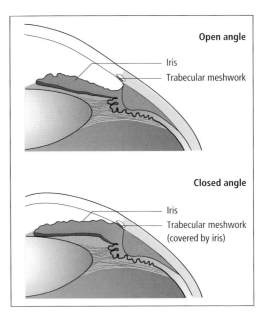

Figure 11.2 Diagram showing the difference between open- and closed-angle glaucoma. Outflow resistance is increased in each case. In open-angle glaucoma, the obstruction is due to structural changes in the trabecular meshwork. In closed-angle glaucoma, the peripheral iris blocks the meshwork.

Pathogenesis

Primary (Chronic) open-angle glaucoma

A special contact lens applied to the cornea (a gonioscopy lens) provides a view of the iridocorneal angle with the slit lamp (Figure 11.3). In primary or chronic open-angle glaucoma, the trabecular meshwork appears normal on gonioscopy but structurally and functionally, it *offers an increased resistance to the outflow* of aqueous. This results in elevated ocular pressure. The causes of outflow obstruction include:

- thickening of the trabecular lamellae, which reduces pore size;
- reduction in the number of lining trabecular cells;
- increased extracellular material in the trabecular meshwork spaces.

A form of glaucoma also exists in which glaucomatous field loss and pathological cupping of the optic disc occurs even though the intraocular pressure is not raised (*normal tension* or *low tension glaucoma*). It is thought that the optic nerve head in these patients

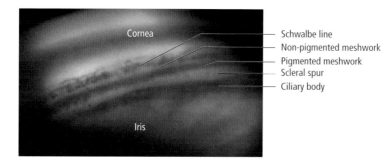

Cornea

Schwalbe line
Non-pigmented meshwork
Pigmented meshwork
Scleral spur
Ciliary body

Iris

Figure 11.3 The iridocorneal angle seen through a gonioscopy lens. The pigmented meshwork is the site of active aqueous drainage.

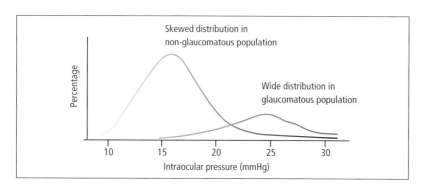

Figure 11.4 The distribution of intraocular pressure in a normal and glaucomatous population.

is unusually susceptible to the intraocular pressure and/or has an intrinsically low blood supply (Figure 11.4).

Conversely, intraocular pressure may be raised without evidence of visual damage or pathological optic disc cupping (*ocular hypertension*). These subjects may represent the extreme end of the normal range of intraocular pressure; however, a small proportion (between 1% and 5% per year) will subsequently develop glaucoma.

An elevation of intraocular pressure is, however, found in the majority of cases of glaucoma.

Angle-closure glaucoma

Primary angle-closure glaucoma (PACG) may be acute, subacute or chronic. This condition occurs in small eyes (i.e. often hypermetropic) which therefore have shallow anterior chambers and a narrow drainage angle.

In the normal eye, the point of contact between the pupil margin and the lens offers a slight resistance to aqueous flow from the posterior into the anterior chamber (relative pupil block) – as a result, there is a pressure drop between the posterior and anterior chamber which drives physiological flow. In acute angle-closure glaucoma, *sometimes in response to pupil dilation,* when the peripheral iris may be bunched up in the angle, this resistance is increased

and the increased pressure gradient bows the iris forward and closes the drainage angle. Aqueous can no longer drain through the trabecular meshwork and ocular pressure rises, usually abruptly. This peripheral iris contact ultimately leads to adhesions, called *peripheral anterior synechiae* (PAS), which consolidate the obstruction.

Acutely the severely reduced drainage of aqueous deprives the whole cornea of nutrition and the posterior cornea of its oxygen supply. This causes a catastrophic failure of endothelial pumping function and a massive degree of corneal oedema and clouding. This is amplified by the raised intraocular pressure and results in a profound fall in vision.

A full-blown attack of acute angle-closure glaucoma may be preceded by subacute episodes of angle closure, associated with transient rises of pressure, headaches and the experience of *coloured haloes around bright lights.* These *rainbows* are due to the presence of mild corneal epithelial oedema which separates the regularly arranged basal epithelial cells so that they act as a diffraction grating. Any patient presenting with a history of headaches should be asked about the presence of *rainbows around lights*, which are a key symptom of such prodromal attacks. Acute attacks are more common in dim light, when the pupil is dilated.

Chronic angle-closure glaucoma may also occur, when extensive PAS causes a gradual elevation of intraocular pressure associated with glaucomatous optic nerve head damage, pathological cupping and visual field loss. It may be asymptomatic until significant changes have occurred.

Some asymptomatic patients may be encountered with shallow anterior chambers and narrow iridocorneal angles (without PAS) who are at risk of developing glaucoma although when examined the pressures are normal and there are no signs of glaucomatous damage. Such patients are termed primary angle-closure suspects (PACS). A further group of patients may have evidence of angle closure on gonioscopy (with PAS) and a raised pressure but again no signs of glaucomatous damage. These patients are classified as having primary angle closure (PAC).

Secondary glaucoma

In secondary glaucoma, the rise of intraocular pressure is due to trabecular meshwork obstruction from other causes. The trabecular meshwork may be blocked by:

- blood (*hyphaema*), following blunt trauma;
- inflammatory cells (*uveitis*);
- pigment released from the iris (*pigment dispersion syndrome*);
- deposition in the trabecular meshwork of material produced by the epithelium of the lens, iris and ciliary body (*pseudoexfoliative glaucoma*);
- drugs increasing the resistance of the meshwork (*steroid-induced glaucoma*).
- blunt trauma to the eye causing structural damage to the drainage angle (*angle recession*).

Angle closure may also account for some cases of secondary glaucoma:

- in neovascular glaucoma, abnormal iris blood vessels (*rubeosis iridis*) obstruct the angle and cause the iris to adhere to the peripheral cornea, closing the angle. This may accompany any cause of extensive retinal ischaemia, such as proliferative diabetic retinopathy or central retinal vein occlusion which result in the forward diffusion of vasoproliferative factors such as vascular endothelial growth factor (VEGF) from the ischaemic retina (Figure 11.5; see Chapter 13).
- a large choroidal melanoma may push the iris forward, approximating it to the peripheral cornea and causing an acute attack of angle-closure glaucoma.
- a cataract may swell, pushing the iris forward to close the drainage angle.
- uveitis may cause the iris to adhere to the trabecular meshwork.

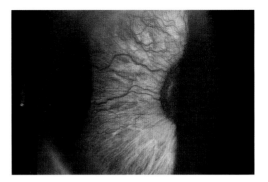

Figure 11.5 The appearance of the rubeotic iris. Note the irregular pattern of the new blood vessels on the surface.

In all cases of secondary glaucoma, it is important to take a full drug history. As well as mydriatic drops, some systemic medications, (for example anticholinergics, some antidepressants and topiramate, an anti-epileptic drug) may be associated with the development of angle closure.

Raised episcleral venous pressure is an unusual cause of glaucoma but may be seen in *carotid-cavernous sinus fistula*, where a connection between the carotid artery or its meningeal branches and the cavernous sinus causes a marked elevation in orbital venous pressure. It is also thought to be the cause of the raised intraocular pressure in patients with the *Sturge–Weber syndrome*.

Chronic (primary) open-angle glaucoma

Epidemiology

Chronic (or primary) open-angle glaucoma affects 1% of the population over the age of 40, affecting males and females equally. The prevalence increases with age to nearly 10% in the over-80 population. There may be a family history although the mode of inheritance is often unclear.

Genetics

First-degree relatives of patients with chronic open-angle glaucoma have up to a 16% chance of developing the disease themselves. Inheritance of the condition is complex. A juvenile form of open-angle glaucoma (presenting at between 3 and 40 years of age) is caused by mutations in the *myocilin gene* (GLC1A), which maps to the long arm of chromosome 1. A different set of mutations in the same gene may be associated with some cases of chronic open-angle glaucoma and other genes, such as *optineurin* (GLC1E) and *WDR36* (GLC1G), may also play a role. The optineurin gene is predominantly associated with normal tension glaucoma (see later). It is likely that an interaction between these genes and others yet to be identified is required for glaucoma to develop. Genome-wide association studies have found several other genes that may be important in glaucoma.

History

The symptoms of glaucoma depend on the rate at which the intraocular pressure rises. Chronic open-angle glaucoma is associated with a slow rise in pressure and is symptomless until the patient becomes aware of a visual deficit or the diagnosis is made by chance. Many patients are diagnosed when the signs of glaucoma are detected by an optometrist (opportunistic screening).

Examination

In patients with chronic open-angle glaucoma, the eyes are white and the corneas clear. Assessment of a glaucoma suspect requires a full slit-lamp examination and involves:

- Measurement of ocular pressure with a tonometer. The mean, normal pressure is 15.5 mmHg. The limits are defined as two standard deviations above and below the mean (11–21 mmHg). In chronic open-angle glaucoma on presentation, the pressure is typically in the 22–40 mmHg range. In acute angle-closure glaucoma, it rises above 60 mmHg.
- Measurement of the thickness of the cornea with a pachymeter. The measured value of the intraocular pressure must be adjusted according to the corneal thickness (see Chapter 3).
- Examination of the iridocorneal angle by *gonioscopy*, to confirm that an open angle is present.
- Exclusion of other ocular disease that may be a cause of a secondary glaucoma.
- Examination of the optic disc and determination of whether it is *pathologically cupped*. Cupping is a normal feature of the optic disc (Figure 11.6a). The disc is assessed by estimating the ratio of the vertical height of the cup to that of the disc as a whole

(the cup:disc ratio). In the normal eye, the cup:disc ratio is usually no greater than 0.4. There is, however, a considerable range and the size of the cup is related to the size of the disc. It is greater in bigger discs and less in smaller discs.

In chronic glaucoma, axons leaving the optic nerve head die. The central cup expands and the outer rim of nerve fibres (*neuroretinal rim*) becomes thinner (Figure 11.6b, c). The nerve head becomes atrophic. The vertical cup:disc ratio becomes greater than 0.4 and the cup deepens. If the cup is deep but the cup:disc ratio is lower than 0.4, then chronic glaucoma is unlikely, unless the disc is very small. Notching of the rim, implying focal axonal loss, may also be a sign of glaucomatous damage (Figure 11.6d). Defects in the nerve fibre layer of the retina may also be apparent and determine the location and area of visual field loss.

Much research is being directed towards accurate methods for analysing and recording the appearance of the disc and the retinal nerve fibre layer. One involves scanning the disc with a confocal ophthalmoscope to produce an image of the disc. The neuroretinal rim area can be calculated from the image (Figure 11.7). Other techniques (optical coherence tomography (OCT)) record the thickness of the nerve fibre layer around the optic disc, an indicator of nerve fibre loss. These new technologies may help to detect changes over time, indicating whether progressive damage to the optic nerve is still occurring despite treatment.

Visual field loss in glaucoma is due to the death of optic nerve axons. Field testing (perimetry, see Chapter 3) is used to establish the presence of islands of field loss (scotomata) and monitor the progression of optic nerve damage (Figure 11.8). It is known that a significant proportion of optic nerve fibres can be lost before a field loss becomes apparent. This has stimulated the search for more sensitive means of assessing visual function with different forms of perimetry (e.g. a blue target on a yellow

---

Symptoms and signs of chronic open-angle glaucoma

- Symptomless in its early stages.
- A white eye and clear cornea.
- Raised intraocular pressure.
- Visual field defect.
- Pathologically cupped optic disc (glaucomatous optic atrophy).

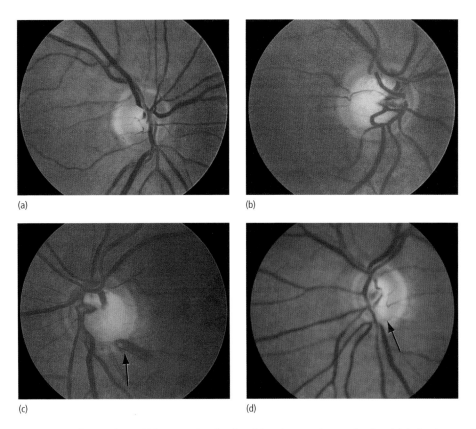

(a) (b)

(c) (d)

Figure 11.6 Comparison of (a) a normal optic disc, (b) a glaucomatous optic disc. (c) A disc haemorrhage (arrowed) is a feature of patients with normal tension glaucoma. (d) A glaucomatous notch (arrowed) in the disc.

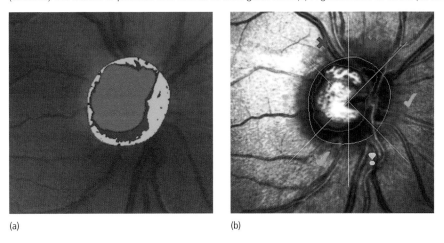

(a) (b)

Figure 11.7 (a,b) A scanning laser ophthalmoscope (Heidelberg) picture of the optic nerve head. The thin green circle in (b) outlines the optic nerve head, allowing the machine to calculate the area of the cup (red in (a)) and neuroretinal rim in different sectors of the disc. (c) An OCT of the retinal nerve fibre layer (RNFL). The scan measures the thickness of the RNFL at a uniform distance from the centre of the optic disc (the outer red circle on the left-hand image). This is then converted to a straight line and compared to an age-matched population and shown graphically (lower right-hand picture). The lower red area of the graph indicates an RNFL that is likely to be abnormally thin (arrowed). The two diagrams of the optic nerve on the left show the area of abnormal RNFL as it relates to the optic nerve. (d) The optic disc picture shows a focal defect of the neuroretinal rim inferiorly (arrowed). This corresponds to the thinning of the RNFL shown on the scan (arrows).

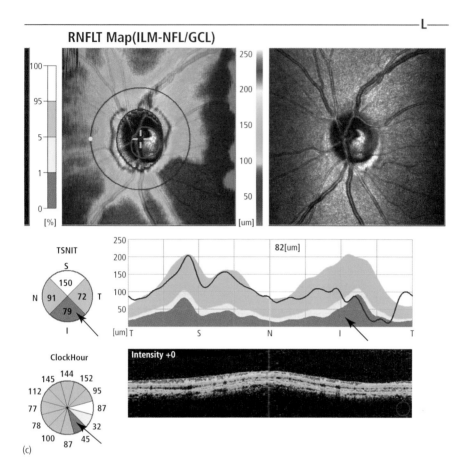

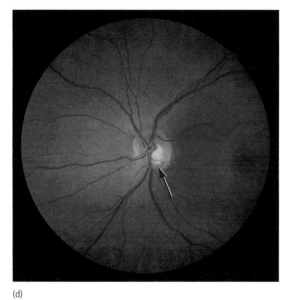

(c)

(d)

Figure 11.7 (Continued)

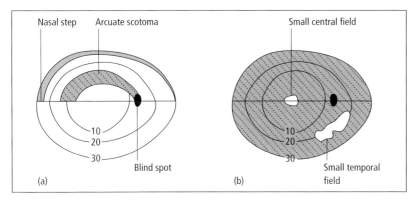

Figure 11.8 The characteristic pattern of visual field loss in chronic open-angle glaucoma. Visual field of the right eye. (a) An upper arcuate scotoma, reflecting damage to a cohort of nerve fibres entering the lower pole of the disc (remember – the optics of the eye determine that damage to the lower retina creates an upper field defect). A nasal step is another classical glaucomatous field defect. (b) The field loss has progressed: a small central island is left (tunnel vision), and sometimes this may be associated with sparing of an island of vision in the temporal field.

background instead of a white target on a white background and testing sensitivity to motion in the peripheral visual field).

Treatment

Treatment is aimed at reducing intraocular pressure. The level to which the pressure must be lowered varies from patient to patient and is that which minimizes further glaucomatous visual loss. This requires careful monitoring in the outpatient clinic. Three modalities of treatment are available:

1 medical treatment;
2 laser treatment;
3 surgical treatment.

In the United Kingdom, guidelines have been published by NICE (National Institute for Health and Clinical Excellence) http://www.nice.org.uk/guidance/ng81 on the treatment of glaucoma, with suggested therapeutic regimens. Each form of treatment has its complications, and therapy must be aimed at minimizing these whilst maximizing effectiveness.

Medical treatment

Topical drugs commonly used in the treatment of glaucoma are listed in Table 11.1. In chronic open-angle glaucoma, the prostaglandin analogues are becoming the first-line of treatment. They act by increasing the passage of aqueous through the

uveoscleral pathway. Topical adrenergic beta-blockers may further reduce the pressure by suppressing aqueous secretion. Non-selective beta-blockers carry the risk of precipitating asthma through their beta 2-blocking action, following systemic absorption, or they may exacerbate an existing heart block through their beta-1 action. Beta-1-selective beta-blockers may have fewer systemic side effects, but must still be used with caution in those with respiratory disease, particularly asthma, which may be exacerbated even by the small residual beta-2 activity. Pilocarpine may occasionally be used in the treatment of chronic open-angle glaucoma. The requirement for frequent application and side effects including headache, miosis and induced myopia, limit its use however. If intraocular pressure remains elevated, the choice lies between:

- adding additional medical treatment (drops combining two different drugs are available to ease application);
- laser treatment;
- surgical drainage procedures.

To ensure compliance, any drop regimen must be easy to take, once a day therapy is ideal. Treatment should not cause the patient significant side effects. The benefits of treatment, aimed at preventing further visual loss, may not be apparent to the patients and may compromise compliance.

Increasingly eye drops are available in (more expensive) preservative-free form. Preservatives increase the shelf life of the medication. The commonest is Benzalkonium Chloride (BAK) which acts

Table 11.1 Examples and mode of action of drugs used in the treatment of glaucoma.

Drug	Action	Side effects
Topical agents		
Beta-blockers (timolol, carteolol, levobunolol, metipranolol, betaxolol (selective))	Decrease secretion	Exacerbate asthma and chronic airway disease Hypotension, bradycardia, heart block
Parasympathomimetic (pilocarpine)	Increase outflow	Visual blurring in the young, due to induced myopia Darkening of the visual world due to pupillary constriction Initially, headache due to ciliary spasm
Alpha-2 agonists (apraclonidine, brimonidine)	Increase outflow through the uveoscleral pathway Decrease secretion	Redness of the eye Fatigue, drowsiness
Carbonic anhydrase inhibitors (dorzolamide, brinzolamide)	Decrease secretion	Stinging, unpleasant taste
Prostaglandin analogues (latanoprost, travoprost, bimatoprost, tafluprost, unoprostone)	Increase outflow through the uveoscleral pathway	Increased pigmentation of the iris and periocular skin Lengthening and darkening of the lashes, conjunctival hyperaemia Rarely, macular oedema, uveitis
Systemic agents Carbonic anhydrase inhibitors (acetazolamide)	Decrease secretion	Tingling in limbs Depression, sleepiness Renal stones Stevens–Johnson syndrome

Side effects occur with variable frequency. Systemic effects are due to systemic absorption of the drug.

as a detergent lysing cell membranes and killing bacteria. They may, however, cause ocular surface disease resulting in:

- Ocular irritation, foreign body and burning sensations.
- Tearing.
- Light sensitivity.
- Visual blurring.
- Redness of the eye.
- Corneal epithelial damage.
- Intractable dry eye disease

Prescription of preservative-free forms, particularly in those on multiple medications or with pre-existing ocular surface disease, may reduce these symptoms and increase compliance with medication.

Laser trabeculoplasty

This involves placing a series of laser burns in the trabecular meshwork, to improve aqueous outflow.

Whilst effective initially, the intraocular pressure may slowly increase. In the United Kingdom this may be used as a first line treatment.

Surgical treatment

Drainage surgery (*trabeculectomy*) relies on the creation of a fistula between the anterior chamber and the subconjunctival space (Figure 11.9a,b). Aqueous humour leaves the anterior chamber, via a bleb of conjunctiva, into the subconjunctival space. The operation usually achieves a substantial reduction in intraocular pressure. It is performed increasingly early in the treatment of open-angle glaucoma.

Complications of surgery include:

- shallowing of the anterior chamber in the immediate postoperative period risking damage to the lens and cornea;
- intraocular infection;
- possibly accelerated cataract development;

- failure to reduce intraocular pressure adequately;
- scarring causing a longer term rise in IOP;
- an excessively low pressure (hypotony) which may cause macular oedema.

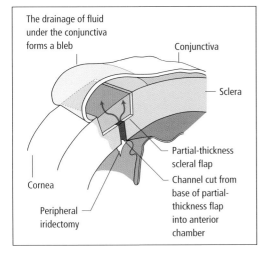

(a)

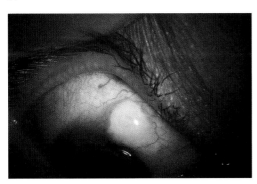

(b)

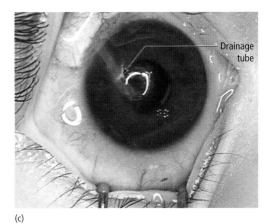

(c)

Figure 11.9 (*Continued*)

Figure 11.9 (a) Diagram showing a section through a trabeculectomy. An incision is made in the conjunctiva, which is dissected and reflected to expose bare sclera. A partial-thickness scleral flap is then fashioned. Just anterior to the scleral spur a small opening (termed a sclerostomy) is made into the anterior chamber to create a low-resistance channel for aqueous. The iris is excised in the region of the sclerostomy (iridectomy) to prevent it moving forward and blocking the opening. The partial-thickness flap is loosely sutured back into place. The conjunctiva is tightly sutured. Aqueous can now leak through the sclerostomy, around and through the scleral flap and underneath the conjunctiva, where it forms a bleb. (b) The appearance of a trabeculectomy bleb. (c) A drainage tube inserted into the anterior chamber allows aqueous fluid to pass to the valve sutured to the sclera.

Evidence suggests that some topical medications, particularly those containing sympathomimetic agents or preservatives, may decrease the success of surgery by causing increased postoperative subconjunctival scarring, resulting in a non-functional drainage channel. In patients particularly prone to scarring, antimetabolite drugs (5-fluorouracil and mitomycin) may be used locally at the time of surgery to prevent subconjunctival fibrosis.

In situations where trabeculectomy surgery has failed or where it is unlikely to be successful due to scarring of the conjunctiva, a drainage tube may be inserted into the anterior chamber (Figure 11.9c). This is connected to a valve placed posteriorly on the sclera, deep to the conjunctiva, from which the aqueous disperses.

Microinvasive Glaucoma Surgery (MIGS)

MIGS is a rapidly developing field. It adds a further surgical means of reducing IOP and may enable some patients to become free of topical medication. It is usually performed at the time of cataract surgery. The reduction in IOP is not usually as great as that achieved by trabeculectomy (in the region of 20%) but there are fewer complications. Techniques employed include:

- Implantation of a micro-stent into Schlemm canal, lowering the resistance to aqueous drainage.
- Excision of part of the trabecular meshwork, opening the aqueous drainage pathway to Schlemm canal.
- Dilation of Schlemm canal, (canaloplasty).

- Implantation of a stent to drain aqueous from the anterior chamber to the subconjunctival space, a similar pathway to trabeculectomy.
- A micro-stent draining aqueous from the anterior chamber into the suprachoroidal space.
- Laser ablation of the ciliary processes endoscopically to reduce aqueous production.

Normal tension glaucoma

Normal tension glaucoma, considered to lie at one end of the spectrum of chronic open-angle glaucoma, can be particularly difficult to treat, although in those with progressive field loss, lowering intraocular pressure is still beneficial. Some patients appear to have non-progressive visual field defects and may require no treatment.

Primary angle-closure glaucoma

Epidemiology

Primary angle-closure glaucoma affects 1 in 1000 subjects over 40 years, with females more commonly affected than males. Patients with angle-closure glaucoma are likely to be long-sighted, because the long-sighted eye is small and the structures of the anterior chamber are more crowded.

History

In acute angle-closure glaucoma, there is an abrupt increase in pressure and the eye becomes photophobic and very painful due to ischaemic tissue damage. There is watering of the eye and loss of vision. The patient may be systemically unwell with nausea and referred abdominal pain, symptoms which may take them to a general casualty department.

Intermittent primary angle-closure glaucoma occurs when an acute attack spontaneously resolves. The patient may complain of ocular pain, blurring of vision and seeing coloured rainbows around lights.

Examination

On examination, visual acuity is reduced, the eye red, the cornea cloudy and the pupil oval, fixed and dilated due to ischaemia (Figure 11.10).

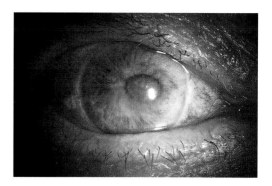

Figure 11.10 The appearance of the eye in angle-closure glaucoma. Note the cloudy cornea and dilated pupil.

Treatment

The acute and dramatic rise in pressure seen in angle-closure glaucoma must be urgently countered to prevent permanent damage to vision. Acetazolamide is administered intravenously and subsequently orally, together with topical pilocarpine and beta-blockers. Pilocarpine constricts the pupil and draws the peripheral iris out of the angle; the acetazolamide and beta-blockers reduce aqueous secretion and the pressure gradient across the iris. These measures often break the attack and lower intraocular pressure. Subsequent management requires that a small hole (*iridotomy* or *iridectomy*) be made in the peripheral iris to prevent further attacks. This provides an alternative pathway for fluid to flow from the posterior to the anterior chamber, bypassing the pupil and thus reducing the pressure gradient across the iris so that it is no longer pushed forwards. This can be done with a Nd-YAG laser or surgically.

If the pressure has been raised for some days, or in chronic angle-closure glaucoma, the iris becomes adherent to the peripheral cornea (*peripheral anterior synechiae* or *PAS*) and the iridocorneal angle may be permanently damaged and obstructed. Additional medical or surgical measures may be required to lower the ocular pressure.

In some patients with cataract, lens extraction with implantation of an intraocular lens may help open the iridocorneal angle and reduce intraocular pressure. This is becoming an increasingly important means of treating angle closure.

Secondary glaucoma

Secondary glaucomas are much rarer than the primary glaucomas. The symptoms and signs depend on the rate at which intraocular pressure rises; most are again symptomless. Treatment broadly follows the lines of the primary disease. In secondary glaucoma, it is important to treat any underlying cause, for example uveitis, which may be responsible for the glaucoma. Neovascular (rubeotic) glaucoma secondary to retinal ischaemia responds to an intra-vitreal injection of an anti-VEGF agent, causing the new vessels on the iris to shrink. This is followed by pan-retinal photocoagulation to reduce VEGF production by the ischaemic retina.

In particularly difficult cases, it may be necessary to selectively ablate the ciliary processes in order to reduce aqueous production. This is done by application of a diode laser to the sclera overlying the processes.

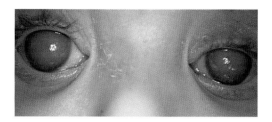

Figure 11.11 The clinical appearance of bilateral buphthalmos.

Childhood glaucoma

Epidemiology

The incidence of congenital glaucoma is highly variable between 1:10,00 and 1:20,000 live births. It is increased in consanguineous marriages. The incidence of juvenile open-angle glaucoma is about 0.38 per 100,000 people.

Genetics

CYP1BI and LTBP2 genes have been linked to primary congenital glaucoma with an autosomal recessive inheritance pattern. Other genes have also been identified. Juvenile open-angle glaucoma has been linked to the MYOC gene and has an autosomal dominant inheritance.

History

Childhood glaucoma covers a diverse range of disease. It may present at birth or be detected within the first year. Symptoms and signs include:

- excessive tearing, photophobia and blepharospasm;
- enlargement of the globe (*buphthalmos*), including an increased corneal diameter, resulting in progressive myopia. Globe enlargement only occurs while the cornea and sclera are plastic, typically under the age of three years;
- splits in Descemet membrane (Haab Striae) and the endothelium due to the corneal stretching;

- a cloudy cornea due to epithelial and stromal oedema as water enters through the breaks (Figure 11.11).

Congenital glaucoma is usually treated surgically. An incision is made into the trabecular meshwork (*goniotomy*) to increase aqueous drainage, or a direct passage between Schlemm canal and the anterior chamber is created (*trabeculotomy*). Trabeculectomy or the implantation of a shunt may be required in some cases.

Prognosis of the glaucomas

The goal of treatment in glaucoma is to stop or reduce the rate of visual damage. It may be that control of intraocular pressure alone is not the only factor that needs to be addressed in the management of glaucoma. The possible role of optic nerve ischaemia has been discussed, and there is interest in developing neuroprotective drugs. Reducing intraocular pressure is currently, however, the mainstay of treatment. Some patients will continue to develop visual loss despite a large decrease in intraocular pressure. Nonetheless, vigorous lowering of intraocular pressure, even when it does not prevent continued visual loss, appears to significantly reduce the rate of progression. If the diagnosis is made late, when there is already significant visual damage, the eye is more likely to become blind despite treatment (Figure 11.12).

If intraocular pressure remains controlled, following acute treatment of angle-closure glaucoma, progressive visual damage is unlikely. The same applies to the secondary glaucomas if treatment of the underlying cause results in a reduction of intraocular pressure into the normal range.

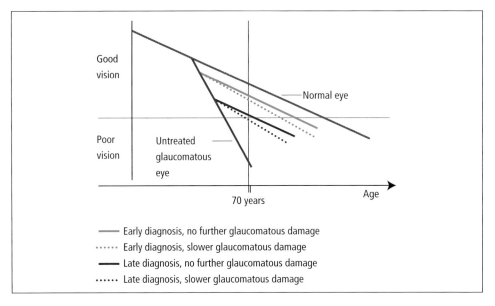

Figure 11.12 All eyes suffer a gradual loss of retinal ganglion cell neurones with aging but death normally precedes a visually significant decline. In glaucoma this loss is speeded up and visual loss occurs (red line). Early diagnosis of the condition with lowering of intraocular pressure results in future age-related neuronal loss only (green line parallel to the normal eye). Even if there is some continued glaucomatous damage the rate is slowed and the patient is unlikely to suffer visual loss during their lifetime (interrupted green line). If the diagnosis is made late (purple lines), arresting the glaucoma completely may still result in visual loss during the patient's lifetime. This emphasizes the need for early diagnosis.

 KEY POINTS

- Chronic glaucoma can be a silent, blinding disease.
- Glaucoma is an optic neuropathy caused by an elevation of intraocular pressure.
- Glaucomatous optic neuropathy is distinguished from that due to other causes by an enlarged optic cup.
- Primary glaucoma is classified according to whether the trabecular meshwork is obstructed by intrinsic changes in the meshwork only (open-angle glaucoma) or by the peripheral iris (angle-closure glaucoma).
- Treatment of glaucoma relies on lowering ocular pressure to reduce or prevent further visual damage.
- In chronic open-angle glaucoma, ocular pressure can be reduced with long-term topical and systemic medications, laser treatment and surgery. Treatment aims to prevent visual loss rather than improve vision and because the patient is asymptomatic in the early stages, compliance with treatment can be difficult.
- Patients who are acutely ill, with a red painful eye and visual loss may have acute angle-closure glaucoma.
- In acute angle-closure glaucoma, urgent therapy with systemic acetazolamide, pilocarpine and ocular hypotensives is needed, followed by iridotomy to break the cycle of angle closure.

Assessment questions
True or False

1. Which of the following statements are true?

a Aqueous is produced by the ciliary processes. The fluid circulates through the pupil and is drained via the trabecular meshwork.

b The uveoscleral pathway accounts for most of the drainage of aqueous.

c The major classification of glaucoma depends on the anatomy of the iridocorneal angle.

d One mechanism of angle-closure glaucoma is an increased resistance to aqueous flow through the pupil. This causes the iris to bow forwards and block the drainage angle.

e Glaucoma is always associated with a raised pressure.

2. A patient is found by his optician to have an arcuate visual field defect, an enlarged optic cup and raised intraocular pressure.

a The most likely diagnosis is acute glaucoma.

b The most likely diagnosis is chronic open-angle glaucoma.

c Treatment is with intravenous acetazolamide.

d Treatment is confined to topical therapy.

e The corneal diameter will be increased.

3. A patient presents to casualty with a painful red eye and a cloudy cornea. The casualty officer suspects he has acute glaucoma.

a He should arrange for him to be seen in the eye clinic in a week.

b The diagnosis would be further confirmed by finding a dilated pupil.

c Treatment is initially with intravenous acetazolamide and pilocarpine eye drops.

d A laser iridotomy should be performed.

e The condition may be caused by a block to the flow of aqueous through the pupil.

4. Symptoms of congenital glaucoma include

a A watering eye.

b Increased corneal diameter.

c A red eye.

d Splits in Descemet membrane.

e Cloudiness of the cornea.

5. Glaucoma surgery (trabeculectomy):

a May be complicated by intraocular infection.

b Is associated with accelerated cataract development.

c Retinal detachment is a common complication of the surgery.

d Reverses damage to the optic nerve caused by glaucoma.

e Success of surgery may be improved by using antimetabolites topically.

6. Match the side effects of treatment with the drug class.

a Exacerbation of asthma.

b Visual blurring in patients with cataract.

c Redness of the eye, increased pigmentation of the periocular skin, darkening of the iris, lengthening of the eyelashes.

d Tingling in the fingers and around the mouth.

   i Beta-blockers.

   ii Prostaglandin analogues.

   iii Parasympathomimetic agents.

   iv Systemic carbonic anhydrase inhibitors.

Answers

1. Which of the following statements are true?

a True. This is the route that most of the aqueous drains through, a small percentage drains via the uveoscleral route.

b False. The uveoscleral pathway accounts for only a small proportion of flow. The conventional pathway across the trabecular meshwork accounts for most of the outflow.

c True. Glaucoma is essentially classified into open- and closed-angle glaucoma.

d True. Termed pupil block this is the cause of acute angle-closure glaucoma.

e False. Some patients develop the typical signs of glaucoma (glaucomatous field loss and disc cupping) but have an intraocular pressure within the normal range.

2. A patient is found by his optician to have an arcuate visual field defect, an enlarged optic cup and raised intraocular pressure.

a False. This is an acute painful condition.

b True. These are the classical signs of chronic open-angle glaucoma.

c False. Intravenous acetazolamide is used to suppress aqueous secretion quickly, in acute glaucoma.

d False. Although this is the commonest treatment, laser and surgical treatments are also possible.

e False. This is only seen in congenital glaucoma.

3. **A patient presents to casualty with a painful red eye and a cloudy cornea. The casualty officer suspects he has acute glaucoma.**

a   False. The patient must be referred immediately for treatment.

b   True. It is likely that the patient has acute closed-angle glaucoma, finding a dilated pupil would help confirm the diagnosis.

c   True. The acetazolamide will reduce the pressure and the pilocarpine will constrict the pupil helping to relieve the angle closure.

d   True. This is the definitive treatment.

e   True. This is the proposed mechanism for this type of glaucoma.

4. **Symptoms of congenital glaucoma include**

a   True. Although most watering eyes in babies are due to non-patency of the nasolacrimal duct (Chapter 7) this is also the presentation of congenital glaucoma. Children are also photophobic and may have blepharospasm.

b   True. These children may have 'beautiful' big eyes.

c   False. The eye is usually white.

d   True. The corneal enlargement is associated with splits in Descemet membrane.

e   True. This is caused by epithelial and stromal oedema.

5. **Glaucoma surgery (trabeculectomy)**

a   True. This is a potential complication of any intraocular surgery.

b   True. Cataract may develop at an increased rate following trabeculectomy.

c   False. Choroidal effusion may be seen immediately following trabeculectomy if the pressure is low but retinal detachment is a rare complication.

d   False. No treatment is known to reverse the damage of glaucoma, but the rate of progression can be reduced with treatment.

e   True. A topical antimetabolite, applied to the sclera and conjunctiva at the time of surgery, reduces scarring and allows a functioning drainage bleb to form.

6. **Match the side effects of treatment with the drug class.**

a   Beta-blockers (i).

b   Parasympathomimetic agents (iii).

c   Prostaglandin analogues (ii).

d   Systemic carbonic anhydrase inhibitors (iv).

12

Retina and choroid

Learning objectives

To understand:

✔ The symptoms of retinal disease.
✔ The cause and treatment of acquired and inherited retinal disease.
✔ The symptoms, signs and complications of posterior vitreous detachment.
✔ The symptoms, signs, complications and treatment of retinal detachment.
✔ The symptoms, signs and treatment of retinal and choroidal tumours.

Introduction

The retina is subject to a great range of disease, both inherited and acquired. Some are common, with significant socioeconomic importance (e.g. age-related macular degeneration, AMD), while others are much rarer (e.g. some of the macular dystrophies). The impact on the individual may be profound in either case. Diseases of the macula, if bilateral, result in a profound reduction in visual acuity. Despite the variety of diseases, the symptoms are relatively stereotyped. These will be described first. In this chapter, both hereditary and acquired disease of the vitreous, neuroretina, retinal pigment epithelium (RPE) and choroid will be discussed. In the chapter which follows, disorders of the retinal circulation will be explored.

Symptoms of retinal disease

Macular dysfunction

The central part of the macula (the *fovea*) is responsible for fine resolution and disorders of this region cause significant visual impairment. The patient may complain of:

- Blurred central vision, with reduced colour perception.
- Distorted vision (*metamorphopsia*) caused by a disturbance in the arrangement of the photoreceptors such as occurs in macular oedema. A reduction of apparent object size occurs (*micropsia*) if the photoreceptors are stretched apart or apparent enlargement (*macropsia*) when photoreceptors are compressed together.
- The patient may notice areas of loss of the central visual field (*scotomata*) if part of the photoreceptor layer becomes covered, for example by blood, or if the photoreceptors are destroyed.

Peripheral retinal dysfunction

The patient complains of:

- Loss of visual field (usually only appreciated clinically when a significant amount of the peripheral retina is damaged). The field loss may be absolute, for example in a branch retinal artery occlusion or relative (i.e. brighter or larger objects are still visible) as in a retinal detachment.
- Some diseases affecting the retina may predominantly affect one type of photoreceptor. Thus, in

Ophthalmology: Lecture Notes, Thirteenth Edition. Bruce James, Anthony Bron, and Manoj V. Parulekar.
© 2024 John Wiley & Sons Ltd. Published 2024 by John Wiley & Sons Ltd.
Companion website: www.wiley.com/go/ophthalmology13e

retinitis pigmentosa, the rods are principally affected so that night vision is reduced (*night blindness*).

Acquired macular disease

Acquired disease at the macula may destroy part or all of the thickness of the retina (e.g. AMD or a macular hole).

If tight junctions of the retinal capillaries that form the *inner blood–retinal barrier* breakdown, fluid may accumulate within the layers of the retina creating cystoid spaces at the macula (*cystoid macular oedema*). This may occur following intraocular surgery, such as cataract surgery.

The neuroretina and RPE may also become separated by diffusion of fluid from the choriocapillaris through an abnormal region of the RPE. This represents a breakdown of the *outer blood–retinal barrier* between the choroid and the retina, and is termed *central serous retinopathy*. It may occur unilaterally, as a potentially reversible disorder particularly in young men.

Age-related macular degeneration

AMD is the commonest cause of irreversible visual loss in the developed world (Figure 12.1).

Pathogenesis

The RPE removes and processes the used discs of the photoreceptor outer segments. Over time, undigested lipid products, such as the age pigment lipofuscin, accumulate in the RPE and the excess material is transferred to Bruch membrane, impairing its diffusional properties. Extracellular deposits form between the RPE and Bruch membrane which can be seen with the ophthalmoscope as discrete, sub-retinal yellow lesions called drüsen. AMD may be classified as follows:

- early AMD. A collection of drüsen in the macula associated with normal vision (Figure 12.1b).
- dry (atrophic or non-exudative) AMD. The neighbouring RPE and photoreceptors show degenerative changes. This may produce a geographic

pattern of atrophy. It is associated with loss of vision.
- exudative (or wet) AMD. New vessels from the choroid, stimulated by angiogenic factors such as vascular endothelial growth factor (VEGF), grow through defects in Bruch membrane and the RPE into the sub-retinal space. Here, they form a *sub-retinal neovascular membrane*. Subsequent fluid exudation or haemorrhage into the sub-retinal space or even through the retina into the vitreous is associated with profound visual loss (Figure 12.1 c). The neuroretina ceases to function if it is detached from the RPE, so these changes may cause marked disruption of macular function even before further retinal damage occurs.

Symptoms

The symptoms are those of macular dysfunction outlined above.

Signs

Early AMD is associated with yellow, well-circumscribed drüsen. In dry AMD, there may be areas of hypo- and hyperpigmentation. In exudative AMD, sub-retinal, or more occasionally pre-retinal, haemorrhages may be seen with retinal elevation. These are caused by a neovascular membrane arising from the choroid (a *choroidal neovascular membrane, CNV*).

Investigation

Diagnosis is based on the appearance of the retina. In patients with a suspected exudative AMD an optical coherence tomograph (OCT), scan is the diagnostic tool of choice (Figure 12.1d). Additionally, OCT angiography or a fluorescein angiogram can delineate the *CNV*.

Treatment

Patients with exudative AMD can be treated with drugs injected into the eye, inhibiting the action of angiogenic factors such as VEGF. These drugs retard angiogenesis and cause regression of existing new vessels. Anti-VEGF agents are currently given by repeated injections into the vitreous cavity although slow release preparations are in development. They reduce visual loss and restore the normal anatomical appearance of the macula. In some patients, vision may improve. This treatment represents a major advance in the therapy of this disease. It does however

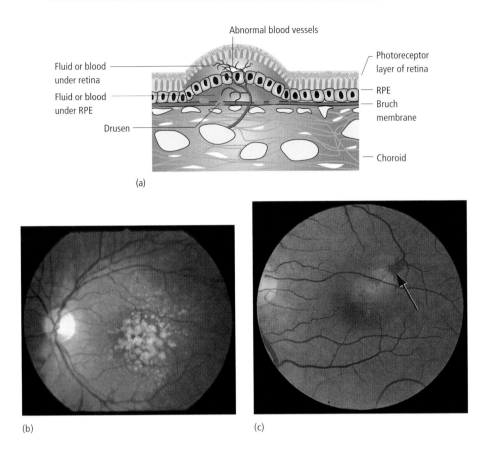

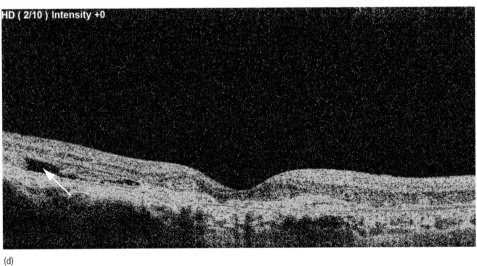

Figure 12.1 (a) The pathogenesis of exudative age-related macular degeneration (RPE, retinal pigment epithelium). (b) dry AMD: note the discrete scattered yellowish sub-retinal drüsen; (c) wet AMD: note the small haemorrhage associated with the sub-retinal membrane (arrowed); (d) OCT scan showing fluid within the retinal layers (arrowed).

require efficient monitoring and injection clinics to be set up. The need for repeated treatment itself has an impact on patients.

Patients with visual loss in one eye (visual acuity < 6/24 from non-exudative or exudative disease) and high-risk features in the fellow eye, or bilateral high-risk features but normal vision (large or confluent drüsen or significant hypo- and hyperpigmentation) may benefit to a small extent from high-dose antioxidant vitamins and zinc, given orally. Smoking itself is associated with an increased risk of developing haemorrhagic, exudative AMD and patients should be encouraged to stop. As UV exposure is believed to be a contributing factor, sun protection may be advised.

Apart from this, there is currently no treatment for non-exudative AMD.

For those with bilateral visual loss, vision is maximized with low-vision aids (see Chapters 4 and 20), including magnifiers and telescopes and closed-circuit television devices (CCTV). The patient must be reassured that although central vision has been lost, the disease will not spread to affect the peripheral vision. Therefore, navigational vision is retained. This is a vital message, since many patients fear that they will become totally blind.

Other degenerative conditions associated with the formation of choroidal neovascular membranes

- Degenerative changes and choroidal neovascular membranes may also occur at the maculae of highly myopic patients and can cause loss of central vision, even in young adulthood.
- Choroidal neovascular membranes may also grow through elongated cracks in Bruch membrane called *angioid streaks* (Figure 12.2). These are seen classically in the rare recessive disorder *pseudoxanthoma elasticum,* and uncommonly, in systemic diseases such as Paget disease and sickle cell disease. Again, there may be a profound reduction in central vision. Vision is also reduced if the crack itself passes through the fovea.

Macular holes and membranes

A well-circumscribed hole may form at the centre of the macular region and destroy the fovea, resulting in a major loss of acuity (Figure 12.3). It results from

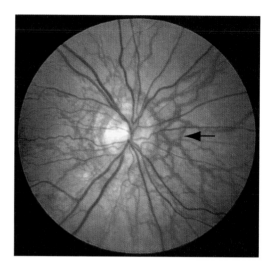

Figure 12.2 The clinical appearance of angioid streaks (arrow) in pseudoxanthoma elasticum. The arrow indicates a streak.

vitreous traction on the thin macular retina (vitreo-macular traction (VMT)). The early stages of hole formation may be associated with visual distortion and mild blurring of vision.

Unlike peripheral retinal holes, macular holes are not usually associated with retinal detachment. Most are idiopathic in origin, but they may be associated with blunt trauma. Where macular traction is evident, vitreous surgery is used to relieve the traction on the retina. The degree of visual improvement depends on the initial vision, the duration of symptoms and the stage (severity) of the macular hole. No other treatment is available.

A pre-retinal glial membrane may form over the macular region, whose contraction causes *puckering* of the retina and again results in blurred and distorted vision. These symptoms may be improved by removing the membrane with microsurgical vitrectomy techniques.

Central serous retinopathy

In this condition, a localized accumulation of fluid between the neuroretina and the RPE separates the two layers and disturbs the photoreceptor layer. It results from a localized breakdown in the normal barrier function of the RPE. It is usually unilateral and typically affects young or middle-aged males. Patients complain of distortion and blurred vision and visual acuity may fall markedly. It may be

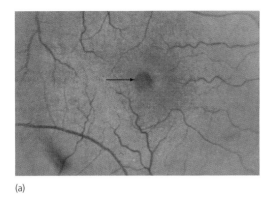

(a)

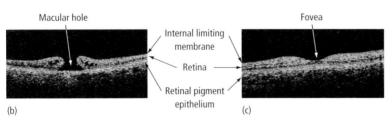

Macular hole

Internal limiting membrane

Retina

Retinal pigment epithelium

Fovea

(b)

(c)

Figure 12.3 (a) The appearance of a macular hole. (b) An OCT scan of the retina showing a macular hole, compared to (c) a normal scan.

associated with steroid use and stress. Examination reveals a dome-shaped elevation of the retina (Figure 12.4a). OCT scan helps confirm the diagnosis (Figure 12.4b).

Treatment is not usually required, as the condition is self-limiting. Occasionally, in intractable cases or those where the vision is severely affected a form of laser (Photodynamic Therapy) may be effective.

Macular oedema

This extracellular accumulation of fluid within the retina is a further cause of distorted and blurred vision (Figure 12.5a). Ophthalmoscopy reveals a loss of the normal foveal reflex and with experience, a cystic appearance to the fovea. If the diagnosis is in doubt, a confirmatory optical coherence tomogram (OCT) scan (Figure 12.5b,c) or a fluorescein angiogram can be performed. The fluorescein leaks into the oedematous retina in a characteristic pattern (see Chapter 3).

Macular oedema may be associated with numerous eye disorders, including:

- intraocular surgery;
- uveitis;
- retinal vascular disease (e.g. diabetic retinopathy and retinal vein occlusion);
- retinitis pigmentosa.

Treatment can be difficult and is dependent on the associated eye disease (see Chapter 13 for diabetic management). Steroids in high doses (oral or

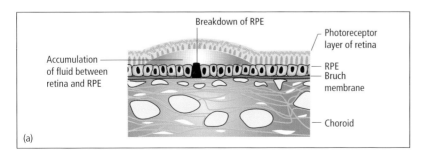

Breakdown of RPE

Photoreceptor layer of retina

Accumulation of fluid between retina and RPE

RPE
Bruch membrane

Choroid

(a)

Figure 12.4 (a) The pattern of fluid accumulation in central serous retinopathy; (b) an OCT scan demonstrating the accumulation of fluid between retina and RPE (black space on the scan arrowed).

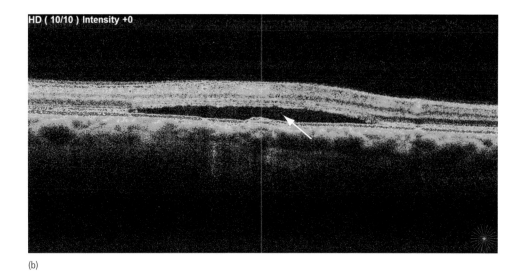

(b)

Figure 12.4 (*Continued*)

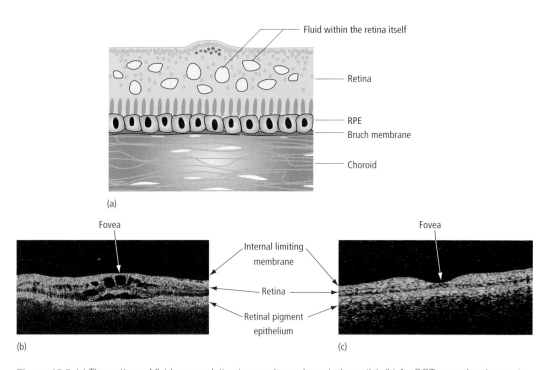

(a)

(b)　　(c)

Figure 12.5 (a) The pattern of fluid accumulation in macular oedema (schematic). (b) An OCT scan showing cysts of fluid in the retina of a patient with macular oedema, compared to (c) a normal scan.

periocular injection) are helpful in macular oedema caused by uveitis; acetazolamide may be helpful in treating patients with macular oedema accompanying retinitis pigmentosa or occurring following intraocular surgery. Non-steroidal anti-inflammatory drops may also have a role in preventing and treating cystoid macular oedema associated with intraocular surgery.

Prolonged macular oedema may result in the formation of a lamellar (partial thickness) macular hole.

Toxic maculopathies

The accumulation of some drugs in the RPE can cause macular damage. These include the antimalarials chloroquine and hydroxychloroquine, used quite widely in the treatment of rheumatoid arthritis and other connective-tissue disorders, which may cause a toxic maculopathy. Chloroquine is the more toxic. Patients on chloroquine require regular visual assessment for maculopathy (Figure 12.6). The maculopathy is initially only detected by accurate assessment of macular function. At this early stage, discontinuation of the drug reverses the maculopathy. Later, a pigmentary, 'target lesion' is seen ophthalmoscopically, associated with metamorphopsia and an appreciable and irreversible loss of central vision. Ocular toxicity is unlikely with a dose of less than 4 mg (chloroquine phosphate) per kg

lean body weight per day or a total cumulative dose of less than 300 g. The screening of patients on hydroxychloroquine at the recommended dose is also advised annually after 5 years of treatment or sooner if higher doses (>5 mg/kg/day) of the drug are used.

Phenothiazines (thioridazine particularly) used in high doses for prolonged periods (to treat psychoses) may cause retinal damage.

Tamoxifen, in high doses, may also cause a maculopathy.

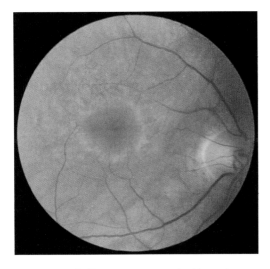

Figure 12.6 Bull's-eye appearance in chloroquine maculopathy.

Vitreous floaters and posterior vitreous detachment

With ageing, the vitreous gel undergoes degenerative changes (earlier in myopes) with liquefaction and the formation of fragments of condensed vitreous. These cast shadows on the retina, giving rise to the common symptom of vitreous 'floaters'. Subjectively, these take the form of spots or cobwebs which obscure vision only slightly and move when the eyes move, reflecting the fluid nature of the vitreous. Symptoms are most marked on bright days, when the small pupil throws a sharper image on the retina.

Sometimes, in older patients or myopes, the vitreous gel collapses and separates from points of retinal attachment, a condition termed *posterior vitreous detachment* (Figure 12.7). This gives rise to acute symptoms of:

- *photopsia* (flashing lights): due to traction on the peripheral retina by the detaching vitreous;
- a shower of floaters – representing condensations within the collapsed vitreous, or sometimes a vitreous haemorrhage caused when the detaching

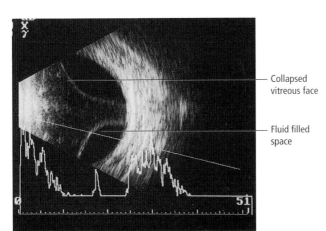

Collapsed vitreous face

Fluid filled space

Figure 12.7 Ultrasound picture showing a posterior vitreous detachment. Note that the vitreous is still attached at the optic disc.

vitreous ruptures a small blood vessel during the formation of a retinal tear or hole.

For this reason, presentation with *recent symptoms* of an acute vitreous detachment is *an indication for full assessment* of the vitreous and peripheral retina with full pupil dilation.

Retinal detachment

A retinal detachment is an ophthalmic emergency requiring urgent diagnosis and treatment.

Pathogenesis

The potential space between the neuroretina and its pigment epithelium corresponds to the cavity of the embryonic optic vesicle. The two tissues are loosely attached in the mature eye and may become separated, to form a retinal detachment, which may be progressive and partial or total:

- Where this is caused by a retinal tear or hole, allowing liquefied vitreous to gain entry to the sub-retinal space, it is termed a *rhegmatogenous* retinal detachment,
- Where it is caused by contracting fibrous tissue on the retinal surface, which pulls off the neuroretina, for example in the proliferative retinopathy of diabetes mellitus, it is termed a *tractional retinal detachment*.

- Rarely, fluid accumulates in the sub-retinal space as a result of an exudative process, which may occur with retinal tumours or during pregnancy-induced hypertension. This is an *exudative retinal detachment*.

Tears in the retina are most commonly associated with the onset of a posterior vitreous detachment. As the gel separates from the retina, the traction it exerts (*vitreous traction*) may become localized and may be sufficient to tear the retina. An underlying peripheral weakness of the retina such as *lattice degeneration* increases the probability of a tear.

Rhegmatogenous retinal detachment

Epidemiology

About 1 in 10,000 of the normal population will suffer a rhegmatogenous retinal detachment (Figure 12.8). The risk is greater in patients who:

- are high myopes;
- have undergone cataract surgery, particularly if this was complicated by vitreous loss;
- have experienced a detached retina in the fellow eye;
- have been subjected to recent severe eye trauma.

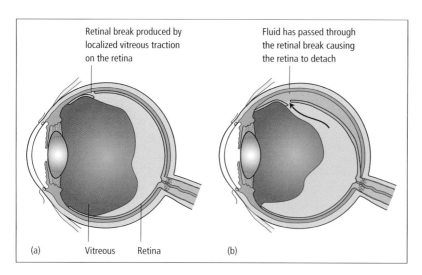

Retinal break produced by localized vitreous traction on the retina

Fluid has passed through the retinal break causing the retina to detach

(a)   Vitreous   Retina   (b)

Figure 12.8 The formation of a rhegmatogenous retinal detachment. (a) The detaching vitreous has torn the retina; the vitreous continues to pull on the retina surrounding the break (vitreous traction). (b) Fluid from the vitreous cavity passes through the break, detaching the neuroretina from the underlying retinal pigment epithelium.

Symptoms

Retinal detachment may be preceded by symptoms of a posterior vitreous detachment, where this has given rise to a retinal hole, including floaters and flashing lights. With the onset of the retinal detachment itself, the patient notices the progressive development of a field defect, often described as a 'shadow' or 'curtain', present at a location opposite to that of the detachment itself – an inferior detachment gives rise to an upper field defect. Progression may be rapid when a superior detachment is present. If the macula becomes detached, there is a marked fall in visual acuity.

Signs

The detached retina is visible on ophthalmoscopy as a floating, diaphanous membrane which partly obscures choroidal vascular detail. If there is a marked accumulation of fluid in the sub-retinal space (a *bullous retinal detachment*), undulating movements of the retina will be observed as the eye moves. A tear in the retina appears reddish pink because of the unobscured view of the underlying choroidal vessels. There may be associated debris in the vitreous comprising blood (*vitreous haemorrhage*) and pigment, or the free-floating lid (*operculum*) of a retinal hole (Figure 12.9).

Management

There are two major surgical techniques for repairing a retinal detachment (Figure 12.10):

1 External (*conventional approach*)
2 Internal (*vitreoretinal surgery*)

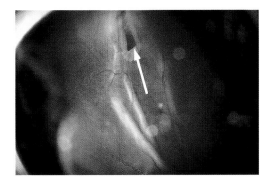

Figure 12.9 The clinical appearance of a retinal detachment. Note the retinal tear (arrowed). The retina has completely detached.

The essential principle behind both techniques is to close the causative break in the retina and to increase the strength of attachment between the surrounding retina and the RPE by inducing inflammation in the region, either by local freezing with a cryoprobe or with a laser. In the external approach, the break is closed by indenting the sclera with an externally located strip of silicone sponge (or plomb). This relieves the vitreous traction on the retinal hole and apposes the RPE to the retina. It may first be necessary to drain an extensive accumulation of sub-retinal fluid by piercing the sclera and choroid with a needle (*sclerostomy*).

In the internal approach, now often the treatment of choice, the vitreous is removed with a microsurgical cutter introduced into the vitreous cavity through the pars plana. This relieves the vitreous traction on the break. Subretinal fluid within the detachment can then be drained through the causative retinal break itself, to reduce the volume of the detachment and laser or cryotherapy applied to the surrounding retina. A temporary internal tamponade is then achieved by injecting an inert, slowly absorbed *fluorocarbon gas* into the vitreous cavity. This has the effect of closing the hole from the inside. Further passage of fluid through the break is thus prevented while the inflammation caused by the laser or cryotherapy securely seals the neuroretina surrounding the hole to the underlying layers. The patient has to maintain a particular head posture for a few days to ensure that the bubble covers the retinal break continuously. Air travel *must be avoided* while the gas is in place because, at the reduced barometric pressure, gas expansion can cause complications such as glaucoma.

Retinal tears unassociated with sub-retinal fluid are treated prophylactically with a laser or cryoprobe to induce inflammation and increase the adhesion between the neuroretina surrounding the tear and the pigment epithelium, thus preventing a retinal detachment. It is always important to check the peripheral retina in the fellow eye, as tears or an asymptomatic retinal detachment may be present here too.

Prognosis

If surgery successfully reattaches the peripheral retina and the macula is attached, the outlook for vision is excellent. If the macula is detached for more than 24 hours prior to surgery, the previous visual acuity will probably not recover completely. Nonetheless, a substantial part of the vision may be restored over several months. If the retina is not successfully attached and the surgery is complicated, then fibrotic changes may occur in the

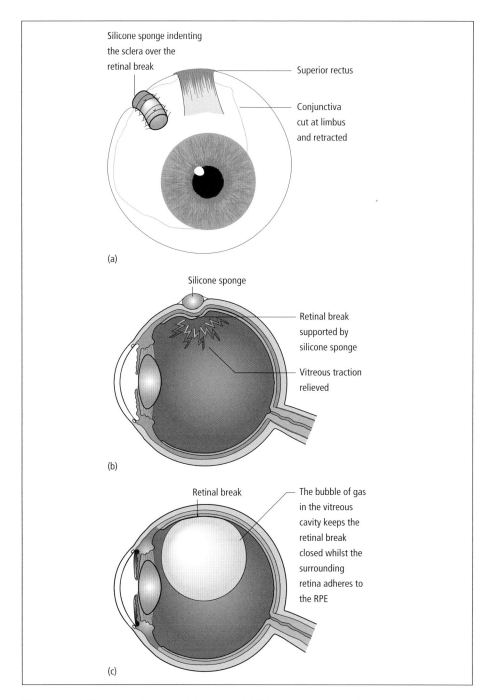

Figure 12.10 The repair of a retinal detachment. (a) External approach: a silicone sponge has been sutured to the globe to indent the sclera over the retinal break following drainage of the sub-retinal fluid and application of cryotherapy. (b) Sagittal section of the eye showing the indent formed by the silicone sponge: the retina is now reattached and traction on the retinal break by the vitreous is relieved. (c) Internal approach: following removal of the vitreous gel and drainage of sub-retinal fluid an inert fluorocarbon gas has been injected into the vitreous cavity.

vitreous (*proliferative vitreoretinopathy, PVR*), which may cause traction on the retina and further retinal detachment. A complex vitreoretinal procedure may yet permit vision to be retained, but the outlook for vision is much poorer.

Tractional retinal detachment

The neuroretina is pulled away from the pigment epithelium by contracting fibrous tissue which has grown on the retinal surface. This may be seen in *proliferative diabetic retinopathy* or may occur as a result of PVR. Vitreoretinal surgery, requiring excision of the contracting bands, is required to repair these detachments. In these cases, it may be necessary to inject silicone oil into the vitreous cavity, temporarily, to hold the retina in place.

Retinoschisis

In retinoschisis, the retina splits into an inner and outer leaf at the outer plexiform and inner nuclear junction. It is usually seen in the lower temporal quadrant of the retina and is often bilateral. The appearance is not dissimilar to a retinal detachment. Rarely, it may cause a retinal detachment when there are holes in both the inner and outer retinal leaves. These patients may require surgery.

Inherited retinal and photoreceptor dystrophies

Retinitis pigmentosa

Retinitis pigmentosa is an inherited disorder of the photoreceptors which has several genotypic and phenotypic varieties. It may occur in isolation or in association with a number of other systemic diseases, such as Usher syndrome, abetalipoproteinaemia and Laurence–Moon syndrome.

Pathogenesis

The disease affects both types of photoreceptors, but the rods are particularly affected. The inheritance may be:

- autosomal recessive (sporadic cases are often in this category);
- autosomal dominant;
- X-linked recessive.

Several forms of retinitis pigmentosa have been shown to be due to mutations in the gene for visual pigment *rhodopsin.*

Epidemiology

The prevalence of this group of diseases is 1 in 4000.

Symptoms

The age of onset, progression and prognosis are dependent on the mode of inheritance. In general, the dominant form is of later onset and milder degree, while recessive and X-linked recessive forms may present in infancy or childhood. Patients notice poor night vision, visual fields become increasingly constricted and central vision may ultimately be lost.

Signs

The three signs of typical retinitis pigmentosa (Figure 12.11) are:

1 peripheral clumps of retinal pigmentation (termed 'bone spicule' pigmentation);
2 attenuation of the retinal arterioles;
3 disc pallor – optic atrophy.

Patients may also have cataracts at an early age and may develop macular oedema.

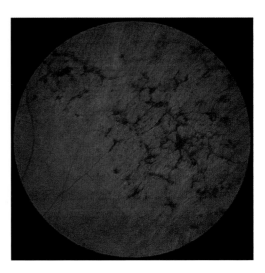

Figure 12.11 The clinical appearance of the peripheral retina in retinitis pigmentosa.

Investigation

A careful family history will help to determine the mode of inheritance (Chapter 2). The diagnosis can usually be made clinically. Electrophysiological tests are also useful in diagnosis. The electroretinogram (ERG) response may be lost early in the disease, when there may be few clinical signs.

Recent work on mapping the genetic loci for the condition has opened new avenues for genetic counselling and determining disease mechanisms.

The possibility of associated syndromes should be borne in mind. Usher syndrome, for example, is a recessive disorder characterized by deafness and retinitis pigmentosa. Retinitis pigmentosa also occurs in mitochondrial disease.

Management

Unfortunately, nothing can be done to prevent the progression of the disease, although there may be possibilities of gene therapy in the future. Associated ocular problems can be treated. Cataracts can be removed, and macular oedema may respond to treatment with acetazolamide. Low-vision aids may be helpful for a period. The possibility of genetic counselling should be discussed with the patient.

Prognosis

X-linked recessive and autosomal recessive disease produce the most severe visual symptoms. About 50% of all patients with retinitis pigmentosa will have an acuity of less than 6/60 by the time they reach 50.

Cone dystrophy

This is less common than retinitis pigmentosa. It is usually autosomal dominant, but many cases are sporadic. Patients present in the first decade of life with poor vision. Examination reveals an abnormal, banded macular appearance which has been likened to a bull's-eye target. No treatment is possible but it is important to provide appropriate help, not only to maximize vision but also to help with educational problems. Genetic counselling should be offered.

Juvenile macular dystrophies

There are a variety of inherited conditions that affect both the RPE and, secondarily, the photoreceptors. All are rare (e.g. the recessive disorder *Stargardt*

dystrophy) and the prognosis for vision is often poor. Once again the social and educational needs of the patient need to be assessed and genetic counselling offered.

Albinism

These patients have defective melanin synthesis. There are two types:

1 *Ocular albinism*, where the lack of pigmentation is confined to the eye. This is X-linked and nearly all of the affected individuals are thus male.
2 *Oculocutaneous albinism*, a recessive disorder where the hair is white and the skin is pale; a few of these patients can manufacture some melanin. There is an autosomal recessive defect in either the enzyme tyrosinase (gene on chromosome 11) or proteins associated with the normal functioning of the enzyme (gene on chromosomes 5, 9 and 15).

Clinically, the iris is blue and there is marked transillumination so that the red reflex is seen through the iris because of the lack of pigmentation (Figure 12.12); this also allows the lens edge to be viewed in silhouette through the iris. The fundus appears abnormal, with lack of a normal foveal reflex, extreme pallor and prominent visibility of the choroidal vessels. There is macular dysfunction and an abnormal projection of retinal axons to the lateral geniculate bodies. Vision is poor from birth and patients have nystagmus.

Some patients will have associated systemic disease (e.g. the Hermansky–Pudlak syndrome, where there is an associated haemorrhagic diathesis, caused by abnormal platelet function, lung and renal disease).

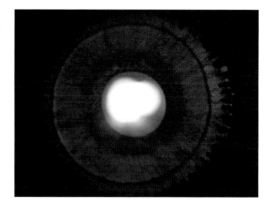

Figure 12.12 Note the transillumination of light reflected from the retina through the albino iris.

Retinal tumours

Retinoblastoma

Retinoblastoma is a malignant tumour arising from the developing retina, typically presenting in the first 2–3 years of life. Cure rates for intraocular retinoblastoma can be as high as 95%. Extraocular spread carries a very poor prognosis, with cure rates below 5–10%. Early diagnosis and prompt treatment is therefore crucial to save life and vision.

The incidence is 1 per 20,000 births. Retinoblastoma tumours result from loss of both copies of the Rb1 gene on chromosome 13. The Rb1 gene is a tumour suppressor gene whose product (pRB) plays a key role in the cell cycle as a negative regulator of cell proliferation. Mutations remove this anti-proliferative action, and predispose to cancer formation. Loss of one normal allele does not cause disease but results in an unstable genetic situation, and the second copy can be lost spontaneously (second hit) resulting in disease.

In somatic cases (60% of all cases), a single retinal cell loses one normal allele of the Rb1 gene during retinal development. Loss of the second normal allele results in disease which is always unilateral. Somatic cases cannot transmit disease to offspring.

In germline cases (40% of all cases), one copy of the Rb1 gene is defective (mutated) at the time of conception from a defective sperm or ovum, and every cell in the body has the defective gene. This can occur as a random event with unaffected parents (sporadic), or either parent might have undergone treatment for retinoblastoma and carry the defective gene, which is passed on to the offspring (inherited) in 50% of cases (autosomal dominant inheritance – see Chapter 2). Such cases can have unilateral or bilateral disease often with multiple tumours. They can genetically transmit the disease to their offspring and are also at risk of developing non-ocular second cancers (50% lifetime risk).

The chance of developing retinoblastoma in a child inheriting the genetic trait is 95% (high but incomplete penetrance – see Chapter 2). Thus, although it occurs frequently in affected families, there may be some unaffected individuals despite carrying the defective gene, and the disease might skip generations.

History

The child may present (at a mean age of 8 months if germline and 25 months if somatic) with:

- A white pupillary reflex (*leukocoria*) due to light scatter from the pale elevated tumour at the

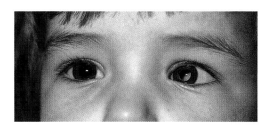

Figure 12.13 Left leucocoria.

posterior pole of the eye (Figure 12.13). Sometimes, the tumour is bilateral on presentation.
- A squint due to reduced vision.
- Occasionally, with advanced tumours, a painful red eye.

Most cases present by the age of 2 years. Inherited retinoblastoma is often bilateral. When the condition is unilateral on presentation and there is no family history, inherited disease is less likely, but not excluded.

Signs

Dilated fundoscopy shows a whitish-pink mass protruding from the retina into the vitreous cavity.

Investigations

The diagnosis is usually a clinical one. Ultrasound B scan exam of the eye confirms the presence of a mass lesion. Cerebrospinal fluid and bone marrow are examined to check for metastatic disease where extraocular spread is suspected.

Treatment

If the eye can be preserved, either cosmetically or functionally, systemic chemotherapy (and sometimes intra-arterial or intra-vitreal injection of chemotherapy) is used to shrink the tumours, along with local treatment such as laser or cryotherapy to eliminate residual tumour. Cryotherapy involves killing the tumour in a series of freeze-thaw cycles applied across the sclera using an externally applied cryoprobe. Laser (thermotherapy) is applied through a dilated pupil to ablate the retinal tumour. Removal (enucleation) of the eye is performed in advanced cases. Radiotherapy is rarely used nowadays. Metastatic disease (either by direct spread through the optic nerve or by a haematogenous route) is treated with high-dose chemotherapy. Regular follow-up and examination of the fellow eye of an affected child is required. Genetic counselling should be offered, and children with a parent who has had a retinoblastoma should be assessed from infancy, shortly after birth. It is possible to detect the mutation by molecular techniques.

Prognosis

This depends on the extent of the disease at diagnosis. Overall, the mortality of the condition is <2% in developed countries, but as high as 50% in some developing countries. Unfortunately, 50% of children with the germinal mutation will develop a second primary tumour (e.g. an osteosarcoma of the femur) or a tumour related to treatment with radiotherapy.

Astrocytomas

These tumours of the retina and optic nerve (Figure 12.14) are seen in patients with certain dominantly inherited systemic disorders:

- tuberous sclerosis;
- neurofibromatosis (less commonly).

They appear as white mulberry-like lesions, are seldom symptomatic and require no treatment. However, their identification may assist in the diagnosis of these important systemic diseases.

Choroidal lesions, including melanoma

Pigmented fundus lesions include:

- areas of old chorioretinitis;
- choroidal naevi;

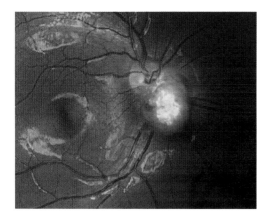

Figure 12.14 The clinical appearance of a retinal astrocytoma.

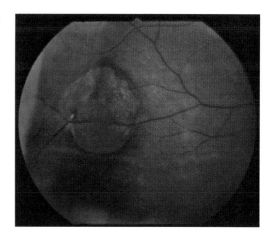

Figure 12.15 The appearance of CHRPE.

- congenital hypertrophy of the retinal pigment epithelium (CHRPE);
- the rarest disorder, malignant melanoma, which has serious implications for life.

CHRPE lesions are darker with better-defined edges than choroidal naevi (Figure 12.15); multiple lesions, changes in both eyes, or lesions with a *comet tail* appearance (Figure 12.16a) may be associated with familial polyposis coli and associated colon cancer and require investigation for this.

Uveal melanomas have an incidence of 6 per million per year in white adults. It is seen very much more commonly in white than in non-white races. It usually presents from middle age onwards (40–70 years). Malignant melanoma may also be seen in the ciliary body and iris, but by far the greatest number are found in the choroid.

Symptoms

The presence of a melanoma may be detected as a coincidental finding during ocular examination (Figure 12.16b, compare to a, CHRPE lesion). Advanced cases may present with a visual field defect or loss of acuity. If situated in the anterior part of the choroid, the enlarging tumour may cause shallowing of the anterior chamber, resulting in secondary angle closure glaucoma. In developed countries, it is unusual for the tumour to be so advanced that it presents with visible destruction of the eye.

Signs

A raised, usually pigmented, lesion is visible at the back of the eye, which may be associated with an area of retinal detachment. The optic nerve may be involved.

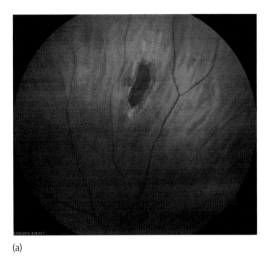
(a)

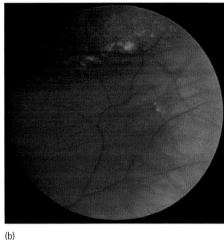
(b)

Figure 12.16 (a) The comet tail appearance of a CHRPE lesion. (b) The clinical appearance of a choroidal melanoma. (*Source:* Courtesy of Kevin Falzon.)

Investigations

The patient is investigated for systemic spread, although this is less usual than in malignant melanoma of the skin. An ultrasound scan of the eye is useful in determining the size of the tumour and can be used both for quantitative assessment and to detect tumour growth over time. Fundus photography is used in follow-up, in the same way. If biopsy or excision is performed, karyotyping is undertaken. Monosomy 3 (partial deletion of the short arm of chromosome 3) is associated with more aggressive tumours and a poor prognosis.

Treatment

A number of therapies are available. The treatment used depends on the size and location of the tumour. Large tumours that have reduced vision, or that are close to the optic nerve, usually require removal of the eye (*enucleation*). Smaller tumours can be treated by:

- local excision;
- local radiation applied to the lesion by an overlying radioactive plaque;
- proton beam irradiation;
- immunotherapy.

Prognosis

This depends very much on the type of tumour (some are more rapidly growing than others) and its location (tumours involving the sclera and optic nerve carry a poorer prognosis). The existence of metastatic lesions at the time of diagnosis carries a poor prognosis.

Some tumours are very slow-growing and have an excellent prognosis. Others, which extend into the optic nerve or through the sclera, are more malignant and result in secondary spread.

Metastatic tumours

These account for the greater part of ocular malignant disease. In women, the commonest site of spread is from the breast; in men, the commonest source is the lung. Symptoms and signs depend on their location in the eye. They appear as a whitish lesion with little elevation, and may be multiple. Treatment is usually by external beam radiotherapy.

🔑 KEY POINTS

- A curtain-like partial loss of vision suggests a retinal detachment and requires urgent ophthalmic assessment.
- Distortion of vision is a sign of macular disease.
- AMD results in loss of acuity but never total loss of vision.
- Leucocoria in a child requires immediate investigation; it may be a sign of retinoblastoma.
- Poor night vision may be a sign of retinitis pigmentosa.

Assessment questions
True or False

1. **Match the symptoms with the likely abnormal part of the retina.**

a Distortion of vision (metamorphopsia).
b Loss of superior visual field.
c Difficulty seeing at night.
   i. The inferior half of the retina.
   ii. The macula.
   iii. The rods.
   iv. The cones.

2. **Age related macular degeneration (AMD)**

a Is the commonest cause of irreversible visual loss in the developed world.
b Is associated with disease of the RPE.
c May be associated with the growth of sub-retinal blood vessels.
d Is caused by a hole forming at the macula.
e The 'dry' type is commonly treated with surgery.

3. **Match the pictures (Figure 12.17) with the diagnoses.**

a AMD.
b Macular hole.
c Retinal detachment.
d Melanoma.
e Retinitis pigmentosa.

4. **Macular oedema**

a Relates to the accumulation of fluid within the macula.
b Causes blurring of vision.
c May be seen following intraocular surgery.
d Is usually associated with the growth of abnormal vessels in the retina.
e Can be treated with steroids.

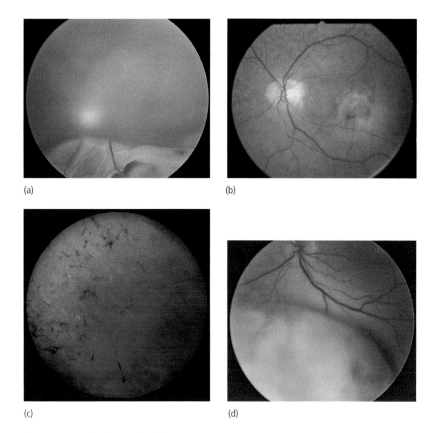

(a)   (b)

(c)   (d)

Figure 12.17 (a–d) See Question 3.

5. **A patient presents with a history of 3 days of floaters, flashing lights and then a dense, curtain-like field loss.**

a   The most likely diagnosis is a retinal vein occlusion.
b   The most likely diagnosis is a retinal detachment.
c   The most likely diagnosis is a posterior vitreous detachment.
d   The patient needs urgent referral to an eye unit.
e   The vision will settle with no intervention.

6. **A 1-year-old child presents with a squint. The doctor notices that the red reflex appears white.**

a   A white pupillary reflex is a normal finding in a child of this age.
b   The child may have a retinoblastoma.
c   The child has albinism.
d   Urgent referral is required.
e   The other eye needs to be assessed.

Answers

1. **Match the symptoms with the likely abnormal part of the retina.**

a   The macula.
b   The inferior half of the retina.
c   The rods.

2. **Age-related macular degeneration (AMD)**

a   True.
b   True. This is a disease of the RPE.
c   True. This is the cause of 'wet' or exudative macular degeneration.
d   False. That is a separate condition, called a macular hole.
e   False. Dry macular degeneration is untreatable. In patients with wet macular degeneration, intravitreal anti-VEGF treatment, and rarely retinal surgery, may prevent visual deterioration.

3. **Match the pictures (Figure 12.15) with the diagnoses.**

a   A retinal detachment.
b   AMD.
c   Retinitis pigmentosa.
d   Melanoma.

4. **Macular oedema**

a   True. See Figure 12.5.
b   True. Visual acuity is affected in macular oedema.
c   True. It may be seen after cataract and other intraocular surgery.
d   False. It is the accumulation of fluid within the retina, there is no associated growth of blood vessels as is seen in exudative AMD.
e   True. Steroids may be given topically but sub-Tenon's injection or intravitreal injection may be required.

5. **A patient presents with a history of 3 days of floaters, flashing lights and then a dense, curtain-like field loss.**

a   False. These are the classical symptoms of a retinal detachment, patients with a retinal vein occlusion would not usually have flashes and floaters.
b   True. These are indeed the classical symptoms.
c   False. Although the symptoms of flashes and floaters suggest a posterior vitreous detachment, the field loss indicates that a hole has been torn in the retina, causing a retinal detachment.
d   True. Surgery will be required to reattach the retina.
e   False. The patient will lose the vision in the eye if urgent treatment is not given.

6. **A 1-year-old child presents with a squint. The doctor notices that the red reflex appears white.**

a   False. Leucocoria always requires urgent examination and investigation. Retinoblastoma is a life-threatening possibility.
b   True. This is a presentation of retinoblastoma.
c   False. The red reflex would be present.
d   True. If there is any doubt that a red reflex is present the child requires urgent ophthalmic assessment.
e   True. Retinoblastoma may be bilateral.

13

Retinal vascular disease

Learning objectives

To understand:

✔ The features of retinal vascular disease.
✔ The classification and treatment of diabetic retinopathy.
✔ The symptoms, signs and complications of retinal arterial and venous occlusion.
✔ The causes, features and treatment of retinopathy of prematurity.

Introduction

The eye is an organ in which much of the microcirculation is readily observed. Vascular disease affecting the eye can thus be seen directly. Furthermore, the eye provides important clues about pathological vascular changes in the rest of the body.

Signs of retinal vascular disease

The signs of retinal vascular disease (Figures 13.1 and 13.2) result from two changes to the retinal capillary microcirculation:

- vascular leakage.
- vascular occlusion.

Leakage from the microcirculation

This results in (Figure 13.2a):

- *microaneurysms:* dilations of the retinal capillaries, seen as small red dots in the retina;

- *haemorrhages:* depending on size, shape and depth in the retina these are termed dot, blot, and, flame-shaped. Haemorrhages (dot and larger blot) caused by leakage of blood from damaged vessels. The flame-shaped haemorrhages arise in the nerve fibre layer which is responsible for the pattern;
- *oedema* of the retina, the result of fluid leakage from damaged vessels;
- *exudates:* formed by lipids, lipoprotein and lipid-containing macrophages – these are yellow in colour, with well-defined margins. May form in a circular (*circinate*) pattern around the leaking vessel.

> ### Classification of diseases affecting the ocular circulation
>
> Diabetic retinopathy
> Central retinal artery occlusion
> Branch retinal artery occlusion
> Central retinal vein occlusion
> Branch retinal vein occlusion
> Hypertensive retinopathy
> Retinopathy of prematurity
> Sickle-cell retinopathy
> Abnormal retinal blood vessels

Ophthalmology: Lecture Notes, Thirteenth Edition. Bruce James, Anthony Bron, and Manoj V. Parulekar.
© 2024 John Wiley & Sons Ltd. Published 2024 by John Wiley & Sons Ltd.
Companion website: www.wiley.com/go/ophthalmology13e

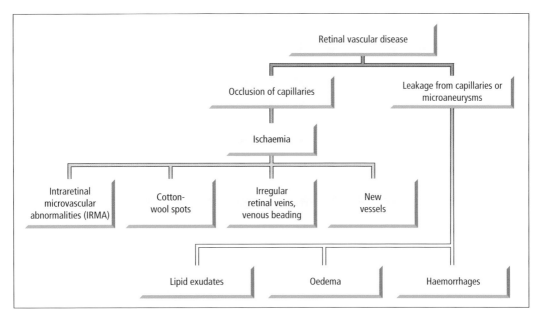

Figure 13.1 The building blocks of retinal vascular disease. Capillary leakage and occlusion often occur together.

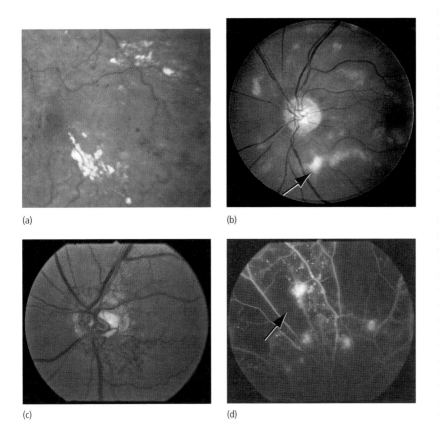

(a)

(b)

(c)

(d)

Figure 13.2 The signs of retinal vascular disease: (a) microaneurysms (seen as small red dots), haemorrhage and exudate; (b) cotton-wool spots; note the yellowish nature and distinct margins of the exudates compared to the less distinct and whiter appearance of the cotton-wool spots (example arrowed); (c) new vessels; here particularly florid and arising on the disc, note also the venous beading: (d) this fluorescein angiogram shows the vascular architecture and demonstrates absent filling of the retinal capillary circulation (dark areas (arrow)). The bright, hazy areas indicate leakage from the new vessels.

Occlusion of the microcirculation

Results in:

- *Cotton-wool spots:* fluffy white focal lesions with indistinct margins, previously termed *soft exudates.* They occur at the margins of an ischaemic retinal infarct due to obstruction of axoplasmic flow and *a build-up of axonal debris in the nerve fibre layer* of the retina. Their visibility depends on nerve fibre layer thickness at that site, so that they are readily seen close to the optic disc, where the nerve fibre layer is thick but not in the periphery, where the nerve fibre layer is thin (Figure 13.2b). They are white in colour because the accumulated axoplasmic particles scatter light, whereas the normal nerve fibre is transparent.
- *New vessels:* Retinal ischaemia releases angiogenic factors, such as VEGF which stimulate the growth of abnormal blood vessels and fibrous tissue onto the retinal surface and forwards into the vitreous. These new vessels are much more permeable than normal retinal vessels, so that they leak dye during retinal fluorescein angiography (Figure 13.2c,d). Their abnormal location predisposes them to break and bleed.
- *Intraretinal microvascular abnormalities (IRMA),* a possible precursor of new vessels. Their presence indicates a risk of progression to proliferative retinopathy. They lie deeper in the retina *between* retinal arterioles and veins and appear as small tortuous spidery vessels, varying in calibre but generally thicker than new vessels and do not grow into the vitreous. They do not leak fluorescein on angiography.
- *Venous beading*, where the diameter of the vein varies intermittently along its length (Figure 13.2c).

Diabetic retinopathy

Diabetes results from a defect in both insulin secretion and action, leading to hyperglycaemia.

Epidemiology

The number of people with diabetes is rising. It is estimated that 438 million people worldwide will have diabetes by 2030. Diabetic eye disease was previously the commonest reason for blind registration in the United Kingdom, in the 30–65 age group. It is now the second commonest cause in this group, below inherited retinal disorders. This may reflect the success of the diabetic screening programme and better glycaemic control.

Type I diabetes (10% of all diabetes) is due to loss of insulin secretion, mostly in young people with particular HLA types. The prevalence in England and Wales is 1.5 per 1000 under the age of 15. The peak age for diagnosis is between 10 and 14 years old. Onset is relatively acute and diabetic retinopathy begins to appear *about 5 years after onset.*

Type II diabetes (90% of all diabetes) occurs in a heterogeneous group of patients and shows a familial bias. Patients usually retain some insulin secretion but develop resistance to its actions. It occurs in an older age group (although is increasingly being seen in younger, overweight people). As type II diabetes may be present for several years prior to diagnosis, retinopathy may be found at presentation and its duration may be unknown.

Within 5 years of diagnosis, 25% of all patients with any type of diabetes will have some form of non-proliferative retinopathy, this rises to 80% at 15 years. Proliferative disease is present in 2% of diabetics at 5 years rising to 15.5% in those who have had diabetes for 15 years or more.

Diabetes is associated with the following ocular events:

- retinopathy;
- cataract: a rare, acute 'snowflake' cataract in youth related to extreme fluctuation in glucose levels, and a greater frequency and earlier onset of age-related cataract;
- glaucoma (neovascular glaucoma and also an association with chronic open-angle glaucoma);
- extraocular muscle palsy due to microvascular disease of the third, fourth or sixth cranial nerves;
- diabetic papillitis.

Pathology

Factors thought to be important in the development of diabetic retinopathy include:

- duration of diabetes;
- poor diabetic control;
- coexisting diseases, particularly hypertension;
- smoking.

The development of retinopathy may also be accelerated by pregnancy, and pregnant patients require careful screening.

Retinal damage results from the vascular pathology, i.e.:

- a decrease in the number of pericytes surrounding the capillary endothelium;

- development of microaneurysms on the capillary network which allow plasma to leak into the retina;
- patchy closure of the capillary network (Figure 13.2d), resulting in capillary non-perfusion, areas of ischaemic retina and the development of arteriovenous shunts (*intraretinal microvascular abnormalities, IRMA*).

History

Diabetic retinopathy should be diagnosed before it becomes symptomatic. All diabetics should have fundoscopy performed at least yearly. Screening for sight-threatening retinopathy (maculopathy and proliferative retinopathy) should begin from 5 years after diagnosis in patients with type I disease, and from the time of presentation in type II diabetes, since its time of onset is unknown. Visual acuity may be reduced gradually by a maculopathy, or suddenly by a vitreous haemorrhage.

Examination

Essentially, visual loss occurs because of severe retinopathy or macular disease. The building blocks of the disease are those of leakage and microvascular occlusion, discussed earlier. The classification of retinopathy is shown in Table 13.1. In the United Kingdom, a separate classification system has been developed for use by the screening service (Table 13.2). This is based on the degree of retinopathy (R1–3) and the presence of maculopathy (M 0 or 1).

Screening

In the United Kingdom, a screening programme using digital retinal photography is employed to review patients on a yearly basis from the age of 12 (more frequently in pregnancy). Patients with a maculopathy, preproliferative or proliferative retinopathy or worse

Table 13.2 The classification of diabetic retinopathy used by the screening service in the United Kingdom.

The grading levels

R Grade	Retinopathy level
Level R0	No retinopathy
Level R1	Background retinopathy
Level R2	Pre-proliferative retinopathy
Level R3A	Active proliferative retinopathy
Level R3S	Stable treated proliferative retinopathy
P1	Evidence of laser photocoagulation
U	Unassessable

M Grade	Maculopathy level
M0	No maculopathy
M1	Maculopathy

Table 13.1 The classification of diabetic retinopathy.

Stage of retinopathy	Description
No retinopathy	There are no abnormal signs present on the retina. *Vision is normal*
Background retinopathy	The earliest and mildest form of retinopathy. Signs of microvascular leakage – microaneurysms, haemorrhage and exudates away from the macula. *Vision is normal*
Maculopathy	Exudates and haemorrhages within the macular region, and/or evidence of retinal oedema, and/or evidence of retinal ischaemia within the macula. *Vision is reduced; sight-threatening*
Preproliferative retinopathy	Evidence of arteriolar occlusions (IRMA, cotton-wool spots). The veins become irregular and may show loops. *Vision is normal*
Proliferative retinopathy	The occlusive changes have led to the release of a vasoproliferative substance from the retina (e.g. VEGF), resulting in the growth of new vessels either on the disc (NVD) or elsewhere on the retina (NVE). *Vision is normal but this is sight-threatening*
Advanced retinopathy	The proliferative changes may result in bleeding into the vitreous or between the vitreous and the retina. The neuroretina may also be pulled from its overlying pigment epithelium by a fibrous proliferation associated with the growth of the new vessels. *Vision is reduced, often acutely, with vitreous haemorrhage. This is a sight-threatening retinopathy*

Note that diabetic maculopathy may coexist with other stages in the classification.

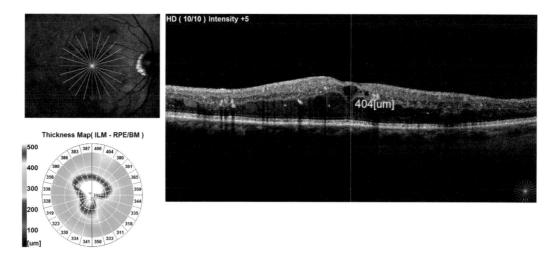

Figure 13.3 An OCT scan showing diabetic macular oedema. Note the cystic spaces in the retina demonstrating the accumulation of fluid on the greyscale picture on the right. The coloured circle represents the thickness of the macula as a contour map. Note the significant thickening in the central foveal region shown as white.

(Figure 13.4a–f) require referral to an ophthalmologist. Any patient with unexplained visual loss should also be referred.

Investigation

For patients with significant disease, an OCT scan of the macula is usually performed to determine if macular oedema is present (Figure 13.3). A fluorescein angiogram (Figure 13.4e) may be performed in some patients to assess the degree of retinal ischaemia and to pinpoint areas of leakage both from microaneurysms and new vessels. OCT angiograms (OCTA) can now also be used to analyse the retinal circulation non-invasively without injection of fluorescein dye.

Treatment

The mainstay of treatment for sight-threatening diabetic retinopathy is laser therapy, although anti-VEGF and steroids injections are playing an increasing part in the treatment of diabetic macular oedema.

Diabetic retinopathy: clinical observations

- Younger patients are more likely to develop proliferative disease.
- Older patients more commonly develop a maculopathy, but because type II disease is more common than type I, it is also an important cause of proliferative disease.

Laser treatment of both the maculopathy and new vessels can be performed on an outpatient basis.

- Diabetic maculopathy is treated by aiming the laser at the points of leakage. The exudate is often seen to be in a circular or circinate pattern, with the focus of leakage or a microaneurysm in the middle. If treatment is effective, the retinal oedema and exudate will resorb, although this may take some months. Increasing use of anti-VEGF injections has reduced the role of laser in the management of diabetic maculopathy.
- Optic disc and retinal new vessels are treated with scattered laser burns to the entire retina (panretinal laser or PRP), leaving an untreated area around the optic disc and around the central region of the macula, to preserve vision (Figure 13.5). The laser treatment ablates areas of ischaemic retina, thus reducing the release of vasoproliferative factors from the retina as a whole. This results in the regression of the new vessels and prevents the development of advanced retinopathy. Such extensive laser treatment affects the visual field, but preserves central vision.

Intravitreal anti-VEGF and steroid treatment

Recently, intravitreal anti-VEGF drugs and more rarely, steroid drugs (in pseudophakic patients), have been found to be beneficial in reducing macular oedema, particularly when it is diffuse or involves the

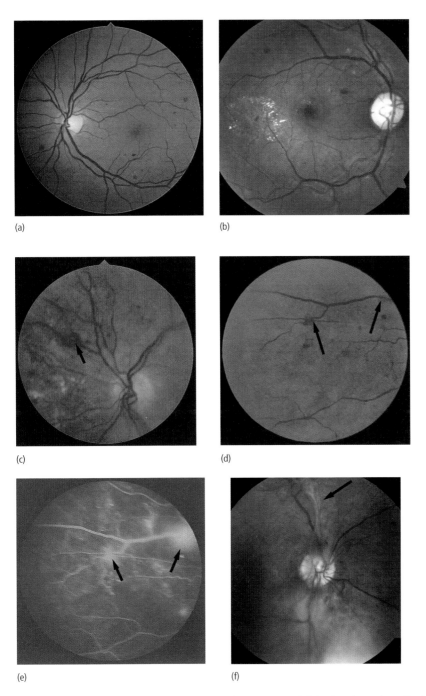

(a)

(b)

(c)

(d)

(e)

(f)

Figure 13.4 The signs of diabetic eye disease. (a) Background diabetic retinopathy, with dot (microaneurysms) and blot haemorrhages away from the macula. (b) Diabetic maculopathy: note the circinate exudate, temporal to the macula. (c) Preproliferative retinopathy with a venous loop (arrow). (d, e) Proliferative retinopathy: new vessels have formed on the retina, their presence demonstrated by leakage of fluorescein (hyperfluorescence) on the fluorescein angiogram; closure of some of the retinal capillary network is demonstrated by its failure to fill with fluorescein (dark appearance on the angiogram). (f) Advanced diabetic retinopathy: the neovascularization has caused a tractional retinal detachment superiorly.

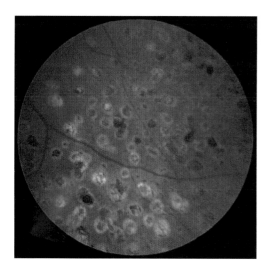

Figure 13.5 Typical appearance of retinal laser burns.

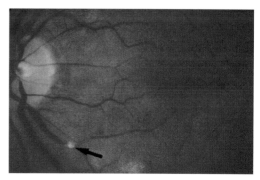

Figure 13.6 The clinical appearance of a cholesterol embolus (arrow). They appear to sparkle when viewed with a direct ophthalmoscope.

fovea. In the United Kingdom, NICE have issued guidelines based on visual acuity and the thickness of the macula (measured on an OCT scan, Figure 13.3) to identify those who will benefit most from anti-VEGF treatment.

Surgery

The development of a vitreous haemorrhage which does not clear quickly, or fibrous traction on the retina causing detachment from the overlying pigment epithelium (tractional retinal detachment), may require surgical treatment. A vitrectomy is performed to remove the vitreous gel and blood and to repair and reattach any detached retina.

Prognosis

Although laser, medical and surgical treatments have greatly improved the prognosis of patients with diabetic retinopathy, the disease may still progress and cause severe visual loss in some patients, potentially leading to blindness.

Arterial occlusion

Pathogenesis

Central and branch retinal artery occlusions are usually embolic in origin. Three types of emboli are recognized:

1 *fibrin–platelet* emboli, commonly from diseased carotid arteries;
2 *cholesterol* emboli, commonly from diseased carotid arteries (Figure 13.6);
3 *calcific* emboli, from diseased heart valves.

History

The patient complains of a sudden painless loss of all or part of the vision. Fibrin–platelet emboli typically cause a fleeting loss of vision as the emboli pass through the retinal circulation (*amaurosis fugax*). This may last for some minutes and then clear. Cholesterol and calcific emboli may result in permanent obstruction with no recovery in vision, although they may also be seen in the retinal vessels of asymptomatic individuals. A central retinal artery obstruction causes ischaemia of the whole retina. It is frequently caused by an embolus, but as it lodges further back in the arterial tree, behind the optic nerve head, it cannot be seen.

Signs

Occasionally, a series of white platelet emboli can be seen passing rapidly through a vessel. More often, a bright yellow, reflective cholesterol embolus is noted, occluding an arterial branch point (Figure 13.6). After a central retinal artery occlusion, the whole retina becomes acutely swollen and white (oedematous (Figure 13.7a)) except at the fovea, which appears as a *cherry-red spot*, because the vascular choroid can be seen through the thin retina at this location. After several weeks, the disc becomes atrophic and white and the arterioles attenuated. The condition may also occasionally be caused by vasculitis of the ophthalmic artery, such as giant cell arteritis (see Chapter 15).

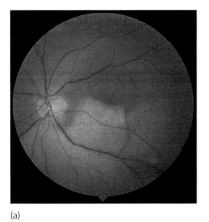

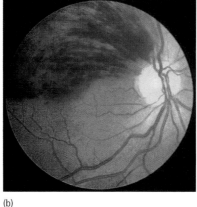

(a)   (b)

Figure 13.7 The contrast between: (a) an inferior branch retinal artery occlusion with a white, oedematous retina below, and (b) a superior branch vein occlusion, with diffuse haemorrhage above.

Investigation

Patients require *an urgent,* careful vascular workup, since disease in the eye may reflect systemic vascular disease and an increased risk of stroke. A search for carotid artery disease should be made by assessing the strength of carotid pulsation and listening for bruits. The presence of ischaemic heart disease, peripheral claudication, hypertension, diabetes and high cholesterol may also be relevant. Doppler ultrasound or magnetic resonance angiography will permit imaging of the carotid arteries. An ESR and CRP should be performed if giant cell arteritis is suspected.

Treatment

Acute treatment of central and branch artery occlusions is aimed at dilating the arteriole to permit the embolus to pass more distally and limit the damage. Results are usually disappointing, although a trial is worthwhile if the patient is seen within 24 hours of onset of the obstruction. The patient is referred to an eye unit, where the following measures may be tried:

- lowering the intraocular pressure with intravenous acetazolamide;
- ocular massage;
- paracentesis (a needle is inserted into the anterior chamber to release aqueous and lower the intraocular pressure rapidly);
- asking the patient to rebreathe into a paper bag firmly applied around the mouth and nose to use the vasodilatory effect of raised carbon dioxide levels.

Systemic treatment

A carotid endarterectomy may be indicated to prevent the possibility of a cerebral embolus if a stenosis of the carotid artery greater than 75% is present. Patients may also benefit from immediate anticoagulant or antiplatelet treatment (e.g. aspirin) if not contraindicated.

Prognosis

Full visual recovery occurs with amaurosis fugax, but more prolonged arterial occlusion results in severe, unrecoverable visual loss.

Venous occlusion

Pathogenesis

Central retinal vein occlusion (CRVO) and branch retinal vein occlusion (BRVO) may result from:

- abnormality of the blood itself (the hyperviscosity syndromes and abnormalities in coagulation);
- an abnormality of the venous wall (inflammation);
- an increased ocular pressure;

There is an association with:

- hypertension;
- hyperlipidaemia;
- diabetes.

History

The patient complains of a sudden partial or complete loss of vision, usually with a slower onset than retinal artery occlusion.

Signs

These contrast markedly with those of arterial occlusion (Figure 13.7b). There is marked retinal haemorrhage and great tortuosity and swelling of the veins. The optic disc appears engorged and swollen. BRVO may originate at the crossing point of an arteriole and a vein, at the site of A/V nipping, where the arteriole has been affected by hypertensive arteriosclerosis.

Subsequently, in an ischaemic retinal vein occlusion, where retinal ischaemia is extensive:

- Abnormal new vessels may grow onto the retina and optic disc, causing vitreous haemorrhage.
- New vessels may grow onto the iris, causing neovascular (*rubeotic*) glaucoma.

Paradoxically, the incidence of retinal neovascularization is greater in CRVO than CRAO, even though the ischaemia is partial in CRVO and more complete in CRAO. This is because the partially ischaemic, functioning retina following CRVO produces more angiogenic factors such as VEGF than a completely ischaemic retina seen in CRAO.

Investigation

Investigation of a CRVO includes a vascular workup and haematological tests to exclude increased blood viscosity. CRVO is also associated with raised ocular pressure, diabetes, hypertension, hyperlidaemia and smoking.

Treatment

Retinal laser treatment is given if the retina is ischaemic, to prevent the development of retinal and iris neovascularization (Figure 13.8, see glaucoma,

Chapter 11). Laser treatment may improve vision in some patients with a BRVO by reducing macular oedema. Intravitreal steroid implants may be used to treat macular oedema, as may anti-VEGF agents. These have fewer complications than steroids (e.g. steroid-induced elevation of intraocular pressure) but have to be given more frequently. Anti-VEGF drugs also have a role in treating iris neovascularization (*rubeosis iridis*).

Prognosis

The vision is usually severely affected in central, and often in branch, vein occlusion and usually does not improve. Younger patients may fare better, and there may well be some visual improvement.

Arteriosclerosis and hypertension

Arteriosclerosis can be observed in the eye as an attenuation of retinal arterial vessel calibre (sometimes referred to as *copper* and *silver wiring*) and by the presence of nipping of the retinal veins where they are crossed by arterioles (A/V nipping). Hypertension, in addition, may cause focal arteriolar narrowing and a breakdown in the blood–retinal barrier, resulting in signs of vascular leakage (haemorrhage and exudate). These are particularly prominent if the hypertension is of renal origin. If severe, the retina may also demonstrate signs of capillary occlusion (cotton-wool spots).

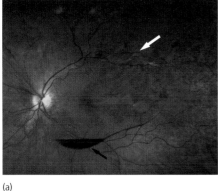
(a)

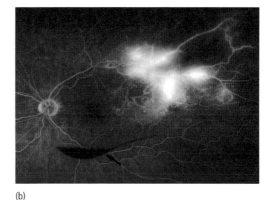
(b)

Figure 13.8 (a) A branch retinal vein occlusion. The retina has developed new vessels (arrowed) due to the ischaemic retina. (b) Note how the new vessels leak on the fluorescein angiogram. The retina peripheral to the leakage is dark due to the reduced capillary circulation in this area. The new vessels have also bled, creating a pool of blood with a horizontal level, lying between the retina and the posterior vitreous face (black arrows).

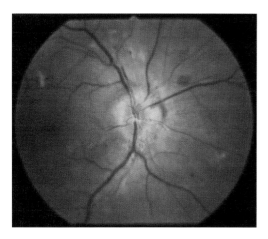

Figure 13.9 The fundus in malignant (now accelerated) hypertension. The disc is swollen, and there are retinal haemorrhages and cotton-wool spots.

In *malignant (now accelerated) hypertension*, very high blood pressure may, in addition, cause swelling of the optic nerve head with peripapillary, linear (nerve fibre layer) haemorrhages (Figure 13.9) and is an indication for urgent referral. The patient may complain of blurring of vision and of episodes of temporary visual loss, which may also occur with severe retinopathy when the macula is affected.

Treatment of the hypertension results in the resolution of the retinal signs over some months. A rapid reduction of systemic blood pressure is avoided, because it may precipitate vascular occlusion.

Retinopathy of prematurity

Retinopathy of prematurity is a vascular response of the retina occurring predominantly in low birth-weight, premature infants exposed to oxygen therapy in the early weeks of life. It may lead to a tractional detachment of the retina and potentially to bilateral blindness.

While improved neonatal care has resulted in an increased survival of premature babies, it has also caused in an increase in the incidence of ROP, particularly in developing countries. The lower the birth-weight and gestation the higher the risk.

Pathogenesis

There is an initial failure of normal retinal vascularization, followed by a phase of aggressive new vessel

formation extending forward into the vitreous and causing traction detachment.

Risk factors associated with retinopathy of prematurity include:

- gestation less than 31 weeks;
- birthweight below 1500 g;
- exposure to supplemental oxygen;
- apnoea;
- sepsis;
- duration of ventilation;
- blood transfusion;
- the presence of intra-ventricular haemorrhage;
- hypotension;
- hypothermia;
- twin pregnancy;
- retinal light exposure.

The incidence of the condition in infants weighing less than 1500 g is between 34% and 60%. The risk of occurrence is reduced by regulating the level of oxygen exposure.

Signs

The retinal appearance depends on the severity of the condition (Figure 13.10, Figure 13.11), but it includes:

- new vessels;
- the development of retinal haemorrhage;
- increased tortuosity and dilation of the retinal vessels.

In severe disease, blindness can result from:

- bleeding into the vitreous;
- retinal detachment.

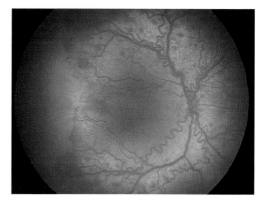

Figure 13.10 The fundus appearance in retinopathy of prematurity. Note the tortuosity of the retinal vessels. Small retinal haemorrhages can be seen superiorly while the peripheral retina is avascular. (*Source:* Courtesy C.K. Patel.)

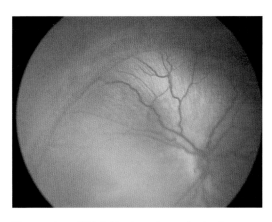

Figure 13.11 Widefield colour photo of retina in a premature infant showing vascularized ridge demarcating vascularized and avascular retina. Note dilated retinal vessels indicating 'plus disease'.

Treatment

At-risk infants are screened on a regular basis. Most cases of ROP resolve and treatment is indicated for severe vision-threatening disease (threshold ROP). The severe complications of the condition can be reduced by applying laser to the avascular retina. Injections of anti-VEGF agents into the vitreous cavity are increasingly used, particularly in systemically unwell babies.

Sickle-cell retinopathy

Patients with sickle-cell haemoglobin C disease (SC disease) and sickle-cell haemoglobin with thalassaemia (SThal) develop a severe form of retinopathy. This is unusual in homozygous sickle-cell disease (SS), where the retinopathy is more confined. Signs include:

- tortuous veins;
- peripheral haemorrhages;
- capillary non-perfusion;
- pigmented spots on the retina;
- new vessel formation, classically in a peripheral 'sea fan' pattern, which may occur as a result of peripheral retinal artery occlusion.

New vessels may cause vitreous haemorrhage and traction retinal detachment. As with diabetes, this may require treatment with laser photocoagulation and vitrectomy. Laser has a limited role in management. Management of the underlying, sickle disease

for example the use of hydroxyurea and prompt management of sickle crises is the mainstay of treatment.

Abnormal retinal blood vessels

Abnormalities of the retinal blood vessels may be seen in rare ocular diseases, associated with the development of massive exudate. They may also be an indication of systemic disorders, as in the retinal and optic disc angioma associated with the familial von Hippel–Lindau syndrome. Here, the ocular condition may be associated with angioma in the brain and spinal cord. Patients and their relatives require regular MRI screening.

Abnormalities of the blood

Clotting abnormalities may be responsible for occlusion of any blood vessel in the eye (e.g. a CRVO). Similarly, increased viscosity may also cause vessel occlusion. Leukaemia with a greatly raised white cell count may lead to the development of a haemorrhagic retinopathy in which the haemorrhages have white centres (*Roth spots*) (Figure 13.12). These may also be a feature of bacterial endocarditis and autoimmune diseases associated with vasculitis.

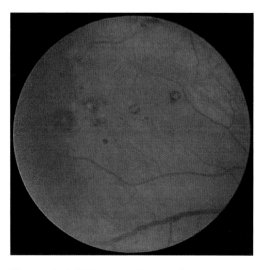

Figure 13.12 White-centred haemorrhages.

KEY POINTS

- Diabetics require regular screening for sight-threatening retinopathy.
- Intravitreal injections of anti-VEGF and steroid are increasingly important in the treatment of diabetic maculopathy.
- Patients with central retinal artery occlusion require urgent referral for cardiovascular examination.
- Children at risk of retinopathy of prematurity require regular screening.

Assessment questions
True or False

1. **Assign each of these signs of retinal vascular disease to either leakage or occlusion.**

a   Haemorrhage.
b   New vessels.
c   Cotton-wool spot.
d   Exudate.
e   Oedema.

2. **A central vein occlusion**

a   Does not usually cause loss of vision.
b   May be associated with the formation of new vessels.
c   May be a cause of neovascular glaucoma.
d   May be associated with hypertension.
e   Produces few abnormal signs in the retina.

3. **Diabetic retinopathy**

a   Is seen in 66% of patients who have had type II diabetes for 20 years.
b   Control of systemic hypertension is important in reducing the severity of the retinopathy.
c   The number of pericytes around the capillaries is increased.
d   Vitreous haemorrhage is associated with the formation of new vessels on the retina or optic nerve head.
e   Circinate patterns of exudates are treated with scattered laser.

4. **Match the pictures (Figure 13.13a–c) with the diagnoses.**

   i.   Diabetic retinopathy.
  ii.   Sickle-cell retinopathy.
 iii.   Bacterial endocarditis.
  iv.   Retinal vein occlusion.
   v.   Retinopathy of prematurity.

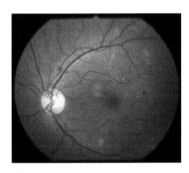

(a)

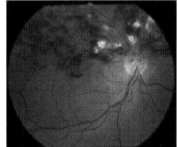

(b)

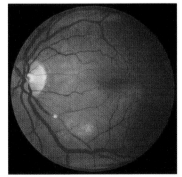

(c)

Figure 13.13 (a–c) See Question 4.

vi. Retinal artery occlusion.

vii. Retinal arteriole embolus.

5. Retinopathy of prematurity

a Is caused by a failure of normal retinal vascularization.

b Is most commonly seen in babies with a low birthweight.

c Is less commonly seen in babies exposed to supplementary oxygen.

d New vessels and haemorrhages may be seen in the retina.

e Retinal detachment may complicate the condition.

Answers

1. Assign each of these signs of retinal vascular disease to either *leakage* or *occlusion*.

a Leakage.

b Occlusion.

c Occlusion.

d Leakage.

e Leakage.

2. A central retinal vein occlusion

a False. It results usually in a significant loss of vision.

b True. This is a serious complication which can lead to vitreous haemorrhage and neovascular glaucoma, see Chapter 11.

c True. New blood vessels may develop in the iridocorneal angle causing neovascular glaucoma.

d True. This may be a predisposing systemic disease.

e False. The retinal veins are swollen and tortuous and there are extensive retinal haemorrhages.

3. Diabetic retinopathy

a True.

b True. This is a very important factor in treating diabetic retinopathy.

c False. The number is decreased.

d True. This is a complication of proliferative diabetic retinopathy when new vessels grow on the retina and/or optic disc.

e False. The laser is applied to the site of leakage, at the centre of the circinate exudate.

4. Match the pictures (Figure 13.13) with the diagnoses.

a Diabetic retinopathy. Note the haemorrhages, exudates and more peripheral cotton-wool spots.

b Retinal vein occlusion. This is a hemi-retinal vein occlusion.

c Retinal arteriole embolus.

5. Retinopathy of prematurity

a True. There is an initial failure of normal retinal vascularization followed by a phase of aggressive new vessel formation.

b True. Low birthweight is a major risk factor.

c False. Supplementary oxygen therapy is a risk factor.

d True. New vessels may form and retinal haemorrhages may be seen.

e True. Retinal detachment is a serious complication of advanced disease.

14

The pupil and its responses

Learning objectives

To understand:

✔ The neural pathways controlling pupillary size and responses.
✔ The causes of pupillary dysfunction.

Introduction

Movements of the pupil are controlled by the parasympathetic and sympathetic nervous systems. The pupils constrict (*miosis*) when the eye is illuminated (parasympathetic activation, sympathetic relaxation) and dilate (*mydriasis*) in the dark (sympathetic activation, parasympathetic relaxation). When the eyes focus on a near object, they converge and the pupils constrict (the *near response*). The pupils are normally equal in size but some 20% of people may have noticeably unequal pupils (*anisocoria*) with no associated disease.

The key to diagnosis of pupillary disorders is to:

- determine which pupil is abnormal;
- search for associated signs.

Disorders of the pupil may result from:

- ocular disease;
- disorders of the neural pathway;
- pharmacological action.

The sympathetic pathway is shown in Figure 14.1. The parasympathetic fibres reach the eye through the third cranial nerve (Figure 14.2).

Ocular causes of pupillary abnormality

Several diseases of the eye cause pupil irregularity and alter pupil reactions:

- anterior uveitis, when posterior synechiae give the pupil an irregular appearance (see Chapter 10);
- the sequelae of intraocular surgery – direct muscle injury;
- blunt trauma to the eye, which may rupture the sphincter muscle, causing irregularity or fixed dilation (*traumatic mydriasis*);
- an acute and severe rise in ocular pressure can cause mydriasis – as in acute glaucoma.

Neurological causes of an abnormal pupil

Horner syndrome

Interruption of the *sympathetic pathway* causes:

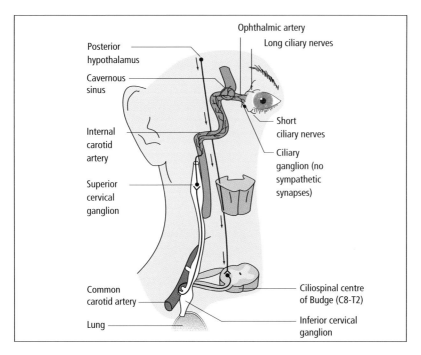

Figure 14.1 The pathway of sympathetic pupillary control. (*Source:* Kanski et al. (1994) / with permission of Elsevier).

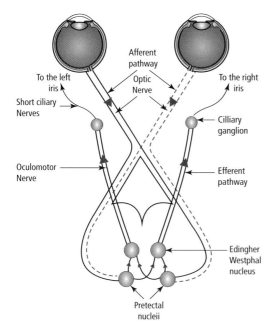

Figure 14.2 The pathway of parasympathetic control.

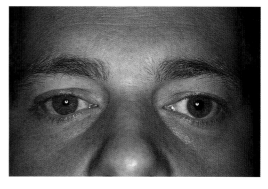

Figure 14.3 A right ptosis and miosis in Horner syndrome.

- A small pupil on the affected side due to loss of the dilator function (Figure 14.3). This is more noticeable in the dark, because the normal pupil of the fellow eye then dilates more than that of the affected pupil.
- A slight ptosis on the affected side, due to denervation of Müller muscle.

- An apparent recession of the globe into the orbit (*enophthalmos*). The reduced palpebral aperture size gives an impression of recession.
- Lack of sweating on the affected side, if the *sympathetic pathway is affected proximal to the base of the skull*. This catches fibres travelling with the branches of the external carotid, which innervate the skin of the face.

Because of its extended course, the sympathetic pathway may be affected by a multitude of pathologies. Examples include:

- *Syringomyelia*, an expanding cavity within the spinal cord, sometimes extending to the medulla (syringobulbia), which compresses the pathway. Typically, it also causes wasting of the hand muscles and loss of sensation.
- *Small-cell carcinoma* at the lung apex which catches the cervical sympathetic chain. Involvement of the brachial plexus gives rise to *pain in the shoulder and arm and to T1 wasting* of the small muscles of the hand (Pancoast syndrome).
- Neck injury, disease or surgery. A dissection of the carotid artery may present as a painful Horner syndrome. This may occur after trauma or spontaneously in collagen vascular disorders e.g. Marfan syndrome. Urgent imaging of the carotid artery is required. The risk of stroke is reduced by administration of anticoagulants (e.g. aspirin).
- Cavernous sinus disease – catching the sympathetic carotid plexus in the sinus.

Horner syndrome may also be congenital, in which case the iris colour may be altered when compared to the fellow eye (*heterochromia*).

Relative afferent pupillary defect (RAPD)

A lesion of the optic nerve on one side blocks the afferent limb of the pupillary light reflex. The pupils are equal and of normal size, but the pupillary response to light directed to the affected side is reduced, while the near reflex is intact. Testing for an RAPD is critical in a patient suspected of having an optic nerve lesion, such as optic neuritis (see Chapter 3). An RAPD may be seen with extensive retinal disease but not with opacities of the cornea or lens.

Light–near dissociation

The key feature is an impaired reaction of the pupils to light, while the near response to accommodation is retained. It is seen with Adie tonic pupil, the Argyll Robertson pupil and with periaqueductal brainstem lesions such as Parinaud syndrome. Other causes include diabetes and multiple sclerosis. There is no condition in which the light reflex is intact but the near reflex is defective.

Adie tonic pupil

This is a not uncommon cause of unequal pupil size (*anisocoria*) in young adults, but has no serious consequences. Onset is subacute and affects females more commonly than males (2 : 1). It is due to a *ciliary ganglionitis* which denervates the parasympathetic supply to the iris and ciliary body. On recovery from the ganglionitis, reinnervation is incomplete and the partially denervated receptors of the iris and ciliary body become supersensitive to muscarinic stimulation. Normally, the ciliary body receives about nine times the number of parasympathetic fibres received by the iris sphincter so the fibres reinnervating the iris sphincter are mainly derived from those previously designated for the ciliary muscle and therefore linked with the accommodative reflex. As the sphincter is partially denervated, its muscarinic receptors are supersensitive to cholinergic agonists.

The consequence is that the pupil:

- is enlarged – because the sphincter is relatively denervated;
- is poorly reactive to light – because few of the innervating fibres were originally destined for the sphincter. Also, because of the irregular fibre distribution, pupil movement in response to light consists of a slow, worm-like (*vermiform*) contraction, on biomicroscopy.

Due to muscarinic supersensitivity of the sphincter, the pupil also:

- shows slow, sustained miosis on accommodation;
- constricts to a single drop of dilute pilocarpine (0.1%), unlike the normal pupil. This is a diagnostic test.

Because the ciliary body is also partially denervated, the ability to accommodate is impaired too and the patient may complain of blurred vision when looking from distance to near, or *vice versa*. Systemically, the disorder is associated with loss of tendon reflexes. There are no other neurological signs.

Argyll Robertson pupil

The pupils are bilaterally small and irregular. They do not react to light but respond to accommodation. The iris stroma has a typical feathery appearance and loses its architectural detail. Classically, it is seen in neurosyphilis. It is suggested that a periaqueductal lesion on the dorsal aspect of the Edinger Westphäl nucleus involves fibres associated with the response to light, but spares those associated with the near response.

Midbrain pupil

Lesions affecting the pretectal nuclear complex in the dorsal region of the midbrain can disrupt retino-tectal fibres while preserving the supranuclear accommodative pathway. This produces mydriasis and a light–near dissociation. Causes include demyelination, infarction, enlargement of the third ventricle and space-occupying tumours such as pinealoma, as part of a *dorsal midbrain (Parinaud) syndrome* (see Chapter 16).

Other causes of pupillary abnormality

In coma, both pupils may become miosed if a pontine lesion is present. The light reflex is preserved but difficult to demonstrate with a small pupil. Remember that patients taking pilocarpine for glaucoma or receiving morphine also show bilateral miosis. Midbrain lesions cause loss of the light reflex with midpoint pupils. Coma associated with a unilateral expanding supratentorial mass, for example a haematoma, results in pressure on the third nerve and dilation of the pupil. Intrinsic third nerve lesions also cause a dilated pupil (see Chapter 16).

The pupil may also be affected by drugs, both topical and systemic (Table 14.1) and in some parts of the world bilateral mydriasis may be caused by the accidental inoculation of plant material into the eye from the Jimson weed (*Datura stramonium*), which contains the belladonna alkaloids atropine and scopolamine ('cornpickers"s pupil'). Occasionally, patients are encountered who have deliberately instilled a mydriatic drop in order to simulate eye disease.

Table 14.1 Drugs having a pharmacological effect on the pupil.

Agent	Action	Mechanism
Topical agents		
Dilates	Muscarinic blockade	Cyclopentolate
		Tropicamide
		Atropine (long-acting)
	Alpha-adrenergic agonist	Phenylephrine
		Adrenaline
Constricts	Muscarinic agonist	Pilocarpine
Systemic agents		
Dilates	Muscarinic blockade	Atropine
	Alpha-adrenergic agonist	Adrenaline
Constricts	Local action and action on central nervous system	Morphine

 KEY POINTS

- Take a good history to help exclude an ocular cause for the pupillary changes and to see if a medical condition or drug history exists which may contribute to the pupillary problem.
- Determine whether it is the small or the large pupil that is abnormal.
- Search for associated signs that may help make a diagnosis.

Assessment questions True or False

1. Pathological miosis is seen in

a Horner syndrome.
b Third nerve palsy.
c Argyll Robertson pupil.
d Coma.
e Systemic and topical atropine treatment.

2. Horner syndrome may be seen in

a Syringomyelia.
b Lung neoplasia.
c Cavernous sinus disease.

d   Myasthenia gravis.

e   Carotid artery dissection.

3.   Light–near dissociation

a   The reaction of the pupils is greater to light than accommodation.

b   May be seen in diabetes.

c   Is seen in Horner syndrome.

d   Is seen in patients with an Argyll Robertson pupil.

e   Is seen following administration of tropicamide drops.

4.   Match the drop to its action: *dilates* (mydriasis) or *constricts* (miosis).

a   Cyclopentolate.

b   Atropine.

c   Pilocarpine.

d   Tropicamide.

e   Phenylephrine.

Answers

1.   Pathological miosis is seen in

a   True. The pupil is small in Horner syndrome; there will also be a small ptosis.

b   False. The pupil is dilated in a third nerve palsy.

c   True. The pupil is small and irregular in an Argyll Robertson pupil.

d   True. Both pupils may be miosed but beware of any associated pharmacological causes of miosis in patients with coma.

e   False. Atropine causes mydriasis.

2.   Horner syndrome may be seen in

a   True.

b   True. An apical lung tumour may catch the cervical sympathetic trunk as it leaves the inferior cervical ganglion.

c   True. The sympathetic pathway may be interrupted here as the nerve travels on the internal carotid artery surrounded by the cavernous sinus.

d   False. This may cause a ptosis but does not affect the pupil.

e   True. This is a cause of a painful Horner syndrome.

3.   Light–near dissociation

a   False. It is the other way round: the pupils react poorly to light – better to accommodation.

b   True. It can be seen in diabetes and multiple sclerosis.

c   False. The pupil is smaller but reacts normally to light and accommodation.

d   True. Argyll Robertson pupils do not react to light.

e   False. The pupil is dilated and unreactive to both stimuli.

4.   Match the drop to its action.

a   Dilates.

b   Dilates.

c   Constricts.

d   Dilates.

e   Dilates.

Reference

Kanski, J.J. et al. (1994). *Clinical Ophthalmology: A Systematic Approach.* Butterworth-Heinemann 3rd Edition.

15

Disorders of the visual pathway

Learning objectives

To understand:

✔ The basic anatomy of the visual pathway.
✔ The field defects produced by lesions at different points along the visual pathway.
✔ The causes, symptoms and signs associated with a swollen optic disc.
✔ The symptoms, signs, treatment and complications of giant cell arteritis.

Introduction

The innermost layer of the retina consists of the nerve fibres originating from the *retinal ganglion cells.* These fibres collect together at the optic nerve head, and form the optic nerve (see Chapter 1). The subsequent course of the visual pathway is shown in Figure 15.1. Diagnosis and location of disease of the optic pathways is greatly aided by study of the differing field defects produced by damage at different sites. It would be useful to read the perimetry section of chapter 3 before progressing further.

The optic nerve

The normal optic nerve head has distinct margins, a pinkish rim and, usually, a pale, central, cup. The central retinal artery and vein enter and leave the globe slightly nasally in the optic nerve head, referred to ophthalmoscopically as the optic disc. The optic disc may be involved in many disorders but has a limited repertoire of responses. Ophthalmoscopically, it may become swollen, or it may become pale in a distinctive way. In glaucoma (Chapter 11), the optic disc cup is enlarged. When assessing the optic nerve head, always compare the two optic discs – this is a useful way of detecting unilateral abnormalities.

The swollen optic disc

The swollen disc (Figure 15.2) is an important and often worrying sign. *Papilloedema* is the term given to disc swelling associated with raised intracranial pressure (ICP). Accelerated hypertension (previously 'malignant' hypertension) and optic disc ischaemia also cause disc swelling. *Papillitis*, a condition with a similar fundoscopic appearance, is due to optic neuritis (inflammation) affecting the nerve head. Visual loss is a typical feature of optic neuritis and ischaemic optic neuropathy but is uncommon with the disc swelling of accelerated hypertension or raised ICP.

Ophthalmology: Lecture Notes, Thirteenth Edition. Bruce James, Anthony Bron, and Manoj V. Parulekar.
© 2024 John Wiley & Sons Ltd. Published 2024 by John Wiley & Sons Ltd.
Companion website: www.wiley.com/go/ophthalmology13e

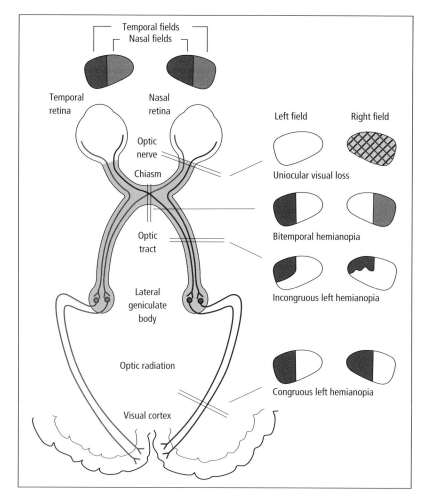

Temporal fields

Nasal fields

Temporal retina

Nasal retina

Optic nerve

Chiasm

Optic tract

Lateral geniculate body

Optic radiation

Visual cortex

Left field

Right field

Uniocular visual loss

Bitemporal hemianopia

Incongruous left hemianopia

Congruous left hemianopia

Figure 15.1 Anatomy of the optic pathway and the field defects produced by lesions at different sites.

The differential diagnosis of disc swelling is shown in Table 15.1. Some normal optic nerve heads may appear to be swollen, due to crowding of nerve fibres entering the disc. This is termed *pseudopapilloedema* and occurs particularly in small, hypermetropic eyes where the nerve entry site is reduced in size. Note also that *myelinated nerve fibres* occurring on the nerve head may be mistaken for optic disc swelling. During development, myelination of the optic nerve begins proximally and spreads centrifugally, to be completed at the lamina cribrosa at term. Occasionally, as a developmental variant, the process extends into the peripapillary retinal nerve fibre layer as a patch of light-scattering, myelinated fibres whose white, feathery, arrangement reflects the organization of the nerve fibre layer. Optic disc drüsen, which are accumulations of proteinaceous amyloid material within the optic nerve head, can also result in a swollen-looking optic disc.

In myopia, it is common to see a pale 'myopic crescent' of peripapillary choroidal atrophy at the temporal margin of the optic disc, allowing the overlying, white sclera to show through. In high myopia, the optic disc may be surrounded by such an atrophic area (*peripapillary atrophy*), which may be confused with disc swelling.

Papilloedema

History

The crucial feature of disc swelling due to raised ICP is that in the short term there is no visual loss. However, in some patients with advanced papilloedema, a fleeting visual loss may occur, lasting seconds, when posture is altered from lying to standing (transient visual *obscurations*). Visual loss (reduced acuity and significant contraction of the visual fields) can occur with chronic papilloedema.

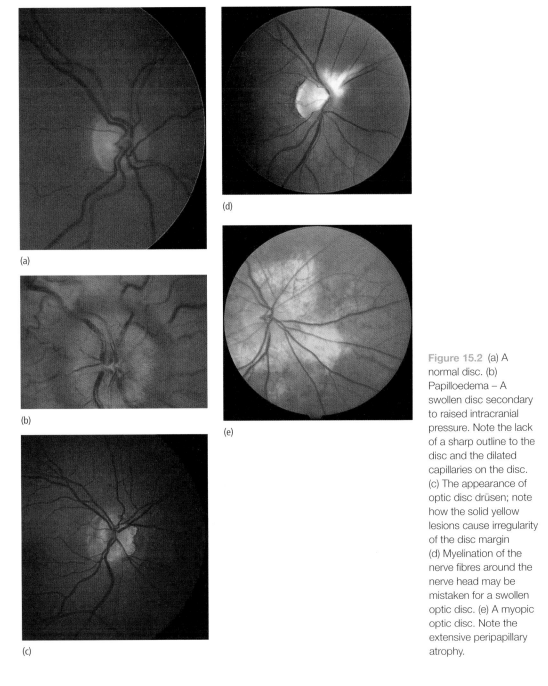

Figure 15.2 (a) A normal disc. (b) Papilloedema – A swollen disc secondary to raised intracranial pressure. Note the lack of a sharp outline to the disc and the dilated capillaries on the disc. (c) The appearance of optic disc drüsen; note how the solid yellow lesions cause irregularity of the disc margin (d) Myelination of the nerve fibres around the nerve head may be mistaken for a swollen optic disc. (e) A myopic optic disc. Note the extensive peripapillary atrophy.

Other important clues to the presence of raised ICP include:

- headache, worse on waking and made worse by coughing;
- nausea, retching;
- diplopia (double vision), usually due to a sixth nerve palsy;
- other neurological signs, if the raised pressure is due to a cranial space occupying lesion – visual field loss; cranial nerve palsy;
- a history of head trauma suggesting a subdural haemorrhage;
- a history of medications sometimes associated with raised ICP (e.g. oral contraceptives, tetracyclines).

Table 15.1 Causes of a swollen optic disc.

Condition	Distinguishing features
Raised intracranial pressure	Vision and field usually normal save for large blind spot. Obscurations (short episodes of visual loss usually on changing posture). Field may be contracted in chronic disease. Colour vision initially normal. No RAPD. No spontaneous venous pulsation of the vein at the disc (but some people with normal intracranial pressure do not have this). Dilated capillaries and haemorrhages on disc. Other symptoms and signs of raised intracranial pressure
Space-occupying lesions of the optic nerve head	Various solid or infiltrative lesions at the nerve head, for example optic disc drüsen (calcified axonal material), gliomas, sarcoidosis and leukaemia, may produce disc swelling. These may be associated with reduced vision, colour vision and field defects. B-scan ultrasound is useful in identifying optic disc drüsen
Papillitis (optic neuritis affecting the optic nerve head)	A swollen optic disc. Exudates around the macula may occasionally be seen. Vision is profoundly reduced. Colour vision is abnormal. RAPD present. A central field defect is present
Accelerated (malignant) hypertension (see Chapter 13)	Reduced vision, haemorrhagic disc swelling. Retinal haemorrhages, exudates and cotton-wool spots away from the nerve head. Check blood pressure!
Ischaemic optic neuropathy	Sudden visual loss, field defect. Colour vision may be normal. RAPD may be present. Spontaneous venous pulsation at the optic disc may be present. May be sectorial swelling only. Haemorrhages on disc and disc margin. Cotton-wool spots may be seen around disc, particularly if caused by giant cell arteritis
Central retinal vein occlusion (see Chapter 13)	Sudden marked visual loss, tortuous veins, gross retinal haemorrhages

Disc swelling must be distinguished from pseudopapilloedema such as optic nerve head drüsen, myelinated nerve fibres and the peripapillary atrophy of high myopia.

RAPD, relative afferent pupillary defect; see Chapter 3.

Signs

- The optic disc is swollen, its edges are blurred and the superficial capillaries are dilated and thus abnormally prominent. The disc appears more pink than normal. The central retinal vein is dilated and there is *no spontaneous venous pulsation*. This has a physiological basis. The central retinal vein is exposed to cerebrospinal fluid (CSF) in the subarachnoid space of the optic nerve as it leaves to join the veins of the orbit. Normally, venous pressure in the retinal veins at the nerve head is just above ocular pressure. Venous pulsation occurs because the vein collapses briefly with each rise in ocular pressure caused by arterial inflow during systole. When the CSF pressure is higher than the ocular pressure, as occurs in papilloedema due to raised ICP, the pressure in the veins at the disc rises above the ocular pressure and spontaneous venous pulsation is lost. Absence of spontaneous venous pulsation is seen in 5–20% of those with normal nerve heads, but in this case, venous collapse at the nerve head can be induced by light pressure on the globe through the lids.
- A large blind spot will be found on visual field testing, corresponding to the swollen nerve head. In chronic papilloedema, the field may become constricted. A field defect may, however, be caused by the space-occupying lesion causing the papilloedema.
- Abnormal neurological signs may indicate the site of a space-occupying lesion.

Investigation

CT and MRI scanning will identify any space-occupying lesion or enlargement of the ventricles. Following neurological consultation (and normally after a scan), a lumbar puncture will enable ICP to be measured.

Treatment is dependent on findings.

Idiopathic intracranial hypertension

ICP may be elevated and disc swelling presents with no evidence of intracranial abnormality and no dilation of the ventricles on the scan. This is termed *idiopathic intracranial hypertension* (previously, benign intracranial hypertension) and usually presents in overweight women in the second and third decades. It may also be caused by exposure to certain drugs such as isotretinoin (for acne), tetracyclines and less certainly, the contraceptive pill. Patients complain of headache and may have obscurations of vision and sixth nerve palsies. No other neurological problems are present. Acute permanent visual loss is not a feature of papilloedema. If however the nerve remains swollen for a prolonged period, there will be a progressive contraction of the visual field. It is thus important to reduce ICP. This may be achieved:

- with medications such as oral acetazolamide;
- by ventriculoperitoneal shunting;
- by optic nerve decompression. Here, a small hole is made in the sheath surrounding the optic nerve to allow the drainage of CSF into the orbit and reduce the pressure of CSF around the anterior optic nerve.

Space-occupying lesions (i.e. tumours and haemorrhage) and hydrocephalus require neurosurgical management.

Optic neuritis

Inflammation or demyelination of the optic nerve results in optic neuritis. This is termed *papillitis* if the optic nerve head is visibly affected and *retrobulbar neuritis* if the optic nerve is affected more posteriorly, with no visible disc swelling.

History

There is:

- an acute loss of vision that may progress over a few days and then slowly improve;
- pain on eye movement in retrobulbar neuritis because rectus muscle contraction pulls on the optic nerve sheath;
- a preceding history of viral illness in some cases.

Between 25% and 70% of patients with optic neuritis will have, or will develop, symptoms or signs of central nervous demyelination due to *multiple sclerosis* (MS).

Examination

This reveals:

- reduced visual acuity;
- a *central scotoma* on field testing;
- reduced colour vision, red desaturation and reduced brightness sensitivity;
- a relative afferent pupillary defect (RAPD) due to reduced optic nerve conduction (see Chapter 3);
- a normal disc in retrobulbar neuritis; a swollen disc in papillitis.

Diagnosis and treatment

Although optic neuritis may occur as an isolated event with full recovery, some cases are due to MS. Other conditions such as *neuromyelitis optica* (NMO, an autoimmune condition where the spinal cord and optic nerves become inflamed) must also be considered.

The diagnosis of MS is a clinical one but while an MRI scan can identify 'silent' plaques of CNS demyelination, the patient must be suitably counselled before a scan is performed. Blood tests to detect anti MOG antibodies and aquaporin 4 antibodies may be indicated in atypical cases to diagnose NMO. Referral to a neurology service may be advisable for counselling and full neurological evaluation.

A short course of systemic steroid treatment may speed up visual recovery and prevent irreversible visual loss in some types of optic neuritis (e.g. NMO).

Prognosis

Vision slowly recovers over several weeks, although subtle defects may persist. In MS, repeated episodes, occurring in either eye, may lead to optic atrophy, a decline in vision and persistent scotomata. Very occasionally, in atypical cases, vision may not recover.

Ischaemic optic neuropathy

Pathogenesis

The anterior optic nerve may become ischaemic if the posterior ciliary vessels are compromised as a result of degenerative vaso-occlusive or vasculitic disease of the arterioles. The resulting disc swelling is due to an *anterior ischaemic optic neuropathy*.

Symptoms

The patient complains of a sudden loss of vision or visual field, often on waking, since the blood pressure falls and vascular perfusion of the eye decreases during sleep. If accompanied by pain or scalp tenderness, the diagnosis of *giant cell arteritis* must carefully be considered. Ischaemic optic neuropathy is the usual cause of blindness in that disease.

Giant cell arteritis

This is an autoimmune vasculitis occurring in patients generally over the age of 60. It affects arteries with an internal elastic lamina, which therefore includes the ophthalmic artery, but not the retinal artery. It may present with any combination of:

- sudden loss of vision;
- scalp tenderness (e.g. on combing);
- pain on chewing (*jaw claudication*);
- shoulder pain;
- malaise.

Signs

There is usually (Figure 15.3):

- a reduction in visual acuity;
- a field defect, typically an absence of the lower or upper half of the visual field (altitudinal scotoma);
- a swollen and haemorrhagic disc with normal retina and retinal vessels (remember, the blood supply to the anterior optic nerve and retina are different) – in arteritic ischaemic optic neuropathy, the disc may be pale;
- a small normal fellow disc with a small cup in non-arteritic disease;
- a tender temporal artery, a sign suggestive of giant cell arteritis. The pulse may also be reduced.

Investigations

If giant cell arteritis is present, the erythrocyte sedimentation rate (ESR) and C-reactive protein are usually grossly elevated. However, in 1 in 10 patients, the ESR is normal. Platelets may also be raised. Temporal artery biopsy shows a granulomatous arteritis with multinucleated giant cells, but this may be absent where only a small specimen is obtained or because the disease has skipped a length of the artery. Giant cell arteritis can also present as a central retinal artery occlusion secondary to an arteritis of the ophthalmic artery.

Investigation of the patient with ischaemic optic neuropathy includes:

- blood pressure check;
- a full blood count to exclude anaemia;
- blood sugar check;
- ESR and C-reactive protein to check for giant-cell arteritis.
- a temporal artery biopsy when there are clinical features of GCA, or no evident vascular risk factors in elderly patients.

Both hypertension and diabetes may be associated with non-arteritic ischaemic optic atrophy. It may also be seen in patients suffering acute blood loss, for example haematemesis, where it may occur some days after the acute bleed. Hypotensive episodes e.g. during surgery or from overtreatment of hypertension may also give rise to ischaemic optic neuropathy. Occasionally, clotting disorders or autoimmune disease may cause the condition.

Treatment

If giant cell arteritis is strongly suspected, treatment must not be delayed while the diagnosis is confirmed. High-dose steroids must be given, intravenously and orally, and the dose tapered over the ensuing weeks on the basis of symptoms and the

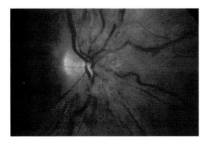
(a)

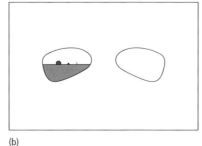
(b)

Figure 15.3 (a) The clinical appearance of the optic disc and (b) one form of field defect (altitudinal) seen in ischaemic optic neuropathy.

response of the ESR or C-reactive protein. The usual precautions must be taken, as with any patient on steroids, to exclude other medical conditions that might be unmasked or worsened by the steroids (e.g. tuberculosis, diabetes, hypertension and an increased susceptibility to infection). Steroids *will not reverse the visual loss* but can prevent the fellow eye being affected.

There is unfortunately no treatment for non-arteritic ischaemic optic neuropathy other than the management of underlying conditions.

Prognosis

The second eye may rapidly become involved in patients with untreated giant cell arteritis but this can be prevented by prompt initiation of systemic steroid therapy. Steroid therapy may have to be continued on a prolonged basis and monitored closely.

There is also a significant rate of involvement of the second eye in the non-arteritic form (40–50%). It is unusual for the vision to get progressively worse in non-arteritic ischaemic optic neuropathy, and the visual outcome in terms of both visual field and acuity is very variable. In both conditions, vision does not recover once it has been lost.

Optic atrophy

In optic atrophy, the optic disc is pale due to a loss of RGC axons and a reduced vascularity of the optic nerve head (Figure 15.4, Table 15.2). The vision is usually reduced and colour vision affected. Comparison of the two eyes is of great help in unilateral cases, as this makes the pallor much easier to detect. A relative afferent pupillary defect will be present.

The chiasm

Compressive lesions at the chiasm produce a bitemporal hemianopia when the fibres representing the nasal retina (temporal field) are compressed as they cross in the centre of the chiasm. Patients may present with rather vague visual symptoms, for example:

- Missing objects in the periphery of the visual field.
- When testing vision with a Snellen chart, patients may miss the temporal letters with each eye.
- The bitemporal field loss may cause difficulty in fusing images, causing the patient to complain of diplopia although eye position and movements are normal.
- There may be difficulty with tasks requiring stereopsis such as pouring water into a cup or threading a needle.

The most common lesion is a pituitary tumour (Figure 15.5), and the patient should be asked whether they have symptoms relating to hormonal disturbance. Treatment depends on the type of tumour found; some are amenable to medical therapy but many require surgical excision. A *meningioma* and *craniopharyngioma* may also cause chiasmal compression.

Optic tract, radiation and visual cortex

Lesions of the optic tract and radiation (usually vascular or neoplastic), produce a *homonymous hemianopic field defect*, that is, loss confined to the right- or left-hand side of the field *in both eyes* (Figure 15.6). This pattern of field loss results from involvement of

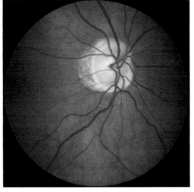

(a)

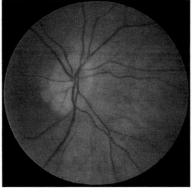

(b)

Figure 15.4 (a) A pale optic disc compared to (b) a normal optic disc.

Table 15.2 Causes of optic atrophy.

Cause	Distinguishing features
Compression of the optic nerve	History of orbital or chiasmal disease. If sectorial, field loss may give a clue to the location of a compressive lesion
Ischaemic optic neuropathy	A history of sudden (unilateral) visual loss in the past
Retinal artery occlusion	The retinal vessels are attenuated
Retinal vein occlusion	Engorged retinal veins; retinal haemorrhage
Glaucoma (see Chapter 11)	The optic disc is pathologically cupped
Papilloedema and chronic elevation of ICP	The visual fields are contracted
Optic neuritis	There may be a history of previous loss of vision. Symptoms and signs compatible with multiple sclerosis may be present
Inherited optic neuropathy	Dominant and recessive forms of optic neuropathy cause blindness in the first few years of life. Leber hereditary optic neuropathy results from a mutation of mitochondrial DNA. It typically affects males in early adulthood, becoming bilateral and causing a bilateral central scotoma
Inherited retinal disease	Retinal disease may result in optic atrophy when accompanied by extensive loss of retinal ganglion cells. It is, for example a feature of retinitis pigmentosa and the rod–cone dystrophies
Toxic optic neuropathy	Optic neuropathy may be due to chemical toxicity, for example from heavy metals, toluene from glue sniffing and some drugs (e.g. isoniazid used in the treatment of tuberculosis). Information should be sought in the history
Nutritional	This may be seen with alcohol abuse or malnutrition and may be due to B12 and micronutrient deficiency

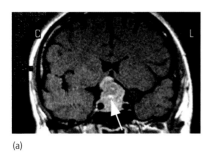

(a)

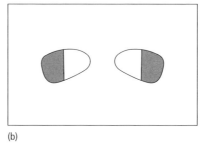

(b)

Figure 15.5 (a) The CT appearance of a pituitary tumour (arrow). (b) The bitemporal visual field loss produced.

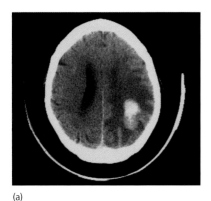

(a)

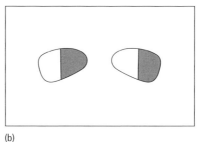

(b)

Figure 15.6 (a) A CT scan showing a left cortical infarct. (b) The complete, congruous right homonymous hemianopia produced by the infarct.

the crossing of the fibres of the chiasm, representing the nasal retina (Figure 15.6). Information from these fibres is projected to the primary visual cortex from the lateral geniculate body (LGB) via the optic tract and radiation. If the extent of field loss is similar in both eyes, a *congruous* defect is said to be present. This occurs when the defect affects the optic radiation or visual cortex; the closer to the visual cortex, the more congruous the field defect. Optic tract lesions produce *incongruous* defects. Neoplasia more commonly affects the radiation in the anterior temporal lobe. The commonest cause of disease in the occipital cortex is a cerebrovascular accident. The visual loss is of rapid onset; a slower onset is suggestive of a space-occupying lesion.

 KEY POINTS

- Careful comparison of the optic discs will help you to detect unilateral optic nerve disease.
- A bitemporal visual field defect suggests a pituitary tumour, compressing the optic chiasm.
- There are several causes of a swollen optic disc; it is not just a sign of raised ICP.
- In a patient of 60 years or older presenting with unilateral headache or sudden loss of vision with a swollen disc, always think of giant-cell arteritis. Urgent treatment may be required.
- Optic atrophy, may also result from retinal disease.

Assessment questions
True or False

1. **Match the field defect to the possible site of disease.**
   a   Unilateral central scotoma.
   b   Congruous left hemianopia.
   c   Bitemporal hemianopia.
   d   Unilateral superior field defect.

e   Incongruous left hemianopia.
   i.   Optic chiasm.
   ii. Visual cortex.
   iii. Optic nerve.
   iv. Optic tract.
   v.   Retina.

2. **A swollen disc may be caused by**
   a   Raised intraocular pressure.
   b   Raised intracranial pressure.
   c   Optic neuritis.
   d   Systemic hypertension.
   e   Central retinal artery occlusion.

3. **Match the pictures (Figure 15.7) to the most probable diagnosis.**
   i.   Optic disc drüsen.
   ii. Glaucoma.
   iii. Pituitary tumour.
   iv. Ischaemic optic neuropathy.
   v.   Retinitis pigmentosa.
   vi. Myelination of the retinal nerve fibre layer.
   vii. Myopia.
   viii. Papilloedema.
   ix. Optic neuritis.

4. **Optic neuritis**
   a   Is associated with a sudden loss of vision that does not progress.
   b   Is painless.
   c   May be part of a systemic neurological disease.
   d   Vision rarely recovers.
   e   Is associated with a reduction in colour vision.

5. **Ischaemic optic neuropathy**
   a   Presents with an acute loss of vision.
   b   On examination the patient has a swollen disc.
   c   May be associated with scalp tenderness and jaw claudication.
   d   Should always be treated with steroids.
   e   May cause an altitudinal field defect.

6. **Optic atrophy may be seen in**
   a   Some retinal diseases.
   b   Compression of the optic nerve.
   c   Diseases of the visual cortex.
   d   Ocular toxicity.
   e   Poor nutrition.

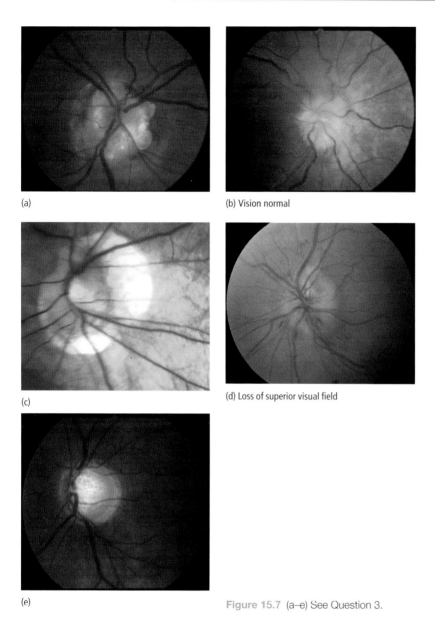

(a)

(b) Vision normal

(c)

(d) Loss of superior visual field

(e)

Figure 15.7 (a–e) See Question 3.

Answers

1. Match the field defect to the possible site of disease.

a Optic nerve or retina.
b Visual cortex.
c Optic chiasm.
d Retina or optic nerve.
e Optic tract.

2. A swollen disc may be caused by

a False. A chronic rise in intraocular pressure will produce pathological cupping of the optic disc.
b True. Papilloedema is a cardinal sign of raised intracranial pressure.
c True. This is then called papillitis; but the optic nerve head appears normal in retrobulbar neuritis.
d True. But only in severe or accelerated hypertension.
e False. It is seen in a central retinal vein occlusion and in ischaemic optic neuropathy.

3. Match the pictures (Figure 15.7) to the most probable diagnosis.

a   Optic disc drüsen.

b   Papilloedema.

c   Myopia.

d   Ischaemic optic neuropathy.

e   Glaucoma.

4. Optic neuritis

a   False. The visual loss usually progresses over a couple of days.

b   False. There may be pain on eye movement in retrobulbar neuritis.

c   True. It may be due to demyelination and be part of multiple sclerosis.

d   False. With isolated optic neuritis there is usually some degree of recovery.

e   True. This is a useful test in assessing optic nerve disease.

5. Ischaemic optic neuropathy

a   True. This may often be noticed by the patient on waking.

b   True. There may be sectorial swelling of the optic disc.

c   True. The condition may be a feature of giant cell arteritis. It is important to think of this in any senior patient, but there are also non-arteritic vascular causes.

d   False. If it is associated with giant cell arteritis this is the immediate treatment, but non-arteritic disease does not respond to steroids.

e   True. This is the classical field defect (Figure 15.3).

6. Optic atrophy may be seen in

a   True. It may be seen for example in retinitis pigmentosa.

b   True. Compression of the optic nerve causes axonal damage.

c   False. Disc pallor will only be seen in lesions anterior to the lateral geniculate body.

d   True. For example tobacco–alcohol or ethambutol toxicity.

e   True. An example is vitamin B_{12} deficiency.

16

Eye movements and their disorders

Learning objectives

To understand:

- ✔ The actions and control of the six muscles moving the eye.
- ✔ The difference between non-paralytic and paralytic squint.
- ✔ What is meant by binocular single vision.
- ✔ The cause, investigation and treatment of non-paralytic squint.
- ✔ The symptoms, signs and treatment of paralytic squint.
- ✔ The importance of the differential diagnosis of third nerve palsy.
- ✔ Gaze palsy and nystagmus.

To be able to:

- ✔ Perform a cover test.

Introduction

Eye movement abnormailities include

- an abnormal position of the eyes;
- a reduced range of eye movements;
- an abnormality in the character of the eye movements.

Anatomy and physiology

The innervation of the extraocular muscles is discussed in detail in Chapter 1.

There are six extraocular muscles that control eye movement: four recti and two obliques. The medial and lateral rectus control horizontal movements only; the vertical recti predominantly subserve vertical eye movements; the oblique muscles subserve rotation of the eyes (Figure 16.1 and Table 16.1).

The *cardinal positions of gaze* for assessing a muscle palsy are gaze right and left, up and down, and (obliquely), gaze up to the right and left, and gaze down to the right and left (Figure 16.2).

Three cranial nerves supply these muscles (see Chapter 1). The nuclei are found in the brainstem and pons (sixth nerve). Supranuclear pathways link them with other brainstem nuclei (e.g. vestibular) and with gaze centres (*horizontal gaze* in the pons and *vertical gaze* in the midbrain). These *supranuclear pathways* coordinate the movements of the two eyes.

Higher cortical centres control the speed with which the eyes follow a moving target (*smooth pursuit*), and the rapid movements required to take up a

Ophthalmology: Lecture Notes, Thirteenth Edition. Bruce James, Anthony Bron, and Manoj V. Parulekar.
© 2024 John Wiley & Sons Ltd. Published 2024 by John Wiley & Sons Ltd.
Companion website: www.wiley.com/go/ophthalmology13e

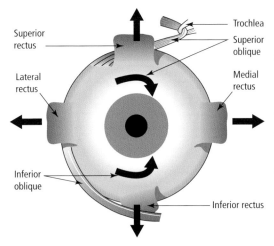

Superior rectus

Lateral rectus

Inferior oblique

Trochlea

Superior oblique

Medial rectus

Inferior rectus

Figure 16.1 The extraocular muscles of the right eye and their principal actions. Upper curved arrow shows incyclorotation, lower curved arrow shows excyclorotation.

new position of gaze (*saccades*). These centres also influence the brainstem nuclei.

The connections of the nuclei ensure that the eyes move together in a coordinated fashion (Figure 16.3). For example, when looking to the right, the right lateral and left medial rectus are equally stimulated and act as *yoke muscles*. At the same time, innervation of the antagonists which move the eyes to the left (the left lateral rectus and the right medial rectus) is inhibited.

Disorders of eye movement

Clinically, eye movement disorders are best described under three headings (which are not mutually exclusive):

1 *Squint* (also called strabismus), where there is non-alignment of the visual axes of the two eyes.

Table 16.1 The actions of extraocular muscles.

Muscle	Primary action	Secondary action	Tertiary action
Medial rectus	Adduction	—	—
Lateral rectus	Abduction	—	—
Superior rectus	Elevation	Incyclorotation	Adduction
Inferior rectus	Depression	Excyclorotation	Adduction
Superior oblique	Incyclorotation	Depression (especially in adduction)	Abduction
Inferior oblique	Excyclorotation	Elevation (especially in adduction)	Abduction

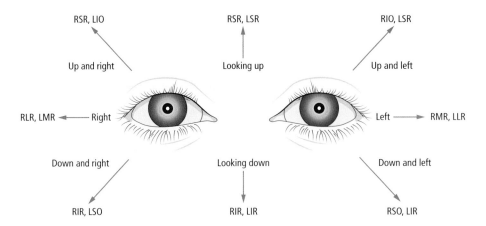

RSR, LIO — Up and right

RSR, LSR — Looking up

RIO, LSR — Up and left

RLR, LMR ← Right

Left → RMR, LLR

Down and right — RIR, LSO

Looking down — RIR, LIR

Down and left — RSO, LIR

Figure 16.2 The muscles responsible for moving the eyes through the cardinal positions of gaze.

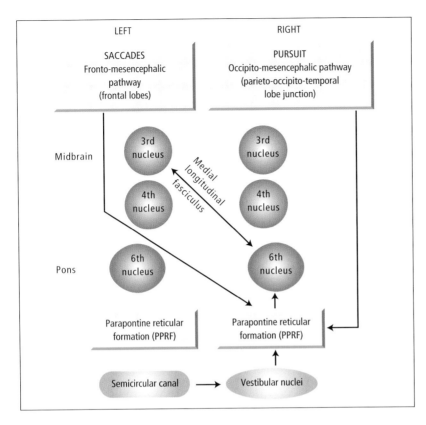

Figure 16.3 The connections of the nuclei and higher centres controlling horizontal eye movements. Vestibular, Saccade and smooth pursuit pathways shown for the right eye only.

Only one eye is directed to the object of regard - the other eye deviates. A squint may be:

a. *Comitant* (sometimes termed *concomitant*): where the angle of deviation remains constant in all directions of gaze and the range of eye movements of both eyes are full (Figure 16.4). This is the common squint seen in childhood.

b. *Incomitant*: where the angle of deviation changes with gaze. This could be due to:

i. underaction of one or more of the eye muscles due to a nerve palsy (*paralytic or paretic* squint) or muscular weakness (*myogenic* squint) as in myasthenia gravis;

ii. mechanical restriction of the muscles - resulting from entrapment of muscles (after orbital fracture), muscle infiltration or scarring (in thyroid eye disease) or an orbital mass.

For a nerve palsy, the squint is greatest in the *field of action* of the affected muscle (i.e. the direction in which that muscle would normally take the globe) (Figure 16.5), while with mechanical restriction, the squint is greatest in the direction *away from* the affected muscle.

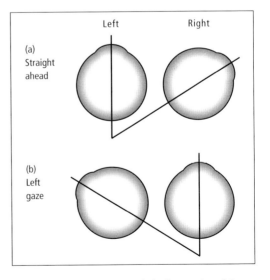

Figure 16.4 Right, non-paralytic divergent squint. (a) The right eye is divergent in the primary position of gaze (looking straight ahead). (b) When the eyes look to the left, the angle of deviation between the *visual axes* of the two eyes (the lines passing through the points of fixation and the foveolae) is unchanged. The same is the case on looking to the right.

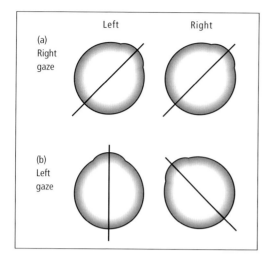

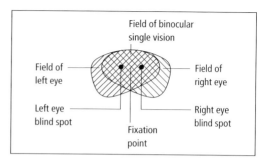

Figure 16.6 Elimination of the blind spot and increase in the field of vision resulting from overlapping visual fields and binocular single vision.

Figure 16.5 Left sixth nerve palsy with paralysis of the left lateral rectus (paralytic squint). (a) With the eyes looking to the right, the visual axes are aligned, there is no deviation between the visual axes of the two eyes. (b) With the eyes looking to the left (the field of action of the left lateral rectus), the left eye is unable to move past the midline as the left lateral rectus is paralysed. This results in a large angle convergent squint.

2 In *gaze palsies,* there is a disturbance of the supra-nuclear coordination of eye movements. Pursuit and saccadic eye movements may also be affected if the cortical pathways to the nuclei controlling eye movements are interrupted.

3 In *nystagmus,* there is an oscillating movement of the eyes due to a disorder of the brainstem nuclei or vestibular apparatus.

The concept of binocular single vision

Normally, (in the absence of a squint), both eyes are directed towards the same object of regard. Their movements are coordinated so that the retinal images of the object fall on almost identical, corresponding points of each retina. These images are fused centrally and are interpreted by the brain as a single image. This is termed *binocular single vision* (Figure 16.6). Because each eye views an object from a different angle, the retinal images do not fall *precisely* on corresponding points of each retina and it is this disparity that permits a three-dimensional percept to be constructed. This is

termed *stereopsis.* The development of stereopsis requires that eye movements and visual alignment are coordinated which occurs over about the first 5 years of life.

Binocular single vision and stereopsis afford certain advantages to the individual:

- They increase the field of vision.
- They eliminate the blind spot since the blind spot of one eye falls in the seeing field of the other.
- They provide binocular acuity, which is greater than monocular acuity.
- Stereopsis provides depth perception and allows an estimation of distance.

If the visual axes of the two eyes are not aligned, binocular single vision is not possible. This results in the following:

- *Diplopia (double vision):* An object is seen to be in two different places.
- *Visual confusion:* Two separate and different objects appear to be super-imposed.

In children, a squint results in suppression of the image in the squinting eye. This is the visual system's protective mechanism against diplopia. If this is prolonged and constant during the sensitive period of visual development (the first 5 years), it may result in permanent reduction in visual acuity in the squinting eye (*strabismic amblyopia*).

Amblyopia will only develop if the squint is constant, consistently affecting one eye (e.g. a right convergent squint). Some children freely alternate fixation, squinting with one eye or the other for an equal time. Such cases do not develop amblyopia, since both eyes are being used in turn and suppression does not occur. However, this means the two eyes are not used together and these children do not develop stereopsis.

History and Examination

History

The presence of a squint in a child may be noted by the parents or detected at preschool or school screening clinics. Older children and adults will be aware of a visible misalignment and may report symptoms of double vision. Squints may be intermittent or constant. There may be a family history of squint or refractive error. The following should be noted:

- When is the squint present – is it constant?
- How long has the squint been present? A long duration may have allowed the amblyopia to become entrenched.
- Past medical, birth and family history of the child.
- Any symptoms e.g. diplopia.

Examination

The patient is examined for external features that may simulate a squint (pseudo-squint) such as:

- *Epicanthus* (a crescentic fold of skin on the side of the nose that incompletely covers the inner canthus) (Figure 16.7) or *telecanthus* (increased distance between the inner canthi), which may simulate a convergent squint.
- Facial asymmetry.

Alignment of the eyes is tested using a pen torch and the cover test. The corneal reflection of a torch-light, held 33 cm in front of the subject, is a guide to eye position (the Hirschberg test). If there is no squint, the light reflex will be central in both eyes. If the subject is squinting, the reflection will be central in the fixating eye and *deviated in the squinting eye* (Figure 16.8).

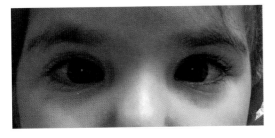

Figure 16.7 A child with epicanthic folds, giving the appearance of a convergent squint. Note the light reflex is central in both eyes.

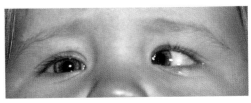

(a)

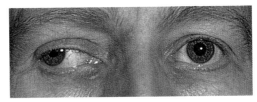

(b)

Figure 16.8 The appearance of (a) a left convergent squint: right eye fixing; and (b) a right divergent squint: left eye fixing. Note the position of the light reflection in each eye.

Before performing the cover test, it is important to understand the concept of *tropia* (manifest squint) and *phoria* (latent squint).

A latent squint (*phoria*) is a tendency of the eyes to lose binocular fixation, so that they drift apart when they are visually dissociated e.g. in the absence of bifoveal visual stimulation by the same object of regard. It is not necessarily an abnormal condition and small phorias can be demonstrated in most people who otherwise have normal binocular single vision. In general, an *esophoria* (a tendency of the eyes to drift inwards) is most common in people with hypermetropia and an *exophoria* (a tendency of the eyes to drift outwards) in those with myopia.

Phorias are usually controlled by unconscious effort. If this effort fails, for instance during fatigue, then a manifest non-paralytic squint (*tropia*), accompanied by diplopia, may occur. This is termed a *decompensation* of the phoria. The effort of maintaining binocular vision by adjusting for the heterophoria may at times be a source of symptoms such as eye-strain and headaches.

A manifest squint (tropia) on the other hand occurs even when both eyes are open and being simultaneously stimulated. One eye is fixing, and the other eye deviating. Tropias appear spontaneously without the need to dissociate the two eyes. Tropias can be constant, or intermittent with variable control.

There are two types of cover tests - the cover–uncover test, and the alternate cover test.

The *cover/uncover test or unilateral cover test* (Figure 16.9) is performed to detect a manifest squint (a tropia):

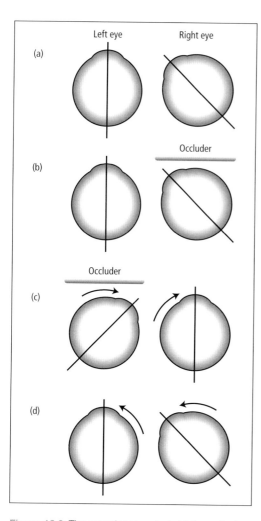

Left eye   Right eye

(a)

Occluder

(b)

Occluder

(c)

(d)

Figure 16.9 The cover/uncover test. (a) A manifest right convergent squint (right esotropia) is present. (b) The right, squinting eye is occluded. There is no movement of the left eye, which maintains fixation. (c) The left eye is occluded. The squinting right eye moves outwards to take up fixation, and the non-squinting eye moves inwards because the movement of the two eyes is linked. (d) The cover is removed from the left eye, which moves outwards to take up fixation; the right eye moves inward to resume its squinting position. (If an alternating squint was present (i.e. each eye retained the ability to fixate), the right eye would maintain fixation and the eyes would not move when the cover was removed.)

After observing to ascertain which eye appears to be deviating (in this case the right eye) the fixing left eye is covered for a few seconds while the subject fixates a target at 6m (Figure 16.9c). The right eye is observed for its reaction. If it moves outwards to take up fixation a right esotropia or convergent squint is

present. If the eye moves inward to take up fixation, a right exotropia or divergent squint is present.

A phoria can be detected with the alternate cover test. At rest, looking at a distant target, the position of the eyes appears normal. The right eye is covered for a few seconds and then the left eye. This is repeated a couple of times. This dissociates the eyes (there is no longer bifoveal stimulation). The right eye is now occluded and uncovered. As the occluder is removed any movement in the right eye is noted. If the eye moved inward to take up fixation an exophoria (latent divergence) is present. If the eye moved outwards to take up fixation an exophoria (latent divergence) is present. The same movements would be seen on uncovering the left eye following dissociation.

Cover tests should be performed both for distance and near targets. Some patients may have both a tropia and a phoria. Vertical tropias and phorias will also be revealed with these cover tests.

In an eye clinic, the squint can be further assessed with the synoptophore (see Chapter 3). This instrument, together with special three-dimensional pictures, can also be used to determine whether the eyes are used together and whether stereopsis is present.

Refractive error is measured following topical administration of cyclopentolate eye drops to paralyse accommodation and dilate the pupil. The eye is then examined to exclude opacities of the cornea, lens or vitreous and abnormalities of the retina or optic disc.

Investigating a squint

The following steps are taken in investigating a squinting child:

- Determination of acuity (see Chapter 3).
- Detection of any abnormality in eye movement.
- Detection and measurement of the squint.
- Measurement of stereopsis.
- Determination of any refractive error.
- Careful examination of the eyes, including a dilated fundus view.

Disorders of eye movements

Disorders of eye movement are discussed below under the three headings.

Squints (comitant and incomitant), gaze palsy and nystagmus.

Comitant squint

- Comitant squints may develop in an otherwise normal child with normal eyes. The cause is obscure but is thought to involve an abnormality in the central coordination of eye movements.
- They may develop in a child with hypermetropia (longsightedness). In a hypermetrope, accommodative effort is required to bring a distant object into focus on the retina; the closer the object to the eye, the greater the accommodative effort required (Chapter 4). A convergent squint develops because of the *increased accommodative effort* required to focus, particularly on near objects. The link (*synkinesis*) between the accommodative and convergence mechanisms leads to an excessive convergence and ultimately to a convergent squint of one eye. Where the squint *only* occurs on attempted focusing on near objects (an accommodative squint), amblyopia does not develop since binocular visual alignment remains normal for part of the time, during distant viewing.
- Comitant squints may develop if there is blurred vision in one or both eyes in early childhood, from any cause. The most common cause is refractive error, when the error is unequal between the two eyes (*anisometropia*). The eye with the greater refractive error and the more blurred vision will squint. Other causes of poor vision in one or both eyes,

cataracts, corneal opacity and retinal disorders, can also result in squint in the eye with the worse vision.

Treatment

The broad principles of treatment for comitant squints include:

- correction of significant refractive error with glasses.
- If amblyopia is present and the vision does not improve with glasses, the better-seeing eye is patched for a few hours each day for a few months (part time occlusion), to stimulate visual development and improve visual acuity in the amblyopic eye. It is important to understand that the purpose of patching is to improve vision in the amblyopic eye; it does not correct the squint. Similarly, squint surgery does not improve the vision in the amblyopic eye, and patching may still be necessary. Patching is only effective in children and not adults. Atropine drops given to the better seeing eye may also be used to stimulate vision in the amblyopic eye.
- *Surgical intervention* to realign the eyes may be required for functional reasons (to restore or establish binocular single vision) or for cosmetic reasons (to improve appearance and prevent a child being singled out at school) (Figure 16.10).

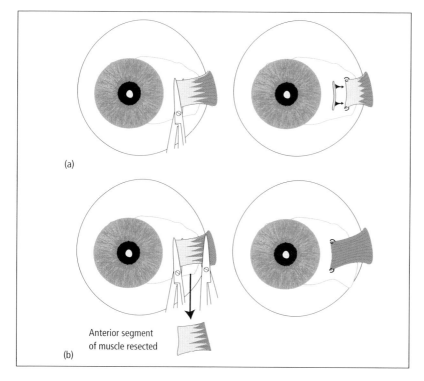

(a)

(b)

Anterior segment of muscle resected

Figure 16.10 The principles of squint surgery. (a) Recession. The conjunctiva has been incised to expose the medial rectus muscle. The muscle is then disinserted and moved backwards on the globe. (b) Resection. Following exposure of the muscle, the anterior tendon and muscle are resected, thus shortening them; the muscle is then reattached to its original position.

The principle of surgery is to realign the eyes by adjusting the position of the muscles on the globe or by shortening the muscle. Access to the muscles is gained by making a small incision in the conjunctiva. Disinserting the muscle and reattaching it further back on the globe (*recession*) reduces its mechanical advantage and weakens its action, causing the eye to move away from the side of that muscle. Removing a segment of the muscle at its insertion *(resection)* and reattaching it to the same location, moves the eye in the direction of the resected muscle.

Glasses and patching can significantly improve vision in the squinting eye. Timely intervention can result in development of stereopsis in the majority of comitant childhood squints.

Incomitant squints

Incomitant squints can be paralytic (due to nerve palsy) or myogenic (due to muscle weakness, or tight or trapped muscles which restrict eye movement).

Paralytic squint

Disorders of the third, fourth and sixth nerves and their central connections give rise to a paralytic strabismus (Figure 16.11). Each nerve may be affected at any point along its course from brainstem nucleus to orbit. Table 16.2 details some causes.

Older children and adults usually complain of diplopia. There may be an abnormal head posture to compensate for the inability of the eye to move in a particular direction.

A sixth nerve palsy results in a convergent squint with failure of abduction of the affected eye.

A fourth nerve palsy results in defective depression of the eye when attempted in adduction. It produces the least noticeable eye movement abnormality. Patients may notice vertical double vision with some torsion of the image, particularly when going downstairs or reading.

A third nerve palsy results in:

- Ptosis. Eye movements can be observed with the upper lid raised manually.
- The eye is directed 'down and out' because of the continued action of the fourth and sixth cranial nerves.
- There is a failure of adduction, elevation and depression of the eye.
- in some cases, a dilated pupil is seen due to involvement of parasympathetic fibres to the iris sphincter;
- pupil involvement in a third nerve palsy can be a feature of extrinsic compression of the nerve.

Posterior communicating artery aneurysm is an important cause of sudden onset of third nerve palsy with pupillary dilatation.

An isolated nerve palsy is often related to coexistent systemic disease. If a posterior communicating aneurysm is suspected, the patient must be sent for neurosurgical review and neuro-imaging. The most common cause of palsy is microvascular disease of a peripheral cranial nerve, associated with diabetes or hypertension. In this case, nerve function often recovers over months.

Orbital disease (see Chapter 5) and disease in the cavernous sinus may also be the cause of multiple nerve palsies involving the third, fourth and sixth nerves, because they are anatomically close together at these locations. A CT or MRI scan will show the lesion (e.g. an orbital metastasis).

Treatment

Diplopia is a very distressing symptom. Untreated diplopia is a contraindication for driving motor vehicles. It can be relieved by fitting *prisms* to the patient's glasses, to realign the retinal images while awaiting recovery of the nerve palsy. Alternatively, the affected eye can be patched. If eye movements fail to improve spontaneously, surgical intervention may be required. Such intervention will seldom restore full eye movements but is aimed at restoring an acceptable field of binocular single vision, that relieves diplopia in the central positions of gaze (i.e. straight ahead and in downgaze), the commonest positions in which the eyes are used.

Myogenic (related to the extraocular muscles)

Thyroid eye disease (Graves disease)

Disorders of the thyroid gland can be associated with an infiltration of the extraocular muscles with lymphocytes and the deposition of glycosaminoglycans in the tissues, leading to proptosis, exposure of the globes and limitation of eye movements. The condition occurs particularly in hyperthyroidism but also in hypothyroidism. The mechanism is believed to be autoimmune.

The patient may sometimes complain of:

- a red painful eye (associated with exposure caused by proptosis). If the redness is limited to part of the eye only, it may indicate active inflammation in the adjacent muscle;
- double vision;
- prominent looking eyes with incomplete lid closure (due to proptosis);

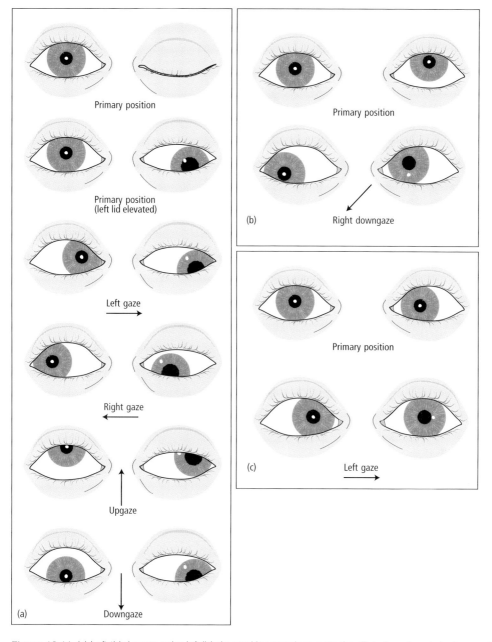

Figure 16.11 (a) Left third nerve palsy left lid elevated by examiner: note the dilated pupil and ptosis as well as the limitation of eye movement. (b) Left fourth nerve palsy: the defect is maximal when the patient tries to look down when the left eye is adducted. (c) Left sixth nerve palsy: the left eye is unable to abduct.

- reduced visual acuity (sometimes associated with optic neuropathy).

  On examination (Figure 16.12a):

- There may be *proptosis* of the eyes (also termed *exophthalmos*) - the eyes protrude from the orbit and appear to *stare*. This is often asymmetrical.

- The conjunctiva may be *chemosed* and the vessels dilated over the muscle insertions.
- The upper lid may be *retracted* so that sclera is visible above the upper border of the cornea, giving the eye a characteristic *staring* appearance. This is due in part to increased sympathetic activity stimulating the sympathetically innervated

Table 16.2 The causes of isolated nerve palsies.

Orbital disease	For example, neoplasia
Vascular disease	Diabetes (a 'pupil sparing' third nerve palsy, there is ptosis and extraocular muscle palsy but no mydriasis)
	Hypertension
	Aneurysm (most commonly a painful third nerve palsy from an aneurysm of the posterior communicating artery. Mydriasis is usually present)
	Carotid-cavernous sinus fistula (also causes myogenic palsy)
	Cavernous sinus thrombosis
Trauma	Most common cause of fourth and sixth nerve palsy
Neoplasia	Meningioma
	Acoustic neuroma
	Glioma
Raised intracranial pressure	May cause a third or sixth nerve palsy (a false localizing sign)
Inflammation	Sarcoidosis
	Vasculitis (i.e. giant cell arteritis)
	Infection (particularly herpes zoster)
	Guillain–Barré syndrome

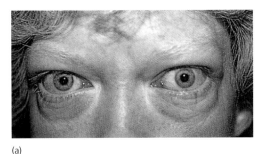

(a)

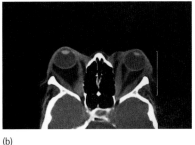

(b)

Figure 16.12 Dysthyroid eye disease: (a) clinical appearance; (b) a CT scan demonstrating muscle thickening.

Müller muscle, arising from the deep surface of the levator muscle.

- The upper lid may lag behind the movement of the globe on downgaze (*lid lag*).
- There may be restricted eye movements.

The inferior rectus is the most commonly affected muscle. Its movement becomes restricted and there is mechanical limitation of the eye in upgaze, which also aggravates the upper lid retraction. Involvement of the medial rectus causes mechanical limitation of abduction, thereby mimicking a sixth nerve palsy. A CT or an MRI scan shows enlargement of the rectus muscles (Figure 16.12b).

Dysthyroid eye disease is associated with two serious acute complications:

1 Excessive exposure of the conjunctiva and cornea with the formation of chemosis (oedematous swelling of the conjunctiva), and corneal ulcers due to exposure and failure of the lids to protect the cornea. The condition may lead to corneal perforation.

2 Compressive optic neuropathy due to compression and ischaemia of the optic nerve by the thickened muscles. This leads to field loss and may cause blindness.

In addition to imaging (CT or MRI scan), other investigations include:

- Thyroid function tests (more commonly hyperthyroid but any thyroid state is possible);
- Thyroid stimulating hormone receptor antibodies (TRAb) are raised in active thyroid eye disease).

Treatment is directed at management of the active disease (immunosuppresion) and of its sequelae.

Corneal exposure and optic nerve compression require urgent treatment with systemic steroids, radiotherapy or surgical orbital decompression.

In the long term, treatment may be needed for the eye movement problems and to improve the cosmetic appearance. A period must elapse while the eye movements stabilize, during which time prisms can be used to manage the diplopia. Once stabilized, if the patient remains symptomatic, surgery on the extraocular muscles can be performed to increase the field of binocular single vision. If desired, surgery to lower the upper lids can be undertaken following the squint surgery. This improves the appearance and achieves better protection of the cornea.

Myasthenia gravis

Myasthenia gravis is caused by the development of antibodies to the acetylcholine receptors of striated muscle. It affects females more than males and although commonest in the 15–50 age group, may affect young children and older adults. Some 40% of patients may show involvement of the extraocular muscles only.

Variation in clinical signs and symptoms over days to weeks, with fatiguability, is the hallmark of myasthenia. Eighty percent of myasthenia affects the eyes only, the remaining 20% may have systemic features such as dysphagia and dysphonia. Variable diplopia and variable ptosis may be present.

The diagnosis can be confirmed by the detection of anti-Acetylcholine receptor (anti-AchR) antibodies in the blood, or by single fibre electromyography of the orbicularis oculi. Injection of neostigmine or edrophonium (cholinesterase antagonists) to temporarily restore normal muscle movement is rarely used now because of the possibility of cholinergic side effects such as bradycardia and bronchospasm (see also Chapter 6).

Patients are treated, in collaboration with a neurologist, with oral pyridostigmine. Systemic steroids, other immunosuppressive agents, and surgical removal of the thymus also have a role in treatment.

Orbital myositis

This inflammation of the extraocular muscles is associated with pain and diplopia, leading to a restriction in the movement of the involved muscle (similar to that seen in dysthyroid eye disease). It is not usually associated with systemic disease, but thyroid abnormalities should be excluded. The conjunctiva over the involved muscle is inflamed. CT or MRI scanning shows thickening of the muscle. If symptoms are troublesome, it responds to a short course of steroids.

Chronic progressive external ophthalmoplegia (CPEO)

CPEO is a rare condition where the movement of the eyes is slowly reduced bilaterally, often symmetrically. It is caused by a mitochondrial DNA mutation affecting muscle function. There is an associated ptosis. Ultimately, eye movement may be lost completely. There may be accompanying retinal dystrophy and heart block.

Brown syndrome

In this condition, elevation of the eye in adduction is restricted due to restriction of the superior oblique muscle. The superior oblique muscle tendon fails to pass smoothly through its trochlear pulley or there is a stiff, inelastic tendon–muscle complex. The exact cause remains unknown. The condition may be congenital or result from orbital trauma or inflammation.

Duane syndrome

This is due to a 'congenital miswiring' or faulty innervation of the medial and lateral rectus muscles. The sixth nerve and/or nucleus may rarely be absent. The lateral rectus receives reduced or absent innervation from the sixth nerve. This is often accompanied by aberrant innervation of the lateral rectus by the third nerve. There is therefore reduced activity of the lateral rectus during attempted abduction, and co-contraction of the medial and lateral rectus during adduction. This results in narrowing of the palpebral aperture on adduction, with retraction of the eye into the orbit (due to simultaneous contraction of medial and lateral rectus muscles). The condition may be unilateral or, more rarely, bilateral. Children do not usually develop amblyopia, because the eyes are aligned in the straight ahead (primary) position, or with a small abnormal head posture (face turn away from the affected lateral rectus). Rarely, surgical intervention is needed if there is a squint or if there is a significant abnormal head posture.

Gaze palsies

Gaze is the coordinated movement of the two eyes together, in a given direction, as in right, left, up or downgaze. It is under the control of *supranuclear* pathways. A gaze palsy is a weakness of gaze resulting from damage to these pathways, connecting the cranial nerve nuclei and higher centres. The more common palsies are briefly described below. The ophthalmologist usually investigates and manages these patients with the help of a neurologist.

Lesions of the paramedian pontine reticular formation (PPRF)

The PPRF controls the horizontal movements of the eyes. Lesions affecting the PPRF are usually associated with other brainstem disease. It may be seen in patients with vascular disease and tumours.

There is a failure of horizontal movements of both eyes to the side of the lesion (a *horizontal gaze palsy*), and deviation of the eyes to the contralateral side in acute cases.

Internuclear ophthalmoplegia

This is caused by a lesion of the *medial longitudinal fasciculus* (MLF) (Figure 16.13). The MLF connects the sixth nerve nucleus to the third nerve nucleus on the opposite side and coordinates their activity in horizontal gaze movements.

It may be affected by demyelination (e.g. multiple sclerosis – usually bilateral) and vascular disease (unilateral).

The patient complains of horizontal diplopia. There is reduction of adduction on the same side as the lesion, and nystagmus of the contralateral, abducting eye (abducting nystagmus).

Spontaneous recovery is usual, although variable in demyelination. An MRI scan may be helpful diagnostically, both to locate the causal brainstem lesion and, in demyelination, to determine whether other plaques are present.

Parinaud syndrome (dorsal midbrain syndrome)

In Parinaud syndrome, a lesion in the dorsal midbrain affects the centre for vertical gaze. It may be seen in patients with demyelination, space-occupying lesions such as a *pinealoma* which presses on the tectum, infarction of the dorsal midbrain or an enlarged third ventricle from hydrocephalus.

The disorder causes deficient (and often painful or uncomfortable) elevation of both eyes, convergence of the eyes and retraction into the orbit associated with nystagmus on attempted elevation (*convergence–retraction nystagmus*) and light–near dissociation of the pupil (the pupil reacts poorly to a light stimulus but constricts normally on accommodation).

Abnormal oscillations of the eyes

Nystagmus

Nystagmus is a repetitive, rhythmic, to and fro movement of one or both eyes. Such movements occur physiologically when viewing a moving object (e.g. looking out of a train window) (*optokinetic nystagmus*) or following stimulation of the vestibular system. When examined closely, they have a slow phase in one direction and a fast phase in the other (*jerk nystagmus*). The nystagmus is described as beating to the side of the fast component. In some cases, the speed of eye movement may be roughly the same in either direction (*pendular nystagmus*). Jerk nystagmus may also be seen at the extreme position of gaze (*terminal or gaze-evoked nystagmus*).

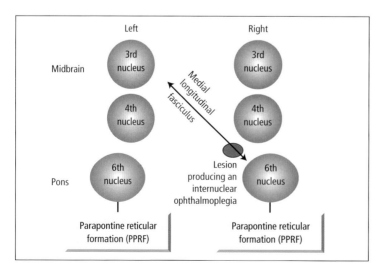

Figure 16.13 The site of the lesion producing an internuclear ophthalmoplegia.

Nystagmus may be present from birth (congenital) or acquired.

Acquired nystagmus

Patients with acquired nystagmus complain that the visual environment is in continual movement (*oscillopsia*).

Acquired nystagmus may result from:

- Cerebellar disease. It is worse when gaze is directed towards the side of the lesion and the fast phase is directed towards the side of the lesion;
- Drugs (such as barbiturates);
- Damage to the labyrinth and its central connections (the vestibular system); a fine jerk nystagmus results – the fast phase of the movement is away from the lesion and it is usually present only acutely.

The pattern of nystagmus may help localize the disease process to certain parts of the brain. An *upbeat* nystagmus (fast phase upwards) is commonly associated with brainstem disease. It may also be seen in toxic states, for example following excess alcohol intake. A *downbeat* nystagmus may be seen in patients with a posterior fossa lesion near the cervicomedullary junction (e.g. a Chiari malformation, where cerebellar tissue is dragged through the foramen magnum). It may also be seen in patients with demyelination, and again may be present in toxic states.

Patients with nerve palsies or weakness of the extraocular muscles may develop nystagmus when looking in the direction of the affected muscle (*gaze-evoked nystagmus*). The fast phase of the movement is in the field of action of the weak muscle.

Congenital nystagmus

Nystagmus can be congenital in origin. It may be due to:

- a defect in the central control mechanisms of eye movements (*congenital idiopathic motor nystagmus*);
- conditions that interfere with visual development within the first few months of life (when steady fixation develops) – for example, bilateral congenital cataracts or glaucoma;
- albinism – the exact mechanism is not understood but may relate to a failure of visual development.

The continuous movement of the eye induces a blur and reduces visual acuity, but congenital nystagmus does not cause oscillopsia. In some cases, nystagmus is damped by accommodation. Some subjects may also find a position of the eyes which reduces the nystagmus to a minimum. (the *null position or null zone*), thus maximizing visual acuity.

Certain forms of congenital nystagmus may benefit from squint surgery to reduce abnormal head posture or improve vision by dampening nystagmus. Drug treatment e.g. with baclofen can help control acquired nystagmus. Unfortunately, most types of nystagmus are not amenable to any form of treatment.

 KEY POINTS

- In analysing eye movement problems, try to determine whether there is an abnormal position of the eyes, a reduction in the range of eye movements, an abnormality in the form of eye movements, or a combination of these events.
- An abnormality in the range of eye movements may reflect muscular, orbital, infranuclear or supranuclear disease.
- An intracranial aneurysm may present as a painful third nerve palsy usually involving the pupil.
- Dysthyroid eye disease may cause exposure of the cornea and optic neuropathy.

Assessment questions True or False

1. **Match the eye muscle to the nerve.**
   a   Lateral rectus.
   b   Superior rectus.
   c   Medial rectus.
   d   Inferior rectus.
   e   Superior oblique.
   f   Inferior oblique.
      i.   Third nerve.
      ii.   Fourth nerve.
      iii.   Sixth nerve.

2. **Which of the following statements are true?**
   a   In a non-paralytic strabismus, the movement of the eyes is reduced.
   b   In a non-paralytic strabismus, the angle of deviation is unrelated to the direction of gaze.
   c   In a paralytic strabismus, the eye movement is reduced.
   d   Nystagmus refers to an oscillating movement of the eyes.
   e   In a horizontal gaze palsy, the patient is unable to look to one side.

3. Amblyopia

a Refers to a developmental reduction in visual acuity.

b May be caused by Duane syndrome.

c May be caused by a previously unidentified difference in refractive correction between the two eyes.

d May be caused by a squint.

e May be treated by patching the amblyopic eye.

4. Nerve palsies affecting the third, fourth and sixth cranial nerves may be seen in:

a Orbital disease.

b Raised intracranial pressure.

c Ischaemia of the cerebral cortex.

d Systemic inflammatory disease.

e Trauma.

5. Internuclear ophthalmoplegia

a Is caused by a lesion of the medial longitudinal fasciculus.

b Manifests as a reduced adduction and contralateral nystagmus in the abducting eye.

c Is manifested by a failure of the eye to elevate in adduction.

d May be caused by demyelination.

e Requires surgical treatment.

Answers

1. Match the eye muscle to the nerve.

a Sixth nerve.

b Third nerve.

c Third nerve.

d Third nerve.

e Fourth nerve.

f Third nerve.

2. Which of the following statements are true?

a False. The eye movements are full but only the dominant eye is directed towards the fixated target.

b True. The angle of deviation will remain the same no matter which direction the eyes are looking.

c True.

d True.

e True. Supranuclear coordination is affected. This may be seen in a patient with an acute cerebrovascular accident.

3. Amblyopia

a True. The poor vision is caused by a failure of visual development.

b False. The eyes are usually aligned in one direction or other, so that binocular vision develops normally.

c True. If the images on the retinas are dissimilar, with one image more blurred than the other, the brain suppresses the more blurred image.

d True. If the visual axes are not aligned, the brain will suppress the image from one eye.

e False. The non-amblyopic eye is patched, to improve vision in the amblyopic eye.

4. Nerve palsies affecting the third, fourth and sixth cranial nerves may be seen in

a True. Any oculomotor palsy or combination of palsies may be seen in diseases affecting the orbital apex where the nerves travel together.

b True. The third and sixth cranial nerve may be compressed along their intracranial course.

c False. This will not affect the cranial nerves.

d True. It may be seen in sarcoidosis, for example.

e True. This is the most common cause of a fourth or sixth cranial nerve palsy.

5. Internuclear ophthalmoplegia

a True. See Figure 16.13.

b True.

c False. This is the description of Brown syndrome.

d True. It is often bilateral in multiple sclerosis.

e False. Spontaneous resolution is usual in patients with a microvascular cause. Recovery is more variable in patients with multiple sclerosis.

17

Trauma

Learning objectives

To be able to:

✔ Take a history in a case of eye trauma.

To understand:

✔ The effects of trauma on the eye and related structures.

✔ The management of penetrating eye trauma.

✔ The management of chemical injury to the eye.

Introduction

Although the eye is well protected by the bony orbit, which itself may be damaged by trauma, it may yet be subject to injury (Figure 17.1). Forms of injury include:

- Foreign bodies which become lodged under the upper lid or on the surface of the eye, especially the cornea.
- Blunt trauma from objects small enough not to impact on the orbital rim (e.g. shuttlecocks, squash balls, champagne corks and knuckles). The sudden alteration of ocular pressure and distortion of the eye may cause severe damage.
- Penetrating trauma, where ocular structures are damaged by a foreign body, which passes through the ocular coat and may be retained in the eye. With the introduction of seat belt laws, the incidence of penetrating injury following road traffic accidents has declined.
- Chemical and radiation injury, where the resultant reaction of the ocular tissues causes the damage.

History

A careful history is essential.

- Use of a hammer and chisel can release a flake of metal which will penetrate the globe, leaving only *a tell-tale subconjunctival haemorrhage* to indicate the site of scleral penetration and suggest a retained foreign body. Pain may be minor and heat, generated by the high velocity, sterilizes the fragment so that infection does not occur. The patient may be unaware of the nature of the injury or its cause. Undetected, such a retained foreign body may have devastating effects on the eye.
- A wire released from tension, or a rose thorn, may penetrate the cornea briefly, sometimes creating a barely visible track.
- A blunt injury to the eye may also result in damage to the orbit (*blow-out fracture*).
- It is vitally important to determine the nature of any chemical that may have been in contact with the eye. Strong alkalis and acids penetrate the

Ophthalmology: Lecture Notes, Thirteenth Edition. Bruce James, Anthony Bron, and Manoj V. Parulekar.
© 2024 John Wiley & Sons Ltd. Published 2024 by John Wiley & Sons Ltd.
Companion website: www.wiley.com/go/ophthalmology13e

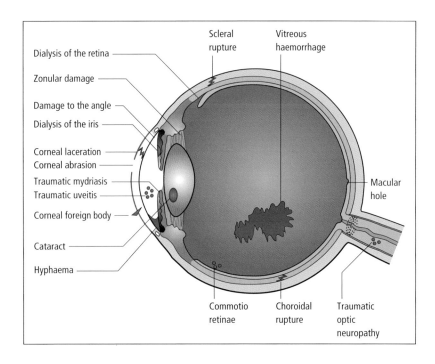

Dialysis of the retina
Zonular damage
Damage to the angle
Dialysis of the iris
Corneal laceration
Corneal abrasion
Traumatic mydriasis
Traumatic uveitis
Corneal foreign body
Cataract
Hyphaema

Scleral rupture
Vitreous haemorrhage
Macular hole

Commotio retinae
Choroidal rupture
Traumatic optic neuropathy

Figure 17.1 The extent of possible traumatic damage to the eye.

anterior tissues of the eye rapidly and may cause irreversible damage.

The patient's symptoms relate to the degree and type of trauma suffered. Pain, lacrimation and blurring of vision are common features of trauma, but mild symptoms may disguise a potentially blinding intraocular foreign body. As in all history taking, it is essential to enquire about previous ocular and medical events.

Examination

Without a slit lamp

The examination will depend on the type of injury. In all cases, it is important that visual acuity is recorded in the injured and *uninjured* eye for medico-legal reasons, among others. Where a penetrating injury is suspected, pressure on the globe must be avoided and it may only be possible to measure vision approximately in the injured eye; the patient may be able to detect light shone through the closed lid and even the direction of the source. The skin around the orbit and eyelids should be carefully examined for a penetrating wound.

Orbital injury

Damage to the orbital walls (a *blow-out fracture*; Figure 17.2) should be suspected if the orbital rim is intact and the following signs are present:

- Emphysema. Air derived from a fractured sinus, crackles when the overlying skin pressed.
- A patch of paraesthesia below the orbital rim suggests *infraorbital nerve* damage. The infraorbital nerve is commonly injured by an orbital blow-out fracture.
- Limitation of eye movements, particularly on upgaze and downgaze, due to trapping of the inferior rectus muscle by connective tissue septa caught in the fracture site in the inferior orbital floor, the wall most commonly fractured.
- Subsequently, the eye may become recessed into the orbit (*enophthalmos*).
- If the lid margin is cut at the medial canthus, it is important to determine if the lacrimal canaliculi are severed. This will cause epiphora.

Further examination of a traumatized eye requires the instillation of a local anaesthetic to facilitate lid opening (benoxinate, lidocaine, amethocaine). If a penetrating eye injury is suspected, *it is important that no pressure is applied to the globe*, to avoid expression of its contents. Blepharospasm can be minimized

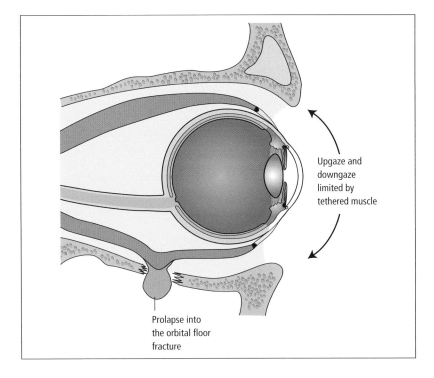

Figure 17.2 A blow-out fracture.

Upgaze and downgaze limited by tethered muscle

Prolapse into the orbital floor fracture

by keeping ambient illumination low. A drop of anaesthetic instilled at the inner canthus with the eyes closed, will find its way onto the ocular surface to achieve anaesthesia. The upper lid can be raised, without pressure on the globe, if a thumb is placed firmly onto the upper orbital rim and then rotated slowly to elevate the lid. With the eye open, the anterior segment can be examined carefully at the slit lamp with a narrow beam of light.

In a child or adult with limited cooperation, examination under general anaesthesia may be indicated to ascertain the extent of injury and plan treatment.

The conjunctiva and sclera

These must be examined for the presence of lacerations. If the history is appropriate, a subconjunctival haemorrhage must be considered as the possible site of a scleral perforation, requiring fundus examination with full mydriasis to exclude a retained intraocular foreign body (Figure 17.3).

Retained, iron-containing foreign bodies may have an insidious and particularly devastating effect on the eye (*siderosis oculi*). A tiny, high-velocity metal fragment, penetrating the ocular coats and retained in the peripheral vitreous cavity, can, with

Symptoms and signs of a penetrating eye injury

- History of high-velocity object hitting the eye.
- Conjunctival or subconjunctival haemorrhage.
- Dark tissue in the cornea or sclera (iris plugging of a penetrating wound).
- Distortion of the pupil.
- Unusually deep anterior chamber.
- Cataract.
- Vitreous haemorrhage.

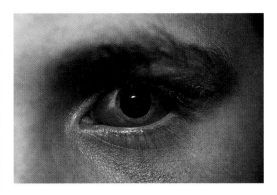

Figure 17.3 A subconjunctival haemorrhage.

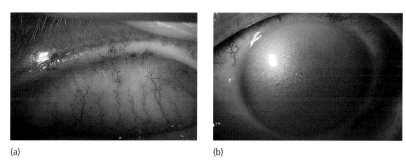

(a)   (b)

Figure 17.4 (a) An everted lid showing ischaemia of the upper tarsal conjunctiva following an alkali burn. (b) A diffusely hazy cornea following an alkali burn.

time, lead to a progressive, pigmentary degeneration of the retina. The mechanism of damage is by the diffusion of ferrous ions throughout the globe and the generation of free radicals in affected tissues, via the Fenton reaction. A discolouration of the iris (*heterochromia*), a dilated and unresponsive pupil (fixed mydriasis) and cataract are late clues to the diagnosis. Failure to detect and remove such a foreign body at the time of injury results in irreversible blindness.

Events of this kind emphasize the need to wear protective goggles when using metal hammers or hammering on metal.

After chemical injury, the conjunctiva may appear white and ischaemic (Figure 17.4). Extensive changes to the corneal limbus, the site of the *epithelial corneal stem cells*, grossly impair corneal healing by retarding epithelial resurfacing. Additional complications such as uveitis, secondary glaucoma and cataract contribute to the overall burden of disease.

The cornea

This is examined for loss of the epithelial layer (abrasion), for lacerations and for foreign bodies (Figure 17.5). Instillation of fluorescein will identify the extent of an abrasion and use of concentrated fluorescein will identify a leak of aqueous through a penetrating wound (see Chapter 3). If the globe appears intact, fine, vertical, linear corneal abrasions may suggest the presence of a *subtarsal foreign body* which can be located by eversion of the upper lid (Figure 3.16) and removed under topical anaesthesia.

Electromagnetic radiation may injure the conjunctiva and the cornea. Unprotected exposure to ultraviolet radiation from an artificial source (such as an arc lamp (*arc eye*) or sunlamp), or a natural source (reflected from snow (*snow blindness*) or water), is the commonest cause of this painful condition. Typically, severe ocular pain starts acutely, 6 hours

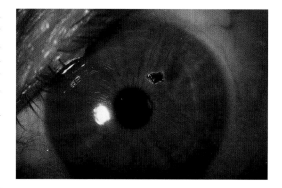

Figure 17.5 A foreign body, embedded in the cornea. (*Source:* Courtesy of Sue Ford, Western Eye Hospital.)

after exposure to the radiation, and the cornea shows diffuse epithelial oedema and punctate keratitis which resolve within 24–48 hours.

The anterior chamber

Blunt trauma may cause haemorrhage into the anterior chamber, where it collects with a fluid level, visible as a *hyphaema* (Figure 17.6a). This is caused by rupture of blood vessels at the root of the iris, or the iris may be torn away from its insertion into the ciliary body (*iris dialysis*) to produce a D-shaped pupil. Hyphaema may also be seen with a penetrating eye injury and the shape of the pupil may be distorted if the peripheral iris has plugged a penetrating corneal wound (Figure 17.6b). The pupil may also show a fixed dilatation as a result of blunt trauma due to injury to the iris sphincter (*traumatic mydriasis*).

The lens

Dislocation of the lens following blunt trauma may be suggested by fluttering of the iris diaphragm on eye

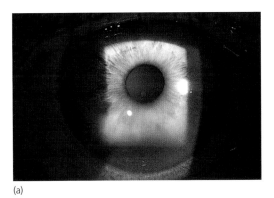
(a)

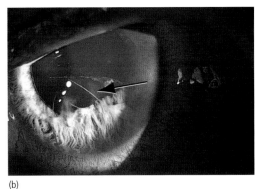
(b)

Figure 17.6 (a) A hyphaema. (b) Penetrating eye injury (note the eyelashes (arrowed) in the anterior chamber and the distorted iris).

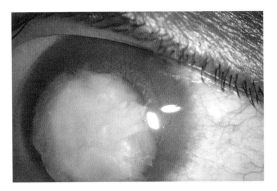

Figure 17.7 The lens in this patient has become disrupted and cataractous following a penetrating injury.

movement (*iridodonesis*). Lens clarity should be assessed against the red reflex after pupil dilatation. Cataracts develop rapidly after direct penetrating trauma (Figure 17.7). Blunt trauma can also cause a posterior subcapsular cataract within hours of injury, which may be transient. A tiny hole in the iris may indicate that a penetrating injury has occurred and a subjacent lens opacity will be found on pupil dilatation.

The fundus

The fundus should be inspected with a direct ophthalmoscope after full mydriasis. If ocular penetration is not suspected, the pupil can be dilated. In a closed eye injury, or *concussion injury,* areas of retinal haemorrhage may be seen with typical patches of white, retinal oedema (*commotio retinae*). A *retinal dialysis* (a separation of the peripheral retina from its junction with the pars plana of the ciliary body) and a

macular hole (see Chapter 12) may also result from blunt trauma. The choroid may also become torn, causing a subretinal haemorrhage which later leads to subretinal scarring. Peripheral retinal changes can only be excluded with indirect ophthalmoscopy or slit-lamp microscopy. If there is no red reflex and no fundus details are visible, this suggests the presence of a vitreous haemorrhage. Where pupil monitoring is indicated following brain injury, it may not be appropriate to dilate the pupils.

The optic disc may be pale from a traumatic optic neuropathy caused by *avulsion* of the blood vessels supplying the optic nerve. Although this is uncommon, it leads to a total loss of vision and no treatment is available.

With a slit lamp

The slit lamp allows a more detailed examination to be performed, which may reveal:

- A shallow anterior chamber compared to the fellow eye, suggesting an anterior penetrating injury with aqueous loss.
- A microscopic hyphaema, where red cells are present, circulating in the anterior chamber, but have not yet settled to form a level.
- The presence of white cells in the anterior chamber (*traumatic uveitis*).
- *Recession* of the iridocorneal angle seen with a gonioscopic contact lens. Here, the ciliary muscle apex is disinserted from the scleral spur and moves posteriorly. This may be seen with blunt trauma and results in raised intraocular pressure, sometimes after a delay of months or years. Conversely a separation of the ciliary body from the scleral spur

may cause a *cyclodialysis cleft* connecting the anterior chamber with the suprachoroidal space causing a low intraocular pressure.

- Raised intraocular pressure measured by applanation tonometry – this may accompany a hyphaema, lens dislocation or, as noted, damage to the chamber angle.

Treatment

Orbital blow-out fracture

If a blow-out fracture is suspected, a CT scan will delineate the bony and soft-tissue injury. If this is not possible, then plain orbital radiographs are performed. Treatment may be delayed until the periorbital swelling has settled. At this later stage, the degree of enophthalmos and the limitation of eye movement can be measured. If the enophthalmos is cosmetically unacceptable or eye movements are significantly limited, then surgical repair of the orbital fracture is indicated. Although some surgeons advocate an early intervention to obtain the best results, many patients require no surgery at all.

Lacerations to the skin and lids

These require careful apposition and suturing, particularly if the lid margin is involved, to retain the lid contour. If one of the lacrimal canaliculi is damaged, an attempt can be made to repair it, but if repair is unsuccessful, usually the remaining tear canaliculus is capable of draining the tears adequately. If both canaliculi are severed, an attempt at repair should always be made.

Corneal abrasion

This results from a glancing blunt injury which shears a patch of corneal epithelium from the basal lamina. It is extremely painful, but normally heals in a few days, depending on its size of the epithelial defect. It is treated with antibiotic ointment, with or without an eye pad. Dilatation of the pupil with cyclopentolate 1% can help to relieve pain caused by spasm of the ciliary muscle.

Recurrent Corneal Erosion

Recurrent corneal erosion is a condition of repeated painful attacks of corneal epithelial detachment, following a non-lacerating corneal injury. Recurrent attacks of extreme, debilitating pain cause marked epiphora and temporary visual loss. The detached epithelium may remain intact, but loose, or be sheared by an extensive erosion. Painful symptoms, persisting for days or weeks, are followed by periods of quiescence.

Despite adequate epithelial resurfacing and an absence of corneal scarring, epithelial adhesion remains impaired, so that the cornea remains vulnerable to further epithelial detachments at the site of injury. Typically, a patient experiences an episode of severe pain on opening the eyes after a night's sleep, as the opening upper lid pulls on the poorly adherent epithelium and triggers an attack. *The history alone should suggest the likely diagnosis.* Between attacks, the cornea may look normal on biomicroscopy but a few, tiny epithelial microcysts, which take up fluorescein in a brilliant and distinctive manner, often mark the affected zone and *can direct the clinician's attention to the region requiring treatment.*

A common cause of recurrent erosion is glancing trauma with a flexible object such as a baby's fingernail, twig or a plastic implement. This scuffs off the corneal epithelium at the site of contact, probably taking with it a layer of the underlying epithelial basement membrane critical for epithelial reattachment once epithelial resurfacing has taken place.

Occasionally, recurrent erosion may occur as a complication of bilateral epithelial basement membrane, or *map-dot-fingerprint* disorder. Here, there is an intrinsic, sometimes inherited, defect in epithelial adhesion which gives rise recurrent erosion attacks after minimal trauma or arising spontaneously; the risk of attacks is bilateral and the disorder is characterized by clusters of epithelial dots or of subepithelial map or fingerprint-like patterns detected by retro-illumination at the slit lamp.

Management

In the first instance, attacks are treated with a simple lubricating ointment at night to reduce friction between the upper lid and the globe. Nightly use of hypertonic agents to draw water from the cornea, such as 5% sodium chloride drops or corn syrup, is also advised. Other conservative measures include the use therapeutic hydrogel contact lenses or gas-permeable scleral lenses. Doxycycline prescribed with steroid eye drops may also be effective.

Where such measures fail, a surgical approach using corneal micropuncture or phototherapeutic (laser) keratoplasty (PTK), to create a subepithelial scar at the site of the original injury, may give long-lasting relief or a permanent cure.

UV injury to the cornea

This responds quickly to topical steroids. Dilation of the pupil with cyclopentolate 1% to overcome the associated spasm of the ciliary muscle and application of a lubricant gel is the standard treatment. Although often given, there is no evidence for the application of topical antibiotics.

Corneal foreign bodies

Corneal foreign bodies should be removed with a needle under topical anaesthesia (Figure 17.8). Where the foreign body contains iron, a rust ring may remain which can be removed with a small, rotating burr. Subtarsal objects can often be swept away with a cotton wool bud from the everted lid. The patient is then treated as for an abrasion. If there is any suggestion that a foreign body may have penetrated the globe, the eye must be carefully examined with dilation of the pupil to allow a good view of the lens and retina. A radiograph of the orbits, with the eyes looking up and then down, or a CT scan, may also be indicated if an intraocular foreign body is suspected. Microsurgical techniques can be used to remove foreign bodies from the eye under direct view.

Corneal and scleral penetrating trauma

Once identified, no further examination of the globe should be performed but a shield should be gently placed over the eye and the patient referred for urgent ophthalmic assessment and treatment. It should be assumed that the patient will need surgery under general anaesthesia and the patient prepared appropriately and kept nil by mouth. These serious injuries, often with grave implications for sight, require careful microsurgical suturing to restore the integrity of the globe. Once the eye has settled from this primary repair, additional operations are often required later to:

- remove a foreign body;
- remove a cataract;
- replace a corneal opacity with a corneal graft;
- repair a detached retina or remove the vitreous gel to prevent detachment.

Occasionally, in severe ocular trauma, the fellow eye may develop a sight-threatening sympathetic ophthalmitis (see Chapter 10).

Uveitis

This responds to treatment with steroids and dilating drops. It may be accompanied by elevated intraocular pressure requiring additional medical treatment.

Hyphaema

This usually settles with rest, but a re-bleed may occur in the first 5–6 days after injury. Children may sometimes require admission to hospital for a few days, while adults can be treated at home, provided they can rest and no complications develop. Steroid eye drops are given for a short time, together with dilation of the pupil. Steroids may reduce the risk of re-bleeds. The commonest complication is a raised ocular pressure, particularly if there is a secondary bleed, which tends to be more severe than the first. It is for this reason that rest is important, although the patient can be ambulant. Raised pressure is due to the accumulation of empty, red cell 'ghosts' in the trabecular meshwork or damage to the drainage angle itself (e.g. angle recession). It usually responds to medical treatment, but occasionally surgical intervention is required. When the hyphaema has settled, it is important that the eye is carefully checked for other complications of blunt trauma. A hyphaema clears more slowly after trauma in patients with sickle cell disease because the hypoxic and acidic environment within the anterior chamber precipitates sickling, and the rigid sickle cells are more difficult to remove via the trabecular meshwork.

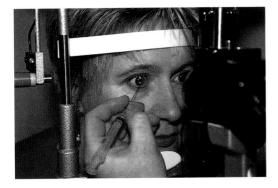

Figure 17.8 Removal of a superficial ocular foreign body at the slit lamp using the dominant hand and the patient's cheek as a rest.

Retinal damage

In *commotio retinae,* the affected zone of retina opacifies and obscures the underlying choroidal detail. It usually resolves, but requires careful observation, since retinal holes may develop in affected areas and may lead to subsequent retinal detachment.

Retinal dialysis, a separation of the retina from the ora serrata, requires surgical intervention to repair any detached retina.

A *vitreous haemorrhage* although it may absorb over several weeks may require earlier removal by vitrectomy. An ultrasound scan is useful in detecting associated retinal detachments when the retina cannot be viewed directly.

Chemical injury

The most important part of the treatment is to *irrigate the eye immediately*, with copious quantities of clean water *at the time of the accident*. Prior instillation of topical anaesthesia may facilitate irrigation. This must be repeated when ophthalmic care is available. It is also important to irrigate under the upper and lower lids to remove solid particles, such as lime. The nature of the chemical can then be ascertained by history and measuring tear pH with litmus paper. Administration of steroid and dilating drops may be required. Vitamin C, given both orally and topically, may improve healing. Systemic and topical anticollagenases may be needed (e.g. tetracyclines).

Extensive damage to the limbus may prevent resurfacing of the cornea with epithelium. A prolonged epithelial defect may lead to a corneal 'melt' (*keratolysis*). Stem cell deficiency is treated later, by limbal *stem cell transplantation,* for instance from the normal, fellow eye or from a donor source. Alternatively or additionally, an overlay of *amniotic membrane* can be applied to the damaged surface, which protects and maintains the underlying tissue and promotes epithelial resurfacing. It is also possible to resurface the cornea by transplanting expanded sheets of corneal limbal or even oral mucosal cells, grown in culture.

Prognosis

The eye heals well following minor trauma and there are rarely long-term sequelae save for the occurrence of the *recurrent corneal erosion* syndrome. Penetrating ocular trauma, however, is often associated with severe visual damage and may require extensive surgery. Long-term retention of iron foreign bodies may destroy retinal function by the generation of free radicals. Similarly, chemical injuries to the eyes can result in severe long-term visual impairment and ocular discomfort. Blunt trauma can cause untreatable visual loss if a retinal hole develops at the fovea. Vision will also be impaired if the choroid at the macula is damaged. In the longer term, secondary glaucoma can develop in an eye several years after the initial insult if the trabecular meshwork has been damaged. Severe orbital trauma may also cause both cosmetic and oculomotor problems.

 KEY POINTS

- Take an accurate history.
- Foreign bodies can often be found under the upper lid.
- Persistent pain in an intact eye suggests a subtarsal foreign body.
- Irrigate chemical injuries immediately with clean water.
- Suspect a perforating eye injury if the pupil is not round, a cataract has developed rapidly or a vitreous haemorrhage is present.
- In a child or adult with limited cooperation, examination under anaesthesia may be needed.
- Patients with ocular trauma should be kept nil-by-mouth in case a general anaesthetic is required.
- Place an eyeshield over an eye suspected of having a penetrating injury.

Assessment questions
True or False

1. **Orbital injury may produce the following signs:**
a Periorbital emphysema.
b Limitation of eye movements.
c Exophthalmos in the longer term.
d A patch of anaesthesia below the orbital rim.
e Hyphaema.

2. **A subconjunctival haemorrhage**
a Is never associated with serious eye disease.
b May cause blood to pass into the cornea.
c Is usually associated with a reduced vision.
d May be associated with some discomfort of the eye.
e Usually settles in a couple of weeks.

3. Chemical eye injuries

a Acids cause more severe damage than alkalis.
b Initial treatment requires copious irrigation of the eye with litres of water.
c May be associated with a melt of the cornea.
d A white eye is a sign that the eye has not been severely affected.
e May be treated with oral and topical vitamin C and tetracyclines.

4. A hyphaema

a Is a fluid collection of white cells in the anterior chamber.
b May be associated with a low intraocular pressure.
c Is treated with restriction of activity.
d If it recurs within a short time, it may result in more severe problems.
e Is treated with steroid drops.

Answers

1. Orbital injury may produce the following signs:

a True. The skin appears to crackle when touch due to the presence of air within it.
b True. There may be swelling of the orbital contents, or the muscle or orbital tissue may become tethered in the orbital fracture.
c False. The eye is usually recessed into the orbit (enophthalmos).
d True. This occurs with an orbital blow-out affecting the floor of the orbit, which damages the infraorbital nerve.
e True. It is always important to look at the eye closely in patients with an orbital fracture.

2. A subconjunctival haemorrhage

a False. In traumatic disease it may overlie a penetrating wound.
b False. The conjunctiva is inserted at the limbus, blood cannot pass into the cornea.
c False. If vision is reduced, another cause must be found.
d True. It may cause slight elevation of the conjunctiva.
e True. It settles spontaneously, treatment is usually not required.

3. Chemical eye injuries

a False. Alkalis diffuse more rapidly and so cause the worst injuries.
b True. The area under the eyelids must also be inspected and irrigated.
c True. Keratolysis is particularly seen with alkali injuries.
d False. This may indicate a severe ischaemic injury by an alkali.
e True. Vitamin C may improve healing, tetracyclines function as anticollagenases.

4. A hyphaema

a False. This is a hypopyon. A hyphaema is a collection of red cells.
b False. It may be associated with a raised intraocular pressure, due to an obstruction of the trabecular meshwork.
c True. This may help to prevent a further bleed.
d True. A re-bleed may result in more significant complications, for example high intraocular pressure.
e True. These will help to reduce any associated inflammation and reduce the incidence of re-bleeds.

18

Tropical ophthalmology: eye diseases in the developing world

Learning objectives

To understand:

✔ The causes of poor vision in developing countries.

✔ How these problems are being addressed.

✔ The clinical presentation and treatment of some major diseases, including trachoma, onchocerciasis and xerophthalmia.

Introduction

Reduction in vision can be divided into distance and near impairment. Globally, the World Health Organisation (WHO) estimates that 2.2 billion people have some form of visual impairment (distance acuity worse than 6/12 or N6 for near). In half of these people, these visual problems could be prevented or treated, the commonest are:

- Undiagnosed refractive error and presbyopia (123.7 million people have reduced vision due to distance refractive error; 826 million due to presbyopia).
- Cataract (65.2 million).
- Glaucoma (6.9 million).
- Corneal opacities, e.g. caused by measles and Vitamin A deficiency (4.2 million).
- Diabetic retinopathy (3 million).
- Trachoma (2.5 million).

43 million people are blind (visual acuity less than 3/60). Although blindness is a global problem, 90% of the blind live in the poorest parts of the developing world. An estimate in 2010, of the age-standardized prevalence of blindness in adults ≥50 years, was ≤0.4% in high-income regions compared to 6%, in western sub-Saharan Africa. Almost 50% of blind people live in China or India.

The prevalence of blindness is greater in women in all regions. Nearly, two-thirds of the world's blind are women. In the developed world, this is partly because women live longer than men, but in the developing world, cultural factors can mean that women are less informed about opportunities for treatment and have fewer resources to pay for and access care. In sub-Saharan Africa and south Asia, the proportion of

Ophthalmology: Lecture Notes, Thirteenth Edition. Bruce James, Anthony Bron, and Manoj V. Parulekar.
© 2024 John Wiley & Sons Ltd. Published 2024 by John Wiley & Sons Ltd.
Companion website: www.wiley.com/go/ophthalmology13e

eligible women who receive cataract surgery may be half that for men.

Reasons for the greater prevalence of blindness in the developing world

- Higher exposure to risk factors.
- Increased susceptibility due to poverty, poor nutrition and ill health.
- Limited treatment facilities and trained personnel in primary and secondary care.
- Poor access to medical care.
- Uneven distribution of preventive programmes.
- Lower awareness and health-seeking behaviour.

Treatment and prevention

Cataract and refractive error are treatable conditions and trachoma and two other major causes of blindness, onchocerciasis and vitamin A deficiency, are entirely preventable. They have each benefited from the adoption of highly successful, cost-effective intervention programmes, instituted over many years. The prevalence of blindness overall, between 1990 and 2010, fell from 3% to 1.9% and that of visual impairment from 14.3% to 10.4%. However, because of population growth and the increase in the ageing population, the absolute number of blind was similar or slightly increased.

Many of the diseases responsible for world blindness have been discussed earlier in this book. This chapter focuses on those diseases that are the major causes of *avoidable (both treatable and preventable) blindness* and on some of the methods for delivering care in the developing world. A valuable account of the major causes of blinding diseases worldwide and of the therapeutic and preventive measures mounted by numerous agencies, will be found on the (International Agency for the Prevention of Blindness IAPB) website.

Providing eye care in the developing world

Availability, accessibility, acceptability and affordability of resources are the key barriers to reducing the burden of poor vision.

The following are the greatest obstacles to success:

- Dealing with environmental and social factors that predispose to disease.
- Covering the cost of providing care.
- Raising awareness of treatment opportunities in affected communities.
- Dispelling the fear of treatment.
- Delivering eye care to remote and widely spread populations.
- Creating a high-quality service that is monitored and constantly improved.
- Sustaining the infrastructure and training requirements of treatment programmes.

Major causes of blindness

Blindness in childhood

- Vitamin A deficiency.
- Trachoma.
- Congenital cataract.
- Ophthalmia neonatorum.
- Congenital glaucoma.
- Congenital malformations.
- Measles.
- Retinopathy of prematurity.
- Other infections (corneal and ocular, for example toxoplasmosis).

It is estimated that there are 1.5 million blind children in the world and that half a million children become blind each year. While they represent about 3% of the world's blind population, they have a lifetime of blindness ahead of them, so the number of 'blind person years' resulting from childhood blindness is only second to cataract (Gogate and Gilbert 2007). Many of the causes of childhood blindness are avoidable.

Blindness in adulthood

Cataract – the world perspective

Cataract is the commonest cause of treatable blindness after refractive error (Figure 18.1). Of the surgical methods available for treatment (see Chapter 9), extracapsular cataract extraction has been the method of choice in the developing world, since it is cheaper than phacoemulsification and not dependent on expensive, high-tech equipment and support costs.

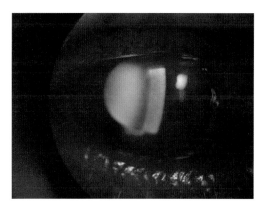

Figure 18.1 Slit-lamp view of a brown, nuclear cataract.

However, increasingly, small incision cataract surgery (SICS) is being adopted (Figure 18.2), which is a low-cost and faster procedure permitting the use of intraocular lens implants. Since sutures are not used, rehabilitation is faster.

The results of surgery are excellent and the challenge is to make it available. The cost of the operation and availability of trained staff, particularly in rural communities, are major problems that have to be overcome. Various models have been developed.

In India, where cataract blindness remains a significant problem, the Aravind Eye Care system has created a highly efficient, high-volume, low-cost, self-financing system for performing cataract surgery. The system uses income from patients who can afford to pay for private surgery, to pay for the poor, who receive free surgery. Patients are screened in eye camps and those in need of surgery or other treatment are referred to hospital.

Several international non-governmental organizations such as Sightsavers, Orbis, Medecins sans

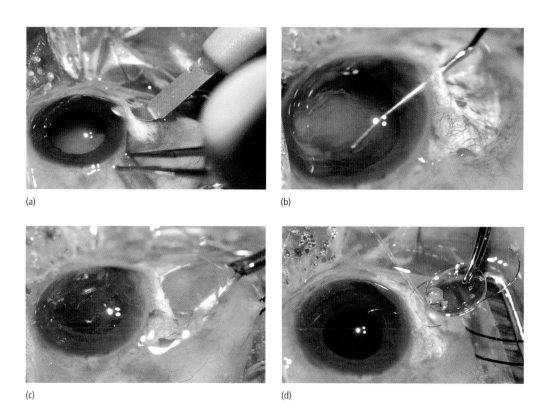

(a) (b) (c) (d)

Figure 18.2 Small incision extracapsular surgery. (a) A tunnel into the eye, via the limbus, is made with a blade. (b) A needle with a bent tip is inserted to make multiple small incisions into the anterior capsule and allow access to the cortex and nucleus of the lens. (c) The nucleus of the lens is expressed through the incision by irrigation. (d) Following aspiration of the soft cortical matter, an intraocular lens is placed in the eye. No sutures to the wound are required, which is self-sealing. (*Source:* Courtesy of Dr. V.R. Vivekanandan, Aravind Hospital, Madurai.)

Frontiers and CBM international, as well as national and regional charities also play an important role in blindness prevention and treatment worldwide.

As with all health programmes, it is important first to understand the epidemiology of the problem in order to determine appropriate resources. There has been increasing emphasis on training local health-care workers to run programmes, with outside aid providing equipment, consumables and training rather than direct surgical input. Additionally, assessment of the outcome of surgery is emphasized, to maximize the quality of care provided and match that in the developed world.

Tropical diseases

Trachoma

Trachoma causes blindness by corneal scarring and is due to infection by *Chlamydia trachomatis*. It was first described in Egypt in the sixteenth century. Active trachoma has not been seen in Europe since the early twentieth century but was present in America until the 1960s. Trachoma is endemic in 48 countries, in Latin America, Africa, the Middle East, Asia and Australasia. Some 157.7 million people living in endemic areas require prophylactic treatment. In 2019, there were 2.5 million people with trachomatous trichiasis, falling from 7.6 million in 2002. Ten percent of the world population are potentially at risk, mostly in dry, hot parts of the developing world (Figure 18.3). It is endemic in rural communities, in areas of water shortage, where living conditions are crowded and sanitation and hygiene are poor. In some communities, 60% of children are affected by active disease.

Transmission is by the transfer of the elementary bodies of the bacteria from one person to another, usually from the nasal and ocular secretions of an infected child. This may involve eye-to-eye transmission with the fingers, the sharing of towels, handkerchiefs and bedclothes, coughing and sneezing. In addition, *eye-seeking flies* (e.g. *Musca sorbens*) act as important vectors, carrying the infective particles from eye or nose, to other individuals.

Initially, follicles (collections of lymphocytes) appear in the superior tarsal conjunctiva (Figure 18.4), followed by papillae. Then, the limbal cornea is invaded by superficial vessels (*pannus*), with the development of peripheral scarring (Figure 18.5). The first infection with *C. trachomatis* does not cause serious disease. Repeated episodes lead to extensive upper tarsal *conjunctival scarring* in children and young adults, and *lid deformity* and *trichiasis*, usually in middle-aged adults, which together exacerbate the

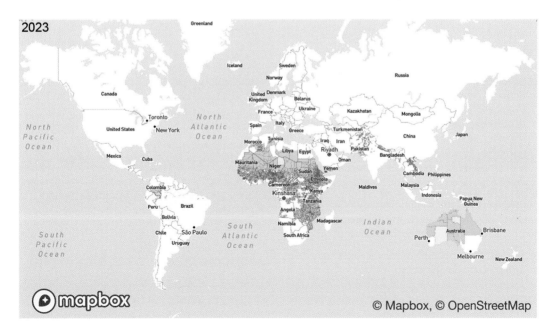

Figure 18.3 The worldwide distribution of trachoma. ©OpenStreetMap

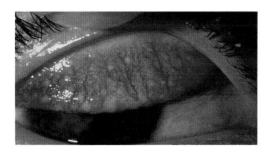

Figure 18.4 Follicles on the upper tarsus of a patient with trachoma. (*Source:* Courtesy of A. Foster.)

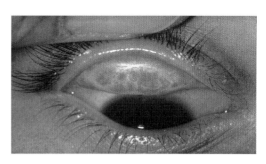

Figure 18.6 Scarring of the tarsal conjunctiva in trachoma. (*Source:* Courtesy of A. Foster.)

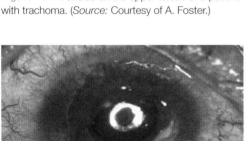

Figure 18.5 Peripheral corneal scarring in trachoma. (*Source:* Courtesy of A. Foster.)

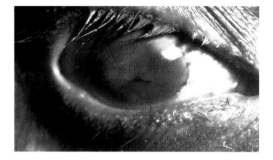

Figure 18.7 Upper lid entropion and corneal scarring in trachoma. (*Source:* Courtesy of A. Foster.)

corneal changes. Continued re-infection leads to chronic corneal scarring and blindness. This results from the following:

- *Dry eye*: Conjunctival scarring blocks lacrimal and meibomian gland duct orifices, leading to reduced tear production and excessive evaporative water loss (Figure 18.6).
- Reduced lubrication through tear deficiency and loss of goblet cell mucin.
- Corneal trauma, due to cicatricial entropion (inturning of the lid margins by tarsal scarring; Figure 18.7) and trichiasis, where aberrant, inturned lashes abrade the cornea. This also predisposes to secondary bacterial and fungal corneal infection, and scarring.

Public health intervention has led to the development of the SAFE strategy, now implemented in at least 32 countries. It involves the following:

- *S*urgery, for entropion, everting the lid to move the lashes away from the globe.
- *A*ntibiotic therapy: A single dose of *oral azithromycin* (20 mg/kg up to 1 g) is effective in treating infected individuals, but the disease must be eradicated from all individuals in a community to prevent re-infection,

and treatment must be repeated yearly. This is expensive, and the disease will recur unless changes are made to the environment in which the organism prospers. This is much harder to achieve.
- *F*ace washing, which reduces transmission of the disease. The flies are less likely to be attracted to the child and the child is less likely to spread *Chlamydia* by direct contact.
- *E*nvironmental change: A clean environment reduces the fly population. Improving the water supply and sanitation with bore holes and pit latrines is important in this respect.

To achieve success, each component of the strategy must be implemented on a community-wide basis. Azithromycin used in this programme continues to be provided without charge by the pharmaceutical company Pfizer.

Onchocerciasis (river blindness)

The filarial nematode, *onchocerca volvulus,* is responsible for this disease, which is found principally in Africa (99%), South America and Yemen (Figure 18.8). In 2017, 220 million people required preventative

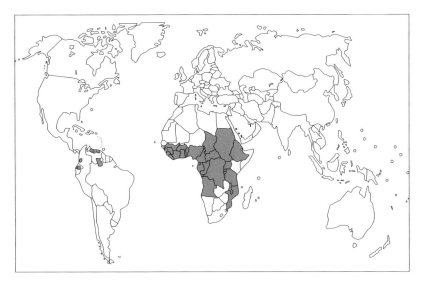

Figure 18.8 The worldwide distribution of onchocerciasis.

anti-helminthic and it was estimated that 1.15 million people had sight loss due to onchocerciasis. Microfilariae in the skin of an affected patient are ingested when the female blackfly (e.g. *Simulium damnosum*) bites a human for a blood meal. The microfilariae develop into infective larvae in the fly, pass to its mouth and are then transmitted to a human with the next bite. Following moulting, the larvae develop into adult worms in the body. They are found in subcutaneous skin nodules (*onchocercomata*) and diagnosis may be made from skin-snip biopsies. Alternatively, antibodies may be detected in the blood and PCR techniques have also been used to detect filarial DNA in skin scrapings. The adult female worm is 30–80 cm long and the male 3–5 cm long. In the human body they have a lifespan of 9–14 years. A female worm may produce 1600 microfilariae a day and generate a body load of 150 million. These migrate in the dermis and its lymphatics and die after a couple of years if they are not taken up into a blackfly.

Microfilariae entering the eye directly from the conjunctiva or the bloodstream are responsible for ocular disease. The living organisms inhibit the host's protective immune response. Clinically, microfilariae are visible in the cornea, anterior chamber, vitreous and retina. Living, mobile, microfilariae may be seen in the anterior chamber on biomicroscopy. In the cornea, a characteristic fluffy, punctate stromal keratitis occurs as an early sign of eye disease, each opacity representing an inflammatory reaction around a dead microfilarium. With increased load, this advances to cause complete corneal opacification (*sclerosing keratitis*) and consequent blindness (Figure 18.9). Uveitis may be associated with anterior and posterior synechiae (Figure 18.10), cataract and secondary glaucoma. Diffuse involvement of the retina and choroid (*choroidoretinitis*) is also a common cause of blindness (Figure 18.11), as is optic neuritis, leading to optic atrophy.

Treatment relies on:

- public health intervention;
- antibiotic therapy (ivermectin).

Water courses provide the breeding grounds for the blackfly, which is why those whose work or daily

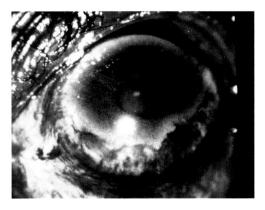

Figure 18.9 Sclerosing keratitis in onchocerciasis. (*Source:* Courtesy of A. Foster.)

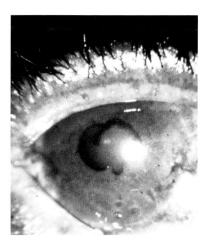

Figure 18.10 Uveitis with synechiae formed between iris and lens in onchocerciasis. (*Source:* Courtesy of A. Foster.)

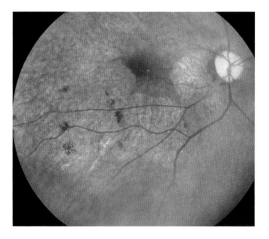

Figure 18.11 The appearance of retinal disease in onchocerciasis. (*Source:* Courtesy of A. Foster.)

life takes them to the banks of rivers are most at risk of infection – hence the name river blindness. Control programmes are aimed at the blackfly vector, by spraying its habitat with larvicides, trapping methods and the removal of vegetation from breeding sites. The onchocerciasis control programme has been successful in the endemic West African region and South America. A low population density in affected areas (principally farming and fishing communities) increases the likelihood of multiple blackfly bites. Protective clothing reduces the possibility of bites but may not always be practical. Vector control programmes are a long-term proposition because the female worm lives for

9–14 years, which perpetuates microfilarial infiltration of the skin.

Ivermectin is a *filaricide* which has revolutionized the treatment of onchocerciasis. It is safe and effective in killing microfilariae and reactions, if they occur, are mild and diminish with repeated dosing. It also reduces the number of adult worms present and their reproductive capability. It is given once a year (150–200 µg/kg), often on a community basis (mass drug administration). Reduction in the number of microfilariae reduces the infectious potential of the blackfly and complements vector control programmes. Over 152.9 million people were treated in 2019 as a result of a donation of the drug by the manufacturer, Merck and collaborations with national and international health organizations. The African programme for onchocerciasis control (APOC) had developed a system whereby the local community is responsible for the delivery of ivermectin treatment. This has now closed but the work continues with the Expanded Special Project for the Elimination of Neglected Tropical Diseases in Africa (ESPEN).

Vitamin A deficiency (xerophthalmia)

Vitamin A is an essential vitamin required for cell maturation and division and the maintenance and protection of mucosal surfaces. Dietary carotenoids from dark, leafy green vegetables, carrots, red palm oil, mangoes and papayas, and so on are absorbed and broken down to release vitamin A (roughly 12 molecules of carotene for every molecule of vitamin A). Preformed vitamin A is available in breast milk, liver, fish oils, eggs and dairy products. Vitamin A is stored chiefly in the liver. Animal sources of the vitamin are often not available in the developing world and environmental factors are crucial to a good diet. Communities may be unaware of the dietary utility of some locally available sources of vitamin A. Social factors are also important, since poor water supply may lead to chronic diarrhoea and malabsorption, which exacerbates any deficiency. Lack of vitamin A increases susceptibility to disease, especially pulmonary infection. Deficiency in vitamin A, when associated with protein malnutrition and febrile illnesses such as measles, gives rise to severe, life-threatening disease.

Vitamin A deficiency causes blinding ocular disease (xerophthalmia) and an increased morbidity and mortality, particularly in growing, preschool children over the age of 1 year, but also in pregnant women, whose nutritional requirement is increased

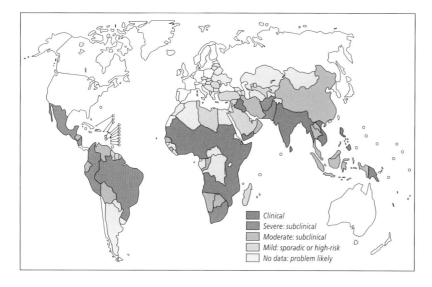

Figure 18.12 The worldwide distribution of vitamin A deficiency.

Legend:
Clinical
Severe: subclinical
Moderate: subclinical
Mild: sporadic or high-risk
No data: problem likely

during gestation and breastfeeding. In countries where vitamin A deficiency is prevalent, 50% of those affected die within 2 years of becoming blind. Improving a child's vitamin A status enhances resistance to infection and decreases the overall risk of mortality by 24% (Mayo Wilson et al. 2011). About 190 million children under 5 years of age suffer from vitamin A deficiency and some 5–10 million develop xerophthalmia each year, with loss of sight in half a million. The peak incidence occurs between 3 and 5 years of age. There is a widespread distribution of clinical and subclinical disease, with much of the clinical disease seen in Africa and South East Asia, with India contributing 85% of cases in South East Asia (Figure 18.12).

The features of xerophthalmia occur in the following sequence with increasing vitamin A deficiency:

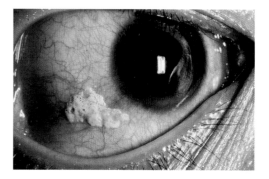

Figure 18.13 The appearance of a Bitot spot. (*Source:* Courtesy of Sommer.)

- *Night blindness:* often the earliest symptom – due to the lack of the visual pigment, rhodopsin.
- *Ocular surface xerosis:* vitamin A deficiency causes a loss of ocular surface wettability due to a reduced expression of epithelial glycocalyx mucins and a loss of goblet cells and their secreted gel mucin. Tear production may also be reduced. This results in:
  - *Conjunctival xerosis:* involving keratinization, thickening and non-wetting of the conjunctiva, frequently with Bitot spots near each limbus (foamy triangular surface plaques containing keratinized cells and saprophytic bacteria) (Figure 18.13).
  - *Corneal xerosis:* involving punctate keratiopathy or diffuse drying of the cornea (Figure 18.14), usually with stromal oedema.
- If untreated, it may progress to:

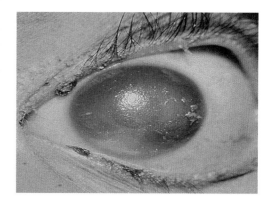

Figure 18.14 Xerosis of the cornea in vitamin A deficiency. (*Source:* Courtesy of A. Foster.)

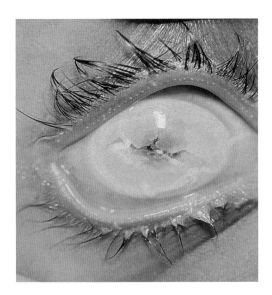

Figure 18.15 Severe corneal disease with ulceration in vitamin A deficiency. (*Source:* Courtesy of A. Foster.)

- *Corneal ulceration* or focal melting (*keratomalacia;* Figure 18.15). This occurs more in severe disease and leads to perforation and *phthisis bulbi* a shrunken, non-functioning eye.

Night blindness, conjunctival and corneal xerosis are usually completely reversed by vitamin A therapy, and even corneal ulceration may be checked, to leave residual scarring.

Treatment with vitamin A supplementation, fortification of food or increasing the natural dietary intake is highly cost-effective (the WHO recommends the provision of two doses of vitamin A annually to children between the ages of 6 and 59 months). A protein-rich diet is also advised. Delivery of supplements is often combined with immunization programmes. Education about breastfeeding, diet and food availability and preparation is also important. Care should be taken in women of childbearing age, as vitamin A in large doses may have teratogenic effects; lower doses are therefore recommended.

Measles

This is an important cause of corneal scarring and childhood blindness and its severity is exacerbated by vitamin A deficiency. During infection with measles, vitamin A stores are significantly depleted, which can result in severe corneal disease (Figure 18.16). Vitamin A deficiency also increases mortality from this disease. Associated exposure

keratopathy, herpes simplex keratitis and other secondary infections may also cause corneal opacification. This may be compounded by treatment with local remedies that traumatize the eye, or cause infection or chemical burns.

More extensive immunization programmes and better control of vitamin A deficiency are helping to reduce the corneal blindness in many low-income countries.

Corneal infection, ulceration and scarring

Infectious keratitis is the fourth leading cause of blindness worldwide, with an incidence in the developing world, that is ten times that in the United States (Pascolini and Mariotti 2012). Scarring occurs due to childhood measles (Figure 18.16), vitamin A deficiency and ophthalmia neonatorum, or the use of traditional eye medicines. In older individuals, where so many people in the developing world are involved in agricultural labour, microbial keratitis initiated by minor eye trauma, is not unusual. Antibiotic treatment of minor eye trauma has an important role in preventing progression to a bacterial keratitis. Community-level prophylaxis in a village setting, treating any corneal abrasion with topical antibiotic ointment within 18 hours of its occurrence can reduce the incidence of bacterial ulcers by 80%.

In northern climates, where agricultural injuries are less frequent, fungal infections are rare. But in tropical zones, fungal keratitis may account for over 80% of infected cases. It is estimated that 1.5 million new cases of unilateral visual impairment due to corneal ulceration occur each year. Treatment can be expensive and is often delayed in the developing world. Some topical antifungal agents are highly toxic and may leave their own sequelae and corneal grafting for central scarring is seldom available.

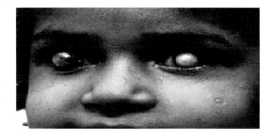

Figure 18.16 Bilateral severe corneal scarring in measles. (*Source:* Courtesy of A. Foster.)

HIV and AIDS

Considering the spectrum of ocular disease associated with HIV and AIDS, CMV retinitis is more unusual in developing countries and herpes zoster more common. However, hotspots for CMV retinitis exist in some endemic regions and rates are highest in southeast Asia, where CMV retinitis has been reported in about one-third of those with CD^{4+} T-lymphocyte count less than 50 cells/μl (Heiden et al. 2007), a stage at which other systemic manifestations will be present. CMV retinitis was the leading cause of irreversible blindness in one hospital-based study from northern Thailand (Pathanapitoon et al. 2007). The visual consequences of CMV retinitis are devastating and although it evolves slowly, detection may be delayed until it is at an irreversible stage. Screening strategies are lacking in the developing world and are greatly needed. A telemedicine approach has been suggested to detect and monitor retinitis, using trained graders and inexpensive smartphone apps for retinal photography.

Treatments which have reduced the severity of opportunistic ocular infections, such as CMV retinitis, in the developed world (see Chapter 10) are becoming available in much of the developing world. In industrialized countries, CMV retinitis is readily treated with oral valganciclovir, which is expensive. The manufacturer Roche has reached an agreement that it will be available at greatly reduced cost in poorer countries, but even this may remain too expensive for many. Repeated intravitreal injections of ganciclovir are an effective low-cost alternative.

Ophthalmia neonatorum

Infection of a child's eye occurring during birth may lead to blindness within the first month of life (see Chapter 8). The infant presents with conjunctivitis and discharge. Although a number of bacteria may be responsible for infection, the two most important are:

- *Neisseria gonorrhoeae,*
- *Chlamydia trachomatis.*

Gonorrhoeal keratitis may progress rapidly to corneal perforation and endophthalmitis. Chlamydial infection is the commonest cause and the associated keratitis, if untreated, may progress to corneal scarring. It can also be associated with a pneumonitis. Because of the systemic implications of these eye infections, both are treated with systemic and topical antibiotics.

Topical instillation of *povidone–iodine* eye drops into the eyes of neonates, at the time of delivery, is a simple and cost-effective means to prevent either disease.

Diabetic retinopathy

This is the next big challenge when the infectious tropical diseases come under control. Although not a tropical disease, it is assuming greater significance in developing countries due to the huge numbers of diabetics in Asia and Africa, diet, lack of awareness, poor glycemic control and absence of retinopathy screening programmes. It is increasingly the focus of WHO, UN and eye care charities worldwide. Following the introduction of a screening programme in the United Kingdom, diabetic retinopathy is no longer the commonest cause of blindness in the working age population.

 KEY POINTS

- 2.2 billion people have some form of visual impairment, 50% with a treatable or preventable cause.
- Of the world's blind population, 90% live in the poorest parts of the developing world.
- Preventable or easily treatable forms of blindness include refractive errors, cataract, trachoma, onchocerciasis and vitamin A deficiency.
- Treatment relies as much on education and environmental changes as on drug therapy.
- Diabetic eye disease is an increasing problem in the developing world.

Assessment questions True or False

1. **Trachoma**
a The global number of people with trachomatous trichiasis is falling.
b In some developing communities, 60% of children have active disease.
c Corneal scarring may result from cicatricial entropion.
d Is treated with ivermectin.
e Follicles are present on the upper tarsus in early disease.

2. **Onchocerciasis**
a Is caused by a bacterium.
b Just over 1 million people had sight loss due to onchocerciasis.
c Is transmitted by the blackfly.

d   Does not affect the cornea.

e   Eye disease is caused by microfilariae.

3. Vitamin A deficiency (xerophthalmia)

a   Affects 190 million children.

b   The peak incidence for xerophthalmia is at age 10–15 years.

c   Does not affect night vision.

d   Bitot spots are a specific sign.

e   The severity of the disease is increased with concurrent measles infection.

Answers

1. Trachoma

a   True.

b   True.

c   True. The lid margin is turned in by tarsal scarring.

d   False. Trachoma is treated with a single dose of azithromycin. This needs to be repeated yearly to prevent re-infection.

e   True. These are collections of lymphocytes preceding papillae formation and corneal vascularization and peripheral scarring.

2. Onchocerciasis

a   False. Onchocerciasis is caused by a filarial nematode.

b   True.

c   True. Microfilariae in the skin are ingested when the female blackfly bites a human for a blood meal.

d   False. It may result in a sclerosing keratitis with complete opacification of the cornea.

e   True. They enter the eye from the conjunctiva or bloodstream.

3. Vitamin A deficiency (xerophthalmia)

a   True.

b   False. The peak incidence is at 3–5 years.

c   False. This is an early sign of the disease.

d   True. Bitot spots are foamy triangular surface plaques containing keratinized cells and saprophytic bacteria.

e   True. There may be increased corneal scarring as vitamin A stores are significantly depleted during measles infection.

References

Gogate P. & Gilbert C. Blindness in children: a worldwide perspective. *Comm Eye Health* 2007; 20(62): pp. 32–33.

Heiden D. *et al*. Cytomegalovirus retinitis: the neglected disease of the AIDS pandemic. *PLoS Med* 2007; **4**: e334.

Mayo W.E. *et al*. Vitamin A supplements for preventing mortality, illness, and blindness in children aged under 5: systematic review and metaanalysis. *BMJ* 2011; **343**: d5094 (Cochrane Review).

Pascolini D. & Mariotti S.P. Global estimates of visual impairment: 2010. *Br J Ophthalmol* 2012; 96(5): pp. 614–618.

Pathanapitoon K. *et al*. Blindness and low vision in a tertiary ophthalmologic center in Thailand: the importance of cytomegalovirus retinitis. *Retina* 2007; **b**(5): pp. 635–640.

19

Eye diseases in children

Learning objectives

To understand:

✔ The milestones in visual development.

✔ The symptoms, signs, causes and treatment of childhood eye disease.

Introduction

Developmental anatomy and embryology

Development of the eye begins early *in utero,* with the optic grooves appearing at 3 weeks, and is largely completed at 7 months of gestation. The visual pathways continue to mature over the next few months *in* and *ex utero.* The globe continues to grow post-natally.

Teratogenic events in the first 3–8 weeks can result in severe eye abnormalities. The choroidal fissure closes at 7 weeks, and incomplete closure can result in chorio-retinal and/or optic nerve colobomas.

Development of vision. The visual milestones

The first few years of life are crucial for visual development. Adequate stimulation of both retinas in the first 6–8 years of life is essential to achieve normal visual acuity in adult life (Table 19.1).

Visual deprivation of one or both eyes from any cause can result in *amblyopia* (a 'lazy eye').

Delayed visual maturation (DVM)

The visual pathways can take a few months to mature functionally. Parents often describe the visual responses as 'inconsistent' or a mother may observe that 'my baby appears to look through me rather than at me'.

There is no need for action as long as:

- the eyes are structurally normal;
- there are no abnormal eye movements;
- there are no other developmental concerns.

Such babies can be observed until 6 months age, by which time most cases improve spontaneously. If there is no improvement after this time, a brain scan and electro-diagnostic testing (ERG and VEP) are indicated.

History and examination

The parents of the child will provide a history of the ocular problem from their perspective; otherwise the history is taken as in an adult. The examination of the child's eye often relies on opportunistic observations without specialist instrumentation (see Chapter 3). It is important to gain the child's confidence and distraction of the child with a toy can provide helpful information about visual attention and hand–eye coordination.

Ophthalmology: Lecture Notes, Thirteenth Edition. Bruce James, Anthony Bron, and Manoj V. Parulekar.
© 2024 John Wiley & Sons Ltd. Published 2024 by John Wiley & Sons Ltd.
Companion website: www.wiley.com/go/ophthalmology13e

Table 19.1 The various stages of visual development.

0–3 months	• Briefly holds gaze on an object • Takes interest in (stares at) surroundings, blinks at bright lights • Tracks vertically and horizontally • Makes eye contact at 6–8 weeks; fixes on mother's face
3–6 months	• Follows adults or moving objects with eyes across midline • Displays interest in human faces • Observes own hands • Briefly fixes on and reaches for small objects
7–12 months	• Recognizes objects at home, tracks across the room • Interested in pictures, inspects toys, enjoys hide-and-seek • Responds to smiles and voices, develops stranger anxiety
1–1½ years	• Enjoys picture books and points to pictures • Holds objects close to eyes to inspect
2–3 years	• Recognizes faces in photographs • Begins to inspect objects without touching them • Likes to watch moving objects, such as wheels on a toy vehicle • Watches and imitates other children • 'Reads' pictures in books
3–4 years	• Copies patterns • Recognizes colours • Can close eyes on request and may be able to wink
4–5 years	• Draws a recognizable person and house and names pictures • Uses eyes and hands together with increasing skill • Moves and rolls eyes expressively • Can place small objects into small openings • Demonstrates visual interest in new objects

Assessment of the child includes, external features, eye movements, visual acuity, binocular vision, refraction and a detailed ocular examination.

External examination

Visual inspection of the eyes and eyelids can reveal dysmorphic features like low set or slanted eyelids and palpebral fissures, wide set eyes (*telecanthus*) and lid *coloboma* (a full-thickness defect), abnormal head posture (because of nystagmus or squint), proptosis, ptosis (Figure 19.1), or squint (Figure 19.2 and see Chapter 16). Look also for abnormalities of eye size (for example enlargement of the eye in congenital glaucoma), or developmental abnormalities like *microphthalmos* (small eye).

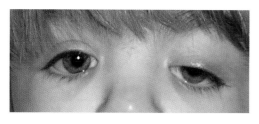

Figure 19.1 Left ptosis. Importantly, the pupil is not completely covered.

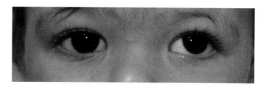

Figure 19.2 Hirschberg test. The corneal light reflex is displaced nasally on the left. The child has a divergent squint.

Assessment of visual acuity

Visual acuity tests for children must be appropriate for the age and development of the child and are indicated in Table 19.2 (see also Chapter 3). The clinic-based tests would form part of the general paediatric assessment and can alert paediatricians and GPs to eye conditions that need referral to an ophthalmologist.

Testing the visual field

This can be a challenge in young children, and formal testing is only possible for the older, cooperative child. Formal tests include automated perimetry

Table 19.2 **Visual acuity tests for children.**

Age	Informal, clinic-based tests for paediatric examination	Formal tests of visual acuity
Neonate	Fixing and following, interest in human faces, response to bright lights	Preferential looking tests (for example Teller Cards) where the child is presented with two cards – one plain and the other with stripes of reducing width (each step representing a level of visual acuity). The expected response is a shift of gaze towards the striped cards. When the child is unable to resolve the stripes, the two cards appear identical. The finest stripes visualized by the child represents the level of visual acuity
Young infants	Interest in human faces, social smile, stranger anxiety, steady fixation, reaching for bright objects	Cardiff acuity cards provide a preferential looking test similar to Teller cards, with familiar objects such as birds instead of stripes
1–2 years	Interest in toys and smaller objects	Kay picture cards have familiar objects like cars and birds, and the child names the object or matches it to the corresponding image on a card held by the parent, by pointing
2–3 years	Visual behaviour when navigating around a room, ability to detect small objects	The Sheridan Gardner test involves single letters rather than rows of letters, and the child points to the corresponding letter on a handheld card
>3 years	Visual behaviour when navigating around room, ability to detect small objects	Snellen or log MAR visual acuity test involves row of letters of reducing size. For pre-school children, the illiterate E or Landolt C test can be used

using the Humphrey instrument or manual perimetry with the Goldmann instrument. For the younger child, tests are more observational, where the clinician places objects (typically bright toys) randomly in various positions in the visual field, and observes the child's response – normally a rapid head and eye movement in the direction of the toy. Valuable information can also be gathered from observing their ability to navigate around obstacles placed in the clinic, for example stepping over or avoiding a large toy placed on the floor.

Testing binocular vision

Binocular vision is the ability of the higher visual centres of the brain to process the visual signals from both eyes simultaneously, to produce a single, three-dimensional visual percept.

It is a function in higher evolved species where the location of the eyes in the head permits an overlap of the visual fields when the eyes are directed at an object of regard. This condition is maximized in humans and in sub-human primates where the eyes are frontally disposed, thus achieving a large binocular visual field. Since each eye views the visual scene from a slightly different angle, the images on each retina have slight hori-

zontal disparity and it is this which creates the three-dimensional percept, carrying depth and distance information, which is the basis of *stereopsis*.

There are several age-appropriate tests to detect the presence and level of binocular vision, such as the Lang, TNO and Titmus tests, the Wirt Fly test and the synoptophore – often referred to by children as 'putting the lion in the cage test'.

There are advantages to having good binocular vision, but lack of binocular vision does not usually limit ability at sport (although catching a ball may be harder) or schooling, and rarely if ever restricts choice of career.

A squint can interfere with the development of binocular vision, and may result in amblyopia. It is desirable to detect and correct a squint early, for this reason.

Direct ophthalmoscopy

The direct ophthalmoscope is a very useful screening tool for the paediatrician as well as the ophthalmologist. It can be used in the clinic, community, or at the bedside. The ophthalmoscope can be held some distance from the child (1–2 ft) to minimize apprehension, enabling a quick assessment of the

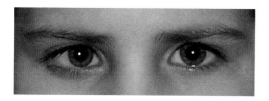

Figure 19.3 Note the faint white opacity in the right pupil. The child has a congenital cataract. Additionally, the eye is microphthalmic with a right convergent squint. All these signs can be detected by simple examination.

clarity of the ocular media by checking the red reflex to identify:

- cataracts;
- corneal opacities and scars;
- retinal conditions such as tumours (retinoblastoma).

See Chapter 3; Figure 19.3.

It is important to remember that it may be more difficult to see a bright red reflex in heavily pigmented fundi (e.g. Asian or Afro-Caribbean eyes) as more light is absorbed and less reflected back. This apparent absence of a red reflex is a common cause of referral to the ophthalmologist. Examining the fundus in a child takes considerable patience and skill. It is easier after pupillary dilatation with eye drops, usually cyclopentolate.

Refraction and the role of the optician and optometrist (general ophthalmic services)

Refractive errors are common in childhood, and significant errors should be corrected with glasses (or contact lenses where appropriate) to provide clear vision, ensure optimum visual and general development and prevent amblyopia.

There may be a higher than normal incidence of refractive errors in:

- Those born prematurely, or showing developmental delay, including that resulting from birth hypoxia.
- Those with multisystem disorders or genetic syndromes such as Trisomy 21.

For younger children, it is usual to assess their refractive status by objective means [retinoscopy (Chapter 3) performed by an ophthalmologist or optometrist]. Older children can be tested subjectively where they look through lenses of different power while viewing the Snellen chart to see which one provides the clearest vision.

The incidence of clinically significant refractive errors requiring the use of spectacle correction in childhood is approximately 5% (the Baltimore Pediatric Eye Disease Study).

Ocular disorders seen in children

The orbit

Proptosis in childhood is an emergency. There are several causes including the following:

- Rhabdomyosarcoma is a malignant tumour of childhood. It commonly affects the orbit and presents with rapidly progressive proptosis (Figure 19.4).
- Bleeding into vascular malformations.
- Infection (orbital cellulitis). Due to the thin bone separating the ethmoid sinuses from the orbit, extension of infection from the ethmoid sinuses resulting in preseptal or orbital cellulitis is commoner in children than adults (Figure 19.5). Treatment is with systemic antibiotics, usually intravenously. See Chapter 5.

A CT or an MRI scan is required in most cases, usually as a matter of urgency.

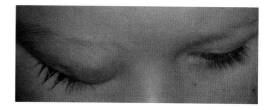

Figure 19.4 Rhabdomyosarcoma. The right eye is proposed compared to the left when looking down at the child's face from above.

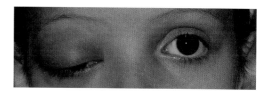

Figure 19.5 Preseptal cellulitis - the lid is swollen but the conjunctiva is white, eye movements full and there is no evidence of optic nerve compromise when the child is examined, differentiating it from orbital cellulitis where the eye appears inflamed, proptosed and eye movements grossly restricted.

Infantile (capillary) haemangioma

These lesions, extending into the lids, typically present within a few weeks of birth. They can grow rapidly and induce astigmatism or ptosis, with resultant amblyopia. Timely treatment with topical (Timolol) or systemic beta-blockers (Propranolol) is essential (see Chapter 5 and Figure 19.6).

Dermoid cysts

These present in infancy and early childhood as well-defined lesions along the supero-temporal, or less commonly, supero-nasal orbital rim. Treatment is with surgical excision (see Chapter 5 and Figure 19.7).

The eyelids

Ptosis

Childhood ptosis can affect one or both lids. Congenital ptosis is present at birth, caused by a weak, poorly developed levator palpebrae superioris muscle. Severe ptosis can obstruct the visual axis and result in amblyopia. Most children instinctively elevate their brows to lift up the lids, or adopt a chin-up head posture, in which case there is no urgent need to correct the ptosis. The treatment is surgical and involves shortening of the levator muscle (resection) or suspending the eyelid from the brow (brow suspension) using material such as silicone or *fascia lata* harvested from the leg (see Chapter 6).

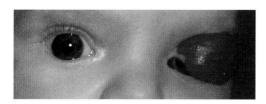

Figure 19.6 A capillary haemangioma.

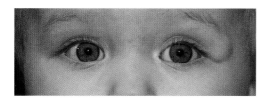

Figure 19.7 A left dermoid cyst is present temporally.

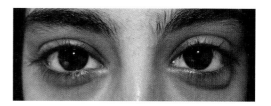

Figure 19.8 Both lower lids appear swollen with multiple chalazia.

Lid lesions

Lid lesions common in childhood are:

- chalazia (hordeolum internum) (Figure 19.8);
- molluscum contagiosum.

  These conditions are described in Chapter 6.

The lacrimal system

Congenital epiphora – specifically refers to watery eyes resulting from congenital obstruction of the nasolacrimal duct. Spontaneous resolution is seen in many cases within the first year of life. Persistent cases can be treated with syringing and probing, with a high success rate.

Conjunctiva, cornea, sclera

Infection

- Ophthalmia neonatorum is a form of infective conjunctivitis. The infection is usually maternally transmitted, from the birth canal, and may be indicative of sexually transmitted disease in the mother (see Chapter 8).
- Childhood conjunctivitis is often viral.
- Recurrent conjunctivitis can occur in the presence of a blocked tear duct.

Allergy

Allergic conjunctivitis is common in childhood. It may be associated with eczema and asthma (atopic tendency). Severe cases can result in considerable morbidity, including corneal scarring and loss of schooling (see Chapter 8).

Keratoconus

This is a corneal disorder that presents in late childhood or adolescence, with progressive, irregular astigmatism, difficult to correct with spectacles but manageable with rigid contact lens wear. It is due to a progressive thinning and ectasia of the corneal stroma that leads to a distinct conical profile of the cornea. Corneal grafting may be indicated in advanced cases, but stromal cross-linking is a newer treatment which can strengthen the corneal lamellae and arrest progression (see Chapter 8).

Corneal dystrophies

Corneal dystrophies can present in early or late childhood. These are discussed in detail in Chapter 8.

Cataract

Childhood cataracts can be present at birth (congenital) or develop during the first few years of life (developmental) (Figure 19.9). The vast majority have a genetic cause, often with a family history of childhood cataract. Other causes include:

- metabolic disorders;
- radiation treatment;
- trauma;
- prolonged steroid treatment (e.g. for nephrotic syndrome).

The management is discussed in detail in Chapter 9.

Uveitis

Juvenile idiopathic Arthritis (JIA)-related uveitis is the commonest cause of uveitis in childhood (see Chapter 10). The presentation of uveitis in children differs from that in adults as it does not cause redness or pain. Consequently, it may be overlooked and children with uveitis or diseases that may cause uveitis need regular screening.

Glaucoma

Congenital glaucoma is a potentially blinding disorder, but prompt diagnosis and treatment can result in very good visual outcomes. It presents with:

- an enlarged eye (bupthalmos);
- photophobia;
- epiphora (beware of diagnosing an obstructed nasolacrimal duct in these children).

Treatment is discussed in Chapter 11.

Retinal and choroidal disease

Retinal disease may become apparent during the investigation of a child with poor vision. Of particular note, in Coats disease and retinoblastoma, a white pupillary reflex (*leucocoria*) may be the presenting symptom. This warrants urgent referral to a specialist.

Important retinal causes of reduced vision in childhood include the following:

- Retinal dystrophies (retinoschisis and rod cone dystrophies).
- Albinism.
- Coats disease (Figure 19.10). This is a form of exudative vascular retinopathy, characterized by abnormally dilated vessels in the peripheral retina that leak blood and blood products. Yellow, cholesterol-rich fluid forms under the retina, resulting in an exudative detachment. It can be difficult to distinguish from retinoblastoma, but an ultrasound B-scan can be used to exclude a mass lesion.
- Astrocytomas are hamartomatous lesions of the retina.
- Retinoblastoma (Figure 19.11) is a malignant tumour of the developing retina and is one of the most successfully treated forms of cancer if detected early (see Chapter 12).

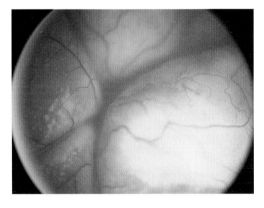

Figure 19.10 The appearance of Coats disease. There is a marked exudative retinal detachment, the folds of retina are almost touching and covering the optic disc.

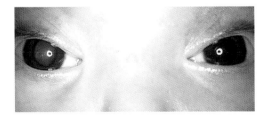

Figure 19.9 The pupils are dilated, note the right pupil is white due to the presence of a cataract.

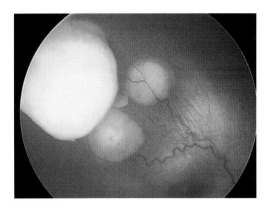

Figure 19.11 Retinoblastoma – the tumours appear white with a solid appearance, contrasting with the flat yellow appearance of Coats disease.

Prematurity and the eye

Prematurity may be associated with eye problems. These include:

- *Retinopathy of prematurity* (*ROP*): Retinal development continues through gestation, and vascularization is completed near term. Premature birth interferes with normal retinal vascularization, with a risk of abnormal retinal vascular proliferation that can cause retinal scarring and/or detachment (ROP, see Chapter 14). Babies born before 32 weeks gestation or of birthweight ≤1500 g are at risk of ROP and undergo regular screening eye examinations in the first few weeks of life. Most cases do not require treatment, but ROP beyond a certain threshold will require prompt laser treatment of the avascular retina to reduce risk of visual loss (Figure 19.12).

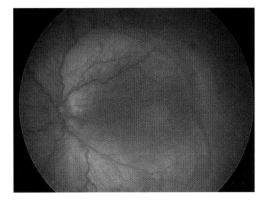

Figure 19.12 Retinopathy of prematurity. Note that the peripheral retina lacks the normal vascular pattern: haemorrhages are also present.

- *Strabismus:* There is a higher than expected incidence of squints in ex-premature children.
- *Refractive errors:* There is a relatively high incidence of refractive errors in ex-premature children, especially high myopia.
- *Cortical visual impairment and developmental delay:* There is a greater incidence of cognitive impairment in children who were born prematurely. This may be associated with visual field defects, visual processing deficits and binocular vision abnormalities.

The visual pathway

Children can develop tumours of the anterior visual pathway:

- Optic pathway gliomas, some of which are related to neurofibromatosis (type 1).
- Extrinsic compression of the optic pathway from supra-sellar tumours (craniopharyngiomas).

These children often present with visual loss or nystagmus.

Squint

This topic is covered in detail in Chapter 16. The salient features are repeated here.

It is not uncommon for the eyes to converge or diverge randomly during the first 2–3 months while the fixation system is still developing. This is referred to as *neonatal ocular misalignment*, and can be kept under observation unless there are concerns about the child's vision. Persistence of ocular misalignment beyond 3 months warrants referral to an ophthalmologist.

A squint may occur in the primary position, that is looking straight ahead, or only in certain directions of gaze. Depending on the direction of misalignment, squints may be horizontal, vertical or both. Some children might appear to have a squint despite accurate ocular alignment. Such cases will have a normal cover test and a normal corneal light reflex test (see Chapter 16). This is referred to as a pseudo-squint, and could be due to abnormal separation of the palpebral apertures, or an unusual facial configuration.

The causes of childhood squint include:

- *Refractive* – due to an underlying refractive error. The commonest situation is a convergent squint associated with a moderate to high, hypermetropic refractive error (also referred to as an *accommodative convergent squint*). Another commonly encountered cause is a high refractive error such as hypermetropia or myopia in one eye only (anisometropia). The eye is amblyopic and drifts in (*convergent*) or out (*divergent*).

- *Non-refractive:* the cause of non-refractive childhood squints is poorly understood, but is believed to be due to defective central control of eye movements. This is the commonest cause, and includes most divergent squints, and infantile esotropia.
- *Mixed:* where there is a refractive and non-refractive element to the squint.
- *Neurogenic:* due to nerve palsy (third, fourth or sixth) or skew deviation following intracranial pathology such as tumours or trauma. Duane syndrome and Moebius syndrome are additional causes of squint where there is an underlying innervational defect.
- *Myogenic:* the cause here is underaction (weakness) or restriction (tightness) of one or more muscles. Common causes are myasthenia, trauma including orbital fractures and orbital masses.
- *Obstruction of the optical media* (e.g. cataract).

The consequences of squint are as follows:

- Adults who develop a new onset squint experience double vision (diplopia). Children rarely develop diplopia since the child's visual system is in development and is immature. Instead, the brain suppresses the image from the squinting eye and the visual acuity fails to develop normally (*amblyopia*). This reduced acuity is reversible if treated in time.
- The presence of a squint, together with the amblyopia disrupts binocular vision. If treated in time, this can be restored, but the defect is sometimes irreversible.
- The child may adopt an abnormal head posture, such as a face turn or head tilt to control the squint.

The treatment of squint requires the following:

- Correction of the refractive error with spectacles or contact lenses.
- Treatment of any underlying medical condition.
- Treatment of the amblyopia – with occlusion (patching) of the better-seeing eye, to encourage the weaker eye to be used, improving visual acuity. In some cases, Atropine drops (penalization) can be used to blur the vision in the better eye, instead of patching.
- Surgery – if spectacles do not correct the squint, to realign the eyes, preserve or restore binocular vision and improve cosmesis.

Any child presenting with a squint should be referred to either:

- a community or hospital orthoptist (a professional specifically trained to assess vision and ocular motility in children in partnership with an ophthalmologist);
- an optometrist.

They should receive an eye examination which *must include testing of the red reflex.*

Sudden onset of squint with diplopia in the older child would merit an *urgent referral.*

For more details on eye movement disorders, see Chapter 16.

Trauma

Trauma to the eye may occur at any age and children may suffer any of the problems discussed in Chapter 17. More specific to children are the ocular signs that may be present in a child who has suffered abuse.

Child abuse

Child abuse is a general term that encompasses several mechanisms of damage to children including neglect, emotional, physical and sexual abuse, and induced illness (Munchausen syndrome or Factitious Induced Illness). Non-accidental injury (NAI) is a term commonly used to describe physical abuse, often involving shaking injury, with or without impact. Other forms include cigarette burns, chemical injuries, and thermal burns (scalding). All children with suspected NAI should receive an eye examination including dilated fundoscopy by an experienced ophthalmologist. The ophthalmologist will look for external evidence of trauma and retinal haemorrhages. Such cases often end up in court, and a careful history with accurate documentation and retinal photography where available, is essential.

 KEY POINTS

- Treat a child with proptosis as an ophthalmic emergency.
- If the pupil is covered in infancy, for example by a ptosis or a capillary haemangioma, amblyopia may develop.
- Ophthalmia neonatorum, which refers to any conjunctivitis that occurs in the first 28 days of neonatal life requires urgent treatment. Swabs for culture are mandatory.
- All children with a white pupil require urgent ophthalmic investigation. An infant with a family history of congenital cataract or a suspected cataract must be seen by an ophthalmologist as a matter of urgency.

- There is a significant risk of glaucoma developing in patients following congenital cataract surgery at an early age.
- Congenital glaucoma presents with enlarged eyes and epiphora.
- Children with juvenile arthritis require regular screening to exclude the presence of uveitis, as it is usually asymptomatic.
- Premature infants require screening for ROP.
- In a child with a squint it is important to exclude intraocular pathology – testing the red reflex is very important.
- A watery eye in a newborn child is commonly due to non-patency of the nasolacrimal duct. Most resolve spontaneously within the first year of life.
- Children with bilateral sight loss require help with their education and development.
- All children with suspected non-accidental injury require an eye examination.

Assessment questions
True or False

1. **A white pupil reflex in a child may be caused by:**
a   Exotropia.
b   Retinoblastoma.
c   Glaucoma.
d   Cataract.
e   Keratoconus.

2. **Proptosis in childhood may be caused by:**
a   Uveitis.
b   Rhabdomyosarcoma.
c   Chalazion.
d   Orbital cellulitis.
e   Coats disease.

3. **A squint may be caused by:**
a   Hypermetropia.
b   Anisometropia.
c   Retinal disease.
d   A non-patent nasolacrimal duct.
e   Ophthalmia neonatorum.

4. **Prematurity may be associated with:**
a   ROP.
b   Squint.
c   Developmental delay.
d   Astrocytoma.
e   Refractive errors.

Answers

1. **A white pupil reflex in a child may be caused by:**
a   False. If marked, there may not be a red reflex on a photograph but examination will confirm it is present.
b   True. This is an important cause of a white pupil reflex.
c   False. Congenital glaucoma may cause opacity of the cornea but not a white pupil reflex.
d   True. A cataract will cause a white pupil reflex.
e   False. This is an abnormality of the cornea.

2. **Proptosis in childhood may be caused by:**
a   False. This is an inflammation within the eye itself.
b   True. Rhabdomyosarcoma results in a rapidly evolving proptosis.
c   False. A Chalazion is a swollen meibomian gland in the lid.
d   True. Here, the proptosis is associated with a red eye, limited eye movements and the child may have a pyrexia.
e   False. Coats disease affects the retina.

3. **A squint may be caused by:**
a   True. Equal hypermetropia in both eyes may cause an accommodative squint.
b   True. If the refractive error in both eyes is significantly different, one eye may become amblyopic and develop a squint.
c   True. Retinal disease in an infant, associated with reduced vision, may cause a squint.
d   False. The watery eye that results from this is unlikely to cause a squint.
e   False. With appropriate treatment, this is an acute illness and should not affect the quality of long-term vision.

4. **Prematurity may be associated with:**
a   True. Babies born before 32 weeks gestation or of birth weight ≤1500 g are at risk of ROP and undergo regular screening eye examination in the first few weeks of life.
b   True. There is a higher incidence of squint in these children.
c   True. There may be developmental delay and cortical visual impairment.
d   False. This is associated with neurofibromatosis.
e. True. Premature infants are more likely to have significant refractive errors.

20

Services for the visually impaired

Learning objectives

To understand:

✔ The nature of visual impairment.

✔ The social help available to the visually impaired.

✔ The reasons for registering a patient in the United Kingdom.

Definitions

The International Classification of Diseases (2018) used by the World Health Organisation (WHO), classifies distance visual impairment as follows for distance:

- *Mild*: visual acuity worse than 6/12 to 6/18.
- *Moderate*: visual acuity worse than 6/18 to 6/60.
- *Severe*: visual acuity worse than 6/60 to 3/60.
- *Blindness*: visual acuity worse than 3/60.

Near vision impairment is defined as an acuity worse than N6 at 40 cm.

Visual loss may be the result of any condition, whether uncorrected refractive error (the commonest problem), disease, trauma, congenital or degenerative.

The definition of blindness, a visual acuity of <3/60 with the best possible refractive correction, can also be met if there is a visual field loss to less than 10°, *in the better eye.*

'Low vision' is defined as visual acuity of <6/18 (that is moderate to severe visual impairment) or a corresponding visual field loss to <10°, *in the better eye* with the best possible refractive correction. The person must also be able to use vision to plan or execute a task.

Key facts

- Worldwide, 43 million people are estimated to be blind (visual acuity less than 3/60).
- An estimate in 2010, of the age-standardized prevalence of blindness in adults ≥50 years, was ≤0.4% in high-income regions compared to levels of up to 6%, in western sub-Saharan Africa.
- Globally, uncorrected refractive errors are the main cause of moderate and severe distance visual impairment that can be corrected and near visual impairment; cataracts remain the leading cause of blindness in middle- and low-income countries.
- The number of people visually impaired from infectious diseases has reduced in the last 20 years.

The causes of visual impairment

Globally, the major causes of visual impairment are:

- uncorrected refractive errors (myopia, hyperopia or astigmatism), 43%;

Ophthalmology: Lecture Notes, Thirteenth Edition. Bruce James, Anthony Bron, and Manoj V. Parulekar.
© 2024 John Wiley & Sons Ltd. Published 2024 by John Wiley & Sons Ltd.
Companion website: www.wiley.com/go/ophthalmology13e

- unoperated cataract, 33%;
- glaucoma, 2%.

Approximately, 90% of visually impaired people live in developing countries.

Effect of visual impairment on motor function, social interactions and cognition

The majority of children with visual impairment have additional disabilities, particularly those with cortical visual impairment. Associated speech, hearing and learning difficulties are not uncommon. Visual impairment in infants and young children will interfere with motor development.

Disorders of the cerebral cortex (cerebral or cortical visual impairment), for example following a stroke, can result not only in poor visual acuity and/or visual field loss but also in deficits of visual processing and cognition.

Colour blindness

The three different photoreceptor cones (Chapter 1) may be deficient in number or function, *dyschromatopsia*. They are described as follows:

Compromised **function of:**

- Red cones, Protanomaly
- Green cones, Deuteranomaly
- Blue cones, Tritanomaly

Absent **function of:**

- Red cones, Protanopia
- Green cones, Deuteranopia
- Blue cones, Tritanopia

Deuteranopia or more commonly deuteranomaly is the usual cause of red–green colour blindness. Protanopia or protonomaly is more unusual. Both are inherited in an X-linked recssive manner. Thus, males (1 in 12) are more commonly affected than females (1 : 200). It affects the ability to detect long and middle wavelengths of the optical spectrum and hence to sense the colours green or red and to discriminate their admixtures. Red and green are colours used in traffic lights and signalling systems.

Impact of colour blindness

- There is very little impact on schooling but it may influence choice of career.
- There is limited impact on the ability to drive and recognize traffic lights because the red–green blind individual can usually distinguish between the extremes of red and green and also uses brightness of light, in a standardized lamp position, as a guide. Newer traffic lights overcome the problem by using a bluish green colour filter.
- Normal colour vision is a pre-requisite for certain professions such as pilots and coastguards.

Children with vision impairment

Every person with visual impairment has the potential to become an independent and productive member of society. It is therefore imperative that adequate resources are made available to ensure that they achieve their full potential. Most local authorities in the United Kingdom offer a sight impairment registration card, which can provide entitlement to certain concessions.

In the United Kingdom, a Certificate of Visual Impairment is completed for a child. This is also useful nationally in planning visual services for children. It is important to provide resources for the whole family of a child with visual impairment. Financial assistance may also be available for those with severe visual impairment. Every local authority in the United Kingdom will have a qualified teacher of the visually impaired (QTVI) and other educational and social care staff trained to provide for the special educational needs of children with visual impairment. The local authority will also provide an education health and care (EHC) plan for young people up to 25 years of age.

The RNIB (Royal National Institute of Blind People) provides a useful guide and advice on its website (www.rnib.org.uk).

Table 20.1 Definition of terms used to describe visual impairment in the United Kingdom.

	Visual acuity	Visual field
Sight impaired	6/60–6/18	Normal field of vision
Sight impaired	≤6/18	Loss of field of vision
Severely sight impaired	3/60–6/60	Normal field
Severely sight impaired	6/60–6/18	Loss of field of vision

Schools for the visually impaired

Most local education authorities in the United Kingdom support schools for the visually impaired. Many of these schools are situated next to schools for sighted children, and visually impaired children receive tutoring in both sectors. Many sight-impaired pupils can receive excellent education in mainstream schools with additional help where needed (integrated schooling).

Adults with visual impairment

In the United Kingdom, people with visual impairment are eligible to be registered as sight-impaired (*partially sighted*) or severely sight-impaired (*blind*) (Table 20.1). This is a process initiated by the consultant ophthalmologist, by completing a Certificate of Visual Impairment (CVI). The process of registration enables the affected individual to access support from social services and entitles them to certain concessions. People who are registered as severely sight-impaired/blind or sight-impaired/partially sighted are not automatically entitled to any welfare benefits; this is subject to age and other circumstances.

The benefits of sight impairment registration in the United Kingdom include the following:

- Financial help (e.g. a disability living allowance).
- Help from the social services (e.g. a specialist assessment leading to an adaptation of living accommodation).
- Public transport travel concessions, railcards, disabled parking schemes for carers.
- Help with access to work.

Living skills

Rehabilitation workers can support sight-impaired individuals in a range of activities in daily life, such as using public transport (mobility officers), cooking and leisure activities.

Low vision aids

Every individual with visual impairment should be referred for low vision assessment and provided with aids where appropriate. This service is provided by many hospital eye departments, some community optometrists, the RNIB and other charities.

Visual aids include hand and stand magnifiers (Chapter 4) and CCTV, now available as digital hand magnifiers. Use of computers with the ability to read text and zoom in on pictures or text is also of great benefit to visually impaired people. Sophisticated magnifying glasses or devices attached to ordinary glasses are also able to read text and, using artificial intelligence, help recognize objects, such as money and faces. These remain expensive however.

Aids may also help with tasks such as filling a cup. Tactile markers can be applied to cooker knobs and other objects to aid location. The settings of electric cookers can be given as a voice message.

Mobile phone apps may help to recognize currency, identify colours, identify objects and navigate. Smart phones also have accessibility settings to facilitate visually impaired users, such as text magnification and much more.

Voice activated technology has also opened up a new range of resources for sight-impaired people by increasing access to the Internet, compiling shopping lists, operating appliances throughout the house and checking the weather.

Guide dogs

The Guide Dogs charity provides approximately 8000 guide dogs in the United Kingdom to assist sight-impaired individuals with mobility and independence.

White cane

A white cane is used by many people who are blind or visually impaired, both as a mobility tool and to make others aware of their visual disability.

Children are usually introduced to using the cane between 7 and 10 years age.

Useful contacts and agencies

- RNIB (Royal National Institute of Blind People) www.rnib.org.uk
- The Royal College of Ophthalmologists www.rcophth.ac.uk
- VIScotland www.ssc.education.ed.ac.uk
- CAF – Contact a Family – for families with disabled children www.cafamily.org.uk

 KEY POINTS

- Every person with visual impairment has the potential to become an independent and productive member of society.
- Patients with visual impairment require a full assessment to determine their needs.

21

Clinical cases

Introduction

These case histories are designed to test your understanding of the symptoms, signs and management of ophthalmic diseases that have been discussed in this book. Answers are given after each case and include references to chapters where additional information may be found.

Clinical cases

Case 1

A 70-year-old woman presents to the eye casualty department with sudden loss of vision in her right eye. She has noted increasing headache and her scalp is tender when she combs her hair. She complains of pain in the jaw when she eats, and tires easily. There is no ophthalmic history but she suffers from peptic ulceration. She takes no regular medications. There is no family history of medical problems.

Examination reveals a visual acuity of counting fingers in the right eye. A relative afferent pupillary defect is present (see Chapter 3). The optic disc appears slightly swollen (Figure 21.1). The left eye is normal.

Questions

- What is the likely diagnosis?
- What is the immediate treatment?
- How would you confirm the diagnosis?
- What other precautions would you take?

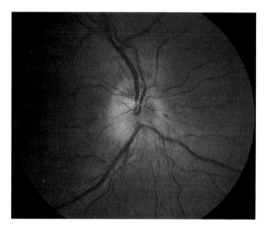

Figure 21.1 The appearance of the optic disc in Case 1.

Answers

The patient almost certainly has giant cell arteritis causing ischaemic optic neuropathy (see Chapter 15). Intravenous steroids must be given *immediately* before any other diagnostic step is taken, for there is a risk of arteritis and blindness in the fellow eye.

An ESR, CRP and temporal artery ultrasound or biopsy will help to confirm the diagnosis.

As the patient is being treated with steroids, it is important to obtain a chest radiograph to exclude tuberculosis (TB) (steroids may reactivate latent TB). Blood pressure and blood glucose must be monitored. The patient should be warned of the other complications of steroid therapy, including immune suppressive effects. Treatment to prevent osteoporosis is required. A positive history of gastric ulceration demands prophylactic treatment with a proton pump inhibitor.

Ophthalmology: Lecture Notes, Thirteenth Edition. Bruce James, Anthony Bron, and Manoj V. Parulekar.
© 2024 John Wiley & Sons Ltd. Published 2024 by John Wiley & Sons Ltd.
Companion website: www.wiley.com/go/ophthalmology13e

Case 2

A 40-year-old man presents with sudden onset of a drooping left eyelid. When he lifts the lid with his finger, he notices that he has double vision. He has a severe headache. He is otherwise fit and well with no past ophthalmic history. He is on no regular medication. There is no family history of medical problems.

Examination reveals normal visual acuity in both eyes. A left ptosis is present. The left pupil is dilated. The left eye is abducted in the primary position of gaze. Testing eye movements reveals reduced adduction, elevation and depression of the left eye. The remainder of the eye examination is normal.

Questions

- What nerve palsy is present?
- What is the most likely cause?
- What is the management?

Answers

The man has a third nerve palsy (see Chapter 16). An aneurysm from the posterior communicating artery pressing on the third nerve must be the initial diagnosis in a *painful* third nerve palsy. The patient requires urgent neurosurgical investigation with a magnetic resonance angiogram (MRA). Urgent neurosurgical intervention may be required. It is also important to check blood pressure and blood glucose. Diabetics may develop a painful third nerve palsy, but the pupil is not always affected (a 'pupil-sparing third nerve palsy').

Case 3

A 55-year-old man presents to his GP with a 5-day history of the sudden onset of floaters in the left eye. These were accompanied by small flashes of light. He has treated hypertension but no other medical problems.

The GP examines the eye and finds a normal visual acuity. Dilated fundoscopy reveals no abnormality.

Questions

- What should the GP advise?
- What is the diagnosis?
- What are the associated risks?

Answers

As the symptoms are acute the GP should arrange for an urgent ophthalmic assessment. The most likely diagnosis is a posterior vitreous detachment.

With careful ophthalmoscopy, it will be possible to identify vitreous opacities in keeping with this diagnosis. The flashing lights are caused by traction of the detached vitreous gel on the retina. A specialized examination of the peripheral retina is needed. A tear may occur in the retina, which in turn may lead to a retinal detachment. Laser applied around the tear while the retina around it is flat can prevent retinal detachment (see Chapter 12).

Case 4

A 75-year-old woman attends the main casualty department with nausea and vomiting. She says that her right eye is painful and red and that her vision is blurred. She is long-sighted and wears glasses for near and distance vision. She is generally fit. There is no family history of medical problems.

On examination, the casualty officer finds the vision to be reduced to counting fingers in the right eye. The eye is red, the cornea appears cloudy, and the pupil is oval and dilated on the affected side. No view of the fundus is obtained.

Questions

- What is the diagnosis?
- How might it be confirmed?
- What is the treatment?

Answers

The lady is long-sighted and has acute angle closure (see Chapter 11). Tonometry would reveal a raised intraocular pressure often has high as 60–70 mmHg (see Chapter 3). If possible through the cloudy cornea, gonioscopy would confirm the presence of a closed angle and a narrow angle in the fellow eye (see Chapter 11). This can also be seen using high-resolution ultrasound or confocal microscopy. The pressure must be lowered with intravenous acetazolamide and topical hypotensive drops, including pilocarpine, to produce miosis. A peripheral iridotomy is then performed, usually with a YAG laser, in both eyes, to prevent further attacks. If she has cataracts, then surgical replacement of her lenses with artificial intraocular lenses can also help to widen the drainage angle.

Case 5

A 28-year-old man presents to his optician with a painful, red right eye. The vision has become increasingly blurred over the last two days. He

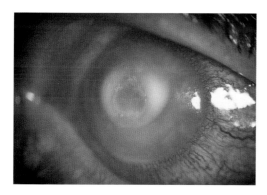

Figure 21.2 The appearance of the eye in Case 5.

wears soft monthly disposable contact lenses, and says he is not very reliable at cleaning his storage containers.

The optician notes that the vision is reduced to 6/60 in the right eye, the conjunctiva is inflamed, and there is a central opacity on the cornea. A small hypopyon (see Chapter 10) is present (Figure 21.2).

Questions

- What is the likely diagnosis?
- What should the optician do?

Answers

The man has a bacterial corneal ulcer secondary to contact lens wear. He requires immediate referral to an ophthalmic casualty unit. The ulcer will be scraped for culture and Gram stain and the contact lens and any lens containers cultured. Intensive, topical, broad-spectrum antibiotics are administered as an inpatient pending the result of the microbiological investigation (see Chapter 8).

Case 6

A mother attends her GP's surgery with her baby, now eight months old. He has had a persistently watery eye since birth. Intermittently, there is a yellow discharge surrounding the eye. The white of the eye has never been red. The baby is otherwise healthy.

Examination reveals a white, quiet, normal eye. Slight pressure over the lacrimal sac produces a yellowish discharge from the normal puncta.

Questions

- What is the diagnosis?
- What advice would you give the mother?

Answers

It is likely that the child has nasolacrimal obstruction due to an imperforate nasolacrimal duct. The mother should be reassured that this often resolves spontaneously. The lids should be kept clean and the region overlying the lacrimal sac massaged gently on a daily basis. Antibiotics are generally not effective. If the symptoms persist after the child's first birthday, the child can be referred to an ophthalmologist for syringing and probing of the nasolacrimal duct (see Chapter 7).

Case 7

A 14-year-old complains of intermittent redness and soreness of the right eye. He has noticed a small lump on the upper lid. The vision is unaffected.

Examination reveals a small, raised, umbilicated lesion on the skin of the upper lid, associated with a follicular conjunctivitis below (Figure 21.3).

Questions

- What is the likely diagnosis?
- What is the treatment?

Answers

It is likely that the lid lesion is a molluscum contagiosum. It is treated by excision (see Chapter 6).

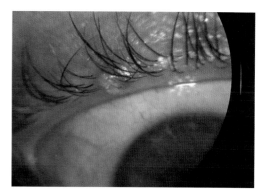

Figure 21.3 The appearance of the lid in Case 7.

Case 8

A 35-year-old man presents to his GP with erythematous, swollen right upper and lower eyelids, worsening over the previous two days. He is unable to open them. He feels unwell and has a temperature.

Examination reveals marked lid swelling, a tender globe and, on manual opening of the lids, proptosis with chemotic injected conjunctiva. Eye movements are limited in all directions. Visual acuity and colour vision are normal, and there is no relative afferent pupillary defect (see Chapter 3). The optic disc and retina also appear normal.

Questions

- What is the diagnosis?
- What is the management?

Answers

The man has orbital cellulitis (see Chapter 5). Blood cultures and a high nasal swab should be performed, together with a CT scan of the orbits and sinuses, to confirm the diagnosis and delineate any abscess. He requires admission to hospital for intravenous antibiotics and close monitoring of his vision, colour vision and pupillary reflexes, as he is at risk of severe optic nerve damage. The ENT surgeons should be informed, as they may be required to drain an abscess. The normal acuity and colour vision suggest that the optic nerve is not compromised at present, but should these signs worsen, urgent surgical drainage will be required.

Case 9

While working in the laboratory a colleague inadvertently sprays his eyes with an alkali solution.

Questions

- What is the immediate treatment?
- What should you do next?

Answers

The eyes must be washed out with copious quantities (litres) of water or saline immediately until the pH is neutralized. Acids and particularly alkalis are very toxic to the eye. Failure to treat immediately may result in permanent, severe ocular damage (see Chapter 17). The patient should then be taken to an eye emergency clinic.

Case 10

A 27-year-old man presents with a 2-day history of a painful red right eye; the vision is slightly blurred and he dislikes bright lights. He is otherwise fit and well, but complains of some backache. He wears no glasses.

Questions

- What is the likely diagnosis?
- What would you expect to find on examination of the eye?
- What treatment would you give?
- What is the eye condition likely to be associated with?

Answers

The patient has iritis (see Chapter 10). Examination would reveal a reduction in visual acuity, redness of the eye that is worse at the limbus, cells in the anterior chamber and possibly on the cornea (keratic precipitates) or a collection at the bottom of the anterior chamber (hypopyon). The iris may be stuck to the lens (posterior synechiae). There may be inflammation of the vitreous and retina. The patient is treated with steroid eye drops to reduce the inflammation and dilating drops to prevent the formation of posterior synechiae. The history of backache suggests that the patient may have ankylosing spondylitis.

Case 11

A 68-year-old lady presents with a 4-day history of a mildly painful red eye and blurring of vision. One year previously she had a corneal graft to the same eye. She is on no medications and is otherwise well.

Questions

- What is the most important diagnosis to rule out?
- What treatment should the patient be given?

Answers

There may be a number of causes of this lady's red eye. A diagnosis of graft rejection must be considered first of all. The patient must be referred to an eye department as an emergency. If a graft rejection is confirmed, she will need intensive treatment with topical steroids to save the graft (see Chapter 8).

Case 12

A 68-year-old hypertensive man noted a fleeting complete loss of vision in one eye lasting for about a minute. He described it as a curtain coming down over the vision. Recovery was complete. There was no pain. Examination reveals no abnormality.

Questions

- What is the diagnosis?
- What treatment would you advise?

Answers

The patient has had an episode of *amaurosis fugax,* most likely caused by the passage of a thrombotic embolus through the retinal circulation. The patient requires treatment with antiplatelet drugs and a cardiovascular work up. The most likely abnormality is a plaque on the carotid artery, which may require an endarterectomy (see Chapter 13).

Case 13

A 60-year-old lady presented to her GP with gradual loss of vision over some months. She noticed that the problem was particularly bad in bright sunshine. The eye was not painful or red. She was otherwise well.

Questions

- What is the probable diagnosis?
- How can the diagnosis be confirmed?
- What treatment may be advised?

Answers

It is likely that the lady has a cataract. These can be readily seen with a slit lamp, but are also well visualized with the direct ophthalmoscope in the red reflex (Figure 21.4). The advantages and possible complications of cataract surgery should be discussed with her once the diagnosis has been confirmed (see Chapter 9).

Case 14

An 80-year-old lady who has already lost the vision in one eye develops distortion and reduction of vision over a few days in her good eye.

Examination reveals an acuity of 6/12, an early cataract and an abnormality at the macula (Figure 21.5).

Questions

- What is the likely diagnosis?
- What treatment may be helpful?

Answers

The rapid onset suggests that the cataract has little to do with the new visual disturbance. It is most likely due to age-related macular degeneration (AMD) (see Chapter 12). In some patients, with wet AMD, where a fibrovascular membrane grows beneath the macula that can be shown on a fluorescein angiogram, anti-VEGF injections into the vitreous may be helpful in preventing further progression and in some cases improving vision.

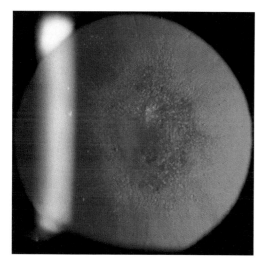

Figure 21.4 A posterior subcapsular cataract, seen in the red reflex by direct ophthalmoscopy in Case 13.

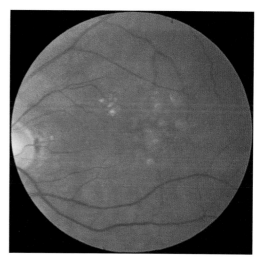

Figure 21.5 The appearance of the macula in Case 14.

Case 15

A 30-year-old builder was using a hammer to hit a steel chisel. He felt something hit his eye and the vision became blurred. He is fit and well and there is no history of medical problems.

On examination by his GP, the vision was reduced to 6/12. A fluorescein staining lesion was seen on the cornea. A small hyphaema was seen in the anterior chamber, and in the red reflex observed with a direct ophthalmoscope a well-delineated lens opacity was seen. The retina appeared normal.

Questions

- What is the cause of the reduced acuity?
- What is the likely origin of the lens opacity?
- What is the possible management of the patient?

Answers

It is likely that a piece of steel travelling at high velocity has penetrated the cornea, traversed the iris (resulting in the hyphaema) and passed into or through the lens (causing the opacity). The relatively good acuity suggests that there has been no damage to the macula. The patient needs to be seen as an emergency in an eye unit. The corneal wound, if self-sealing, will probably not require suturing. The exact location of the foreign body has to be determined. Although it is unlikely to cause an infection (heat generated by the impact of the hammer on the metal may effectively sterilize the fragment), it may cause retinal toxicity if it has entered the vitreous cavity or retina. If it is enclosed in the lens (Figure 21.6), there is less chance of retinal toxicity developing but the patient is at high risk of developing a subsequent cataract that may require an operation. A foreign body that impacts on the retina or the vitreous body requires a vitrectomy to remove it, with careful examination of the retina for tears (see Chapter 17).

Case 16

A 2-year-old child was thought to have a squint by her parents. The finding was confirmed by her GP and she was referred to hospital.

Question

What examination must be conducted in hospital?

Answer

Having taken a full history, an orthoptist will measure the visual acuity of the child, examine the range of eye movements, determine the presence of type of squint with a cover test, trying to assess the degree of binocular vision present. The child will have a refraction performed and glasses prescribed if there is a significant refractive error or a difference in the strength of the lens needed between the two eyes (anisometropia). An ophthalmologist will examine the eye to check that there is no ocular or neurological condition that may account for the squint (see Chapter 16), and can discuss any future need for surgery.

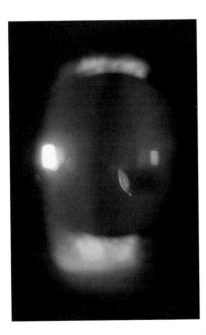

Figure 21.6 The intralenticular foreign body seen in Case 15.

Case 17

A 26-year-old lady presents with a 3-day history of blurring of vision in the right eye. This has become progressively worse. She also has pain caused by moving the eye. She has previously had an episode of weakness in the right arm 2 years ago whenever she took a warm bath, but this settled without treatment. She is otherwise fit and well.

On examination, the vision was 6/60, with no improvement on looking through a pinhole. A central scotoma was present on confrontation. The eye was white and quiet with no abnormality noted save for a right relative afferent pupillary defect (see Chapter 3).

Questions

- What is the diagnosis?
- How could this be confirmed?
- What are the management options?
- What is the prognosis?

Answers

The patient has the typical symptoms and signs of optic neuritis (see Chapter 15). The diagnosis can be supported by an MRI scan to look for additional plaques of demyelination and a visual evoked potential to examine the functioning of the optic nerve. A neurologist may also suggest performing a lumbar puncture, particularly if there is any doubt about the diagnosis. With the possibility of a previous neurological episode, it is likely that the patient has multiple sclerosis. It is of great importance that appropriate counselling is given. Steroid treatment may speed up the recovery of vision but would not change the outcome and the prognosis for recovery of vision over a few months is good.

Case 18

A 79-year-old man presents with a lesion on his right lower lid (Figure 21.7). It has been there for some months and has gradually grown bigger. It is ulcerated and the ulcer shows a pearly margin.

Questions

- What is the lesion?
- How should it be treated?

Answers

This is a basal cell carcinoma. It requires local excision. There is no problem with metastatic spread but local extension could cause severe problems as the tumour grows and infiltrates surrounding structures (see Chapter 6).

Case 19

A 60-year-old man presents with tired sore eyes. He has noted that the eyelids may crust in the morning. Sometimes, the white of the eye is red. The vision is unaffected. He is otherwise fit and well.

Questions

- What is the probable diagnosis?
- What signs would you look for?
- How can this condition be treated?

Answers

The patient has blepharitis (see Chapter 6). Scaling of the lid margins and at the base of the lashes, together with inflammation of the lid margins and plugging of the meibomian glands, may be present (Figure 21.8). Lid cleaning, along with the use of local antibiotic ointment and possibly topical steroids (supervised by an ophthalmologist), will improve, if not alleviate, the symptoms. Heat and lid massage can restore oil flow. Courses of systemic tetracycline may be beneficial in more advanced cases and are in any case used in the treatment of acne rosacea which may be an associated condition.

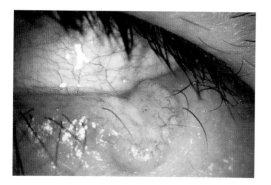

Figure 21.7 The appearance of the lid in Case 18.

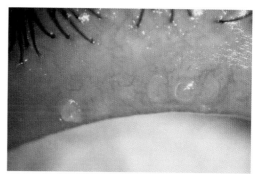

Figure 21.8 Plugging and capping of the meibomian glands in Case 19.

Case 20

A 30-year-old man developed an acute red eye first on the right and then in the left eye, associated with a watery discharge. Vision is unaffected but the eye irritates. He is otherwise fit and well.

Questions

- What is the diagnosis?
- What confirmatory signs would you look for on examination?
- What precautions would you take following your examination?

Answers

The patient has viral conjunctivitis – probably adenovirus – (see Chapter 8). Examination for a preauricular lymph node and conjunctival follicles on the lower tarsus would confirm the diagnosis. This form of conjunctivitis is highly contagious; it is important to ensure that hands and equipment are thoroughly cleaned following the examination, and that the importance of good hygiene is emphasized to the patient.

Case 21

A 26-year-old woman attends the eye casualty on the advice of her optician. She has a 6-week history of headaches and feeling nauseated in the mornings. She has normal vision and a normal examination, except for her optic discs which appear swollen, with blurred margins and no spontaneous venous pulsation.

Questions

- What would be your differential diagnosis?
- What further investigations are needed?

Answers

The description of the optic discs is suggestive of papilloedema from raised intracranial pressure. In the context of recent onset headaches and early-morning nausea, it is important to rule out an intracranial space occupying lesion and an urgent MRI of the brain should be requested. If the scan does not show any pathology, idiopathic intracranial hypertension would be the most likely diagnosis and the

patient should be referred to neurology for lumbar puncture and ongoing management. Optic discs can appear swollen for other reasons including optic disc drüsen (which could be visualized with a B-scan ultrasound of the eyes) and hypermetropia. Spontaneous venous pulsation is absent in around 10% of healthy people.

Case 22

A 65-year-old man presents to his GP complaining that he is struggling to see things on his left-hand side for the last two days. He has a background of hypertension and is found to have an irregular heart rhythm. On examination, the left part of the visual field is missing in both eyes.

Questions

- How would you describe this visual field defect?
- What is the most likely diagnosis?
- What management would be needed?

Answers

The visual field loss described is a left homonymous hemianopia. This would be caused by disruption to the visual pathway anywhere after the optic chasm in the right-hand side of the brain. In the context of his cardiovascular risk factors, this is most likely a cerebral infraction and he should be referred urgently to the stroke team. In addition to imaging of the brain and the carotid arteries, he needs a full cardiovascular work up including an ECG, blood pressure measurement and blood tests to check his glucose and lipids. The stroke physicians would work with the patient to modify these risk factors to reduce the probability of further ischaemic events, this is likely to include anti-platelet agents or anticoagulation.

Case 23

A 30-year-old man presents to the emergency department stating that the sight in his right eye was very blurred when he woke up and he has lots of floaters moving in his vision. He has type 1 diabetes and you see from his notes that he failed to attend his last three diabetic eye screening appointments. The visual acuity in the right eye is counting fingers, it is 6/6 in the left eye.

Questions

- What are the possible causes for his symptoms?
- How should he be managed?

Answers

The most likely cause of these symptoms is a vitreous haemorrhage, possibly associated with diabetic retinopathy or possibly a retinal tear, which may lead to a retinal detachment. As he is a diabetic, this also puts him at risk of vascular pathology including a retinal vein or artery occlusion, this would cause loss of vision but the patient would be unlikely to complain of floaters. This patient should be referred immediately to the ophthalmologists for a full dilated retinal examination. If he has a vitreous haemorrhage, it is likely that he has developed proliferative diabetic retinopathy and would need urgent laser photocoagulation treatment or a vitrectomy. He needs to have his blood glucose and blood pressure checked to ensure that these are adequately controlled.

Case 24

A 2-month-old baby boy who was born overseas is brought to his GP by his parents, who showed them the following photograph (Figure 21.9) and said that they have been told that he needs to have his eyes checked. He was born by normal delivery at full term and is otherwise healthy.

Questions

- What are the possible causes for this appearance?
- Why does this need urgent assessment?

Answers

This shows a white reflex in the left eye. The most likely cause for this is a congenital cataract but the

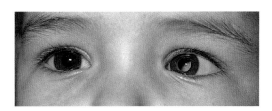

Figure 21.9 Appearance of the eyes in question 24.

most serious pathology to rule out is a retinoblastoma. This child needs urgent ophthalmic review and management to prevent the development of amblyopia.

Case 25

A 54-year-old man attends his GP concerned about his peripheral vision; he had recently hit a parked car while driving. He has large sweaty hands, coarse facial features and tells you that he is struggling to find shoes which fit him.

Questions

- What is the most likely diagnosis?
- How would you explain his visual complaints?

Answers

These are the classic features of acromegaly. Most cases of acromegaly are associated with a pituitary adenoma. A macro adenoma of the pituitary may push upwards on the optic chiasm and put pressure on the decussating fibres from the nasal retinae, which represent the temporal vision in both eyes. This presents as a bitemporal hemianopia on visual field testing.

Useful references

Textbooks

Listed below are some sources that will provide more detailed information about the subjects covered in this book.

Clinical ophthalmology

American Academy of Ophthalmology. Basic and Clinical Science Course (BCSC). 2020–2021. Reviews of ophthalmic subspecialty subjects.

Gervasio K. & Peck T. (2021) *The Wills Eye Manual*. Eighth edition. Wolters Kluwer Health. Concise details on the management of ophthalmic disease.

Salmon J.F. (2019) *Kanski's Clinical Ophthalmology: A Systematic Approach*. Nineth edition. Elsevier. Concise illustrated description of ophthalmic disease.

Deniston A.K.O. & Murray P.I. (2014) *Oxford Handbook of Ophthalmology*. Third edition. Oxford University Press. Concise diagnostic and therapeutic ophthalmic information.

Jackson L.J. (2019) *Moorfields Manual of Ophthalmology*. Third edition. JP Medical Ltd. Concise practical ophthalmic textbook.

Rowe F.J. (2012) *Clinical Orthoptics*. Third edition. Wiley Blackwell. Outlines the examination and diagnosis of eye movement disorders.

Spalton D.J., Hitchings R.A. & Hunter P.A. (2004) *Atlas of Clinical Ophthalmology*. Third edition. Mosby. Illustrated account of ophthalmic disease.

Yanoff M. & Duker J.S. (eds) (2022) *Ophthalmology*. Sixth edition. Elsevier. Large comprehensive textbook from America.

Basic science

Bron A.J., Tripathi R.C. & Tripathi B.J. (1997) *Wolff's Anatomy of the Eye and Orbit*. Eighth edition. Chapman & Hall.

Elkington A.R. (1999) *Clinical Optics*. Third edition. Wiley Blackwell.

Forrester J.V. *et al.* (2020) *The Eye: Basic Sciences in Practice*. Fifth edition. Elsevier.

Snell R.S. & Lemp M.A. (1998) *Clinical Anatomy of the Eye*. Second edition. Blackwell Science.

Review journals

Eye News
Published by Pinpoint Ltd. Provides short practical review articles and information about new developments in ophthalmology.

Survey of Ophthalmology
Published by Elsevier Science. Bi-monthly. Provides in-depth well-referenced review articles on particular topics in ophthalmology.

Progress in Retinal and Eye Research
Published by Elsevier Science. Bi-monthly. Provides in-depth well-referenced review articles on basic science topics in ophthalmology.

Ophthalmic journals

For detailed research articles there are numerous ophthalmic publications; most of the subspecialty fields in ophthalmology have their own journal. Among the leaders in clinical ophthalmology are:

Ophthalmology: Lecture Notes, Thirteenth Edition. Bruce James, Anthony Bron, and Manoj V. Parulekar.
© 2024 John Wiley & Sons Ltd. Published 2024 by John Wiley & Sons Ltd.
Companion website: www.wiley.com/go/ophthalmology13e

American Journal of Ophthalmology

JAMA Ophthalmology

British Journal of Ophthalmology

Eye

Experimental Eye Research

Graefe's Archive for Clinical and Experimental

Ophthalmology

Investigative Ophthalmology and Visual Science (IOVS)

Websites

American Academy of Ophthalmology (www.aao. org). This site contains updates on every aspect of ophthalmology together with treatment guidelines.

Digital Journal of Ophthalmology (www.djo.harvard. edu). Includes clinical case presentations from the large American ophthalmic hospitals.

Examination techniques: www.mrcophth.com. Information on the UK postgraduate examinations and MCQ question bank. Clinical cases.

Eye News (www.eyenews.uk.com). An online version of the journal Eye News with an archive. The Eye Directory lists companies involved in the manufacture of ophthalmic equipment and medicines.

International Council of Ophthalmology (www.icoph. org). Includes a handbook for medical students. Information about educational meetings. Information about eye diseases for patients. A link to the free Atlas of Ophthalmology.

Glaucoma UK. (https://glaucoma.uk). Provides patient-orientated information about glaucoma.

Macular Society (www.macularsociety.org). The website provides patient-orientated information about macular disease.

Moorfields Eye Hospital (www.moorfields.nhs.uk). Describes the facilities of the hospital, courses available, and has information sheets for patients on common eye diseases.

Optic Disc org (www.optic-disc.org). This site is specifically aimed at diseases of the optic disc, including an atlas and tutorials on examination.

Orbis website (www.cybersight.org) includes videos of ophthalmic procedures.

Oxford Eye Hospital (www.ouh.nhs.uk). Details on common ocular emergencies, and patient information sheets on common eye problems.

Retinal Screening (www.gov.uk>guidance.diabetic-eye-screening). Information on the UK national screening programme for diabetic retinopathy.

RootAtlas (www.rootatlas.com). An American site with videos on ophthalmic conditions, examination and treatment.

Royal College of Ophthalmologists (www.rcophth. ac.uk). Includes details of the college's publications and information about ophthalmic disease for patients.

Royal National Institute of the Blind (www.rnib.org. uk). Produces a range of fact sheets for patients.

Organizations producing patient information literature

See some of the websites mentioned above, in addition:

The Royal National Institute of Blind People, 105 Judd Street, London WC1H 9NE, UK. Produces a variety of leaflets on common ocular conditions from the patient's perspective. It is also a most valuable source of information and practical help for visually impaired people.

The Royal College of Ophthalmologists, 18 Stephenson Way, London NW1 2HD, UK; The American Academy of Ophthalmology, PO Box 7424, San Francisco, CA 94120-7424, USA. These organizations produce a range of booklets and guidelines on ophthalmic topics.

Appendix 1: Conversion table for representation of visual acuity

20 ft	6 m	Log MAR
20/630	6/190	+1.5
20/500	6/150	+1.4
20/400	6/120	+1.3
20/320	6/95	+1.2
20/250	6/75	+1.1
20/200	6/60	+1.0
20/160	6/48	+0.9
20/125	6/38	+0.8
20/100	6/30	+0.7
20/80	6/24	+0.6
20/63	6/19	+0.5
20/50	6/15	+0.4
20/40	6/12	+0.3
20/32	6/9.5	+0.2
20/25	6/7.5	+0.1
20/20	6/6	0
20/16	6/4.8	−0.1
20/12.5	6/3.8	−0.2
20/10	6/3	−0.3

Ophthalmology: Lecture Notes, Thirteenth Edition. Bruce James, Anthony Bron, and Manoj V. Parulekar.
© 2024 John Wiley & Sons Ltd. Published 2024 by John Wiley & Sons Ltd.
Companion website: www.wiley.com/go/ophthalmology13e

Appendix 2: Drugs available for ophthalmic use

Detailed information on drugs available for ophthalmic use is available in the regularly updated British National Formulary published by the BMJ group and the Pharmaceutical Press.

Eye drops and ointment are applied to the lower fornix by gently pulling down the lower lid. It is only necessary to apply one drop. Pressure in the medial corner of the eye for at least 60 seconds after application will occlude the lacrimal puncta and canaliculi, reducing the systemic absorption and prolonging the exposure of the eye to the medication.

Many eye drops are available with and without preservatives. Preservatives may cause allergic or toxic reactions in some patients. Single use preparations of drops, particularly those used for diagnostic purposes are also available.

Treatment of infection

Topical antibiotics

Aminoglycosides

Gentamicin (broad spectrum including pseudomonas). Neomycin (in combination with steroid drops). Tobramycin.

Quinolones (broad spectrum)

Ceftazidime.
Ciprofloxacin (corneal ulcers).
Levofloxacin.
Moxifloxacin.
Ofloxacin.
Cefuroxime (prophylaxis following intraocular surgery by infusion into the anterior chamber).
Chloramphenicol (broad spectrum, used to treat superficial eye infections).
Fusidic acid (Staphylococcal infections).

Treatment of chlamydial infections

Azithromycin (trachoma).

Treatment of Acanthamoeba infections

Propamidine isethionate.
Chlorhexidine (specialist formulation).
Polyhexamethylene biguanide (PHMB) (specialist formulation).

Treatment of viral infections

(Herpes simplex.)

Aciclovir.
Ganciclovir (topical and slow release implants available to treat CMV retinitis).
Trifluorothymidine (specialist formulation).

Ophthalmology: Lecture Notes, Thirteenth Edition. Bruce James, Anthony Bron, and Manoj V. Parulekar.
© 2024 John Wiley & Sons Ltd. Published 2024 by John Wiley & Sons Ltd.
Companion website: www.wiley.com/go/ophthalmology13e

Treatment of fungal infections

(Specialist formulation of drops is required.)
Pimaricin (natamycin) 5%.

Treatment of inflammation

Non-steroidal anti-inflammatory preparations

Bromfenac.
Diclofenac.
Flurbiprofen sodium.
Ketorolac trometamol.

Steroid preparations

Betamethasone (also available combined with an antibiotic).
Dexamethasone (also available combined with an antibiotic).
Fluorometholone.
Loteprednol etabonate.
Prednisolone.
Rimexolone.

Intravitreal preparations (dexamethasone, fluocinolone acetonide) are available to treat macular oedema associated with diabetes and retinal vein occlusion.

Mast cell stabilizers

Lodoxamide.
Nedocromil.
Olopatadine (also antihistamine).
Sodium cromoglycate.

Antihistamines

Antazoline.
Azelastine.
Epinastine.
Ketotifen.
Levocabastine.
Olopatadine (also mast cell stabilizer).

Mucolytics

Acetlycysteine.

Mydriatics and cycloplegics

Antimuscarinics

Atropine.
Cyclopentolate hydrochloride (routinely used for therapeutic pupillary dilation).
Homatropine hydrobromide.
Tropicamide (routinely used for diagnostic pupillary dilation).

Sympathomimetics

Phenylephrine hydrochloride.

Ocular hypotensives

Single drops are listed here but combined preparations with two different classes of drop are available.

Beta receptor antagonists

Betaxolol.
Carteolol.
Levobunolol.
Timolol.

Prostaglandin analogues

Bimatoprost (synthetic prostamide).
Latanoprost.
Tafluprost.
Travoprost.

Sympathomimetics

Brimonidine tartrate.
Apraclonidine.

Carbonic anhydrase inhibitors

Brinzolamide.
Dorzolamide.

(Systemically, acetazolamide is used to treat acute elevation of intraocular pressure.)

Miotics

Pilocarpine.

Local anaesthetics

Lidocaine hydrochloride
Oxybuprocaine hydrochloride.
Proxymetacaine hydrochloride (causes less stinging on initial application).
Tetracaine hydrochloride.

Ocular lubricants

Carbomers (polyacrylic acid).
Carmellose sodium.

Hypromellose.
Macrogols (polyethylene glycols).
Polyvinyl alcohol.
Sodium chloride 0.9%.
Sodium hyaluronate.

Eye ointments containing paraffin.

Vascular endothelial growth factor inhibitors

For the treatment of wet age-related macular degeneration, retinal vein occlusion and diabetic macular oedema.

Aflibercept.
Pegaptanib.
Ranibizumab.

Diagnostic preparations

Fluorescein sodium.
Lissamine green.

Index

Ophthalmology: Lecture Notes, Thirteenth Edition. Bruce James, Anthony Bron, and Manoj V. Parulekar.
© 2024 John Wiley & Sons Ltd. Published 2024 by John Wiley & Sons Ltd.
Companion website: www.wiley.com/go/ophthalmology13e